DR. COLBERT'S "I CAN DO THIS" DIET

DON COLBERT, MD

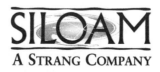

SILOAM
A STRANG COMPANY

Most STRANG COMMUNICATIONS BOOK GROUP products are available at special quantity discounts for bulk purchase for sales promotions, premiums, fund-raising, and educational needs. For details, write Strang Communications Book Group, 600 Rinehart Road, Lake Mary, Florida 32746, or telephone (407) 333-0600.

DR. COLBERT's "I CAN DO THIS" DIET by Don Colbert, MD
Published by Siloam
A Strang Company
600 Rinehart Road
Lake Mary, Florida 32746
www.strangbookgroup.com

Unless otherwise noted, all Scripture quotations are from the New King James Version of the Bible. Copyright © 1979, 1980, 1982 by Thomas Nelson, Inc., publishers. Used by permission.
Scripture quotations marked KJV are from the King James Version of the Bible.

Cover design by Justin Evans
Design Director: Bill Johnson

Visit the author's website at www.drcolbert.com.

International Standard Book Number: 978-1-61638-267-4

The Library of Congress has catalogued the previous edition as follows:

Library of Congress Cataloging-in-Publication Data

Colbert, Don.
  Dr. Colbert's "I can do this" diet / Don Colbert. – "I can do this" diet
      p. cm.
  Includes bibliographical references and index.
  ISBN 978-1-59979-350-4 (hardback) -- ISBN 978-1-59979-546-1 (international
trade pbk.) 1. Reducing diets. 2. Weight loss. I. Title.
  RM222.2.C5523 2010
  613.2'5--dc22
                                        2009040243

E-book ISBN: 978-1-61638-410-4

This book contains the opinions and ideas of its author. It is solely for informational and educational purposes and should not be regarded as a substitute for professional medical treatment. The nature of your body's health condition is complex and unique. Therefore, you should consult a health

professional before you begin any new exercise, nutrition, or supplementation program or if you have questions about your health. Neither the author nor the publisher shall be liable or responsible for any loss or damage allegedly arising from any information or suggestion in this book.

People and names in this book are composites created by the author from his experiences as a medical doctor. Names and details of their stories have been changed, and any similarity between the names and stories of individuals described in this book to individuals known to readers is purely coincidental.

The statements in this book about consumable products or food have not been evaluated by the Food and Drug Administration. The recipes in this book are to be followed exactly as written. The publisher is not responsible for your specific health or allergy needs that may require medical supervision. The publisher is not responsible for any adverse reactions to the consumption of food or products that have been suggested in this book.

While the author has made every effort to provide accurate telephone numbers and Internet addresses at the time of publication, neither the publisher nor the author assumes any responsibility for errors or for changes that occur after publication.

11 12 13 14 15 — 9 8 7 6 5 4 3 2 1
Printed in the United States of America

DEDICATION

E VERY DAY PEOPLE walk into my office hoping to become healthier. Many are obese or overweight dieters frustrated with their inability to keep the pounds off for good or with doctors who can't seem to "fix" their overweight issues. For these patients, I cherish the opportunity to inform them that there is hope—that they *can* lose the weight and become healthier.

Yet every now and then I meet with patients who are on their last line of hope. I can tell by the painful, exasperated, despondent look in their eyes. No matter what they try, no matter how faithful they are to an eating program or how religious an exerciser they have become, no matter what various medications or supplements they've taken, they *still* can't lose weight. Without knowing it, they are metabolically compromised. And yet possibly the saddest part is that they have lost hope.

Because of what they and countless others have gone through, I dedicate this book to all who are metabolically compromised. To those who feel hopeless, helpless, and with no way out, I pray this book offers information that will become your beacon in the night. To those who feel lost in your journey toward a healthy life, my desire is that this book serves as a road map to redirect you to a future filled with wellness. I want you to lose weight, regain your health, and feel great again. I want you to dream again and daily forgive yourself, accept yourself, and love yourself.

ACKNOWLEDGMENTS

I WOULD LIKE TO thank the people at Strang Communications for once again helping to make this book a success: Stephen Strang, Tessie DeVore, Barbara Dycus, Debbie Marrie, Debbie Moss, and many others. A special thanks to Marcus Yoars for his contribution in making *Dr. Colbert's "I Can Do This" Diet* a fun and easy read. I would also like to thank my brother-in-law, David Holland, for assisting me with some of the research for this book, as well as Melissa Garcia and my entire staff at Divine Health Wellness Center for their support. I would also like to thank my good friend, Lee Viersen, for his passion and insights regarding diet and exercise. Last but certainly not least, thanks to my wife, Mary, who lived this program with me and has helped me present it to many churches and organizations over the years.

CONTENTS

INTRODUCTION

C OME FLY WITH DreamFlight…because we get you there at least 5 percent of the time."
Would you choose to fly on an airline that had this kind of motto? Of course not! With a track record of arriving safely at a destination only 5 percent of the time, you wouldn't dare set foot on one of their planes. Yet every day, dieters embark on a new diet with the same success rate.

Some hop on board the latest hyped-up, low-fat, wonder-working program that has made it past the late-night infomercial phase to become a *New York Times* best seller. Still others prefer a more adventurous journey with a no-carb miracle pound-shedder that has a host of B-list celebrities touting its amazing results. Of course, almost all who set out to lose weight via one of these diets swear that it will be absolutely, *positively* the last one they'll ever try.

It seems everyone is looking for the "Diet to End All Diets." Sadly, they're looking for something that doesn't exist. Why? Because in the long run, dieting just doesn't work. Some reports indicate that only 2 percent of all dieters manage to lose weight and keep it off for good; others claim it's closer to 5 percent. Although those figures are hotly contested, what we do know for certain is that even those researchers who support dieting concur that diets fail at least 80 to 90 percent of the time.[1] After a year, the overwhelming majority of dieters regain whatever weight they've lost. Worse still, almost two-thirds end up weighing even more within four or five years than before they started their diet.[2]

By now you might be thinking this is an odd way to begin a diet book. You're probably wondering, "Dr. Colbert, why would you even write a diet book if diets don't work? Why should I bother trying to lose weight if it will most likely come back?"

SUCCESS FOR LIFE

I'll be honest with you: If you are just looking to continue that pattern of following here-today, gone-tomorrow fad diets, you might as well put down this book now. Go ahead, you have my permission. Why? Because I am not a fan of diets. In fact, I think dieting, over the long haul, is one of the surest ways to become frustrated, discouraged, fed up, and even depressed about losing weight. How do I know this?

1

Because after treating more than forty thousand patients over the past twenty-five years, I have observed some definitive commonalities among those who repeatedly attempted to lose weight, only to gain it back. I have also found a medically verifiable answer that leads to lifetime success in this area.

That's a big statement, I know. I have yet to find it in any diet book—or at least any that can back it up with proof. Virtually every diet assures you that you can lose weight following its principles, techniques, and plan. Yet most, if not all, stop short of making long-term promises. Why do you think that is? Could it be they know that over the course of several months, years, even decades, it becomes impossible to stick to their guidelines?

It seems the industry has caught on. We are currently seeing a trend among weight-loss books that claim to be anything but a diet. They have finally realized that people are tired of jumping from one trendy diet to another, only to lose a few pounds here that eventually—*always*—find their way back.

So what makes *Dr. Colbert's "I Can Do This" Diet* any different from those books? As a medical doctor, I deal every day with getting results—verifiable results that prove a patient is on his way to long-term health, not just fixing an immediate problem. And that is what this book is about. You will learn:

- How to overcome your hidden obstacles to weight loss, such as insulin resistance, neurotransmitter imbalance, hormonal imbalance, and delayed food sensitivities
- How to design a meal plan for YOUR body, including snacking, cooking, eating out, shopping, supplements, and more
- The secret about calories that will boost your metabolism and make weight loss easier

Dr. Colbert's "I Can Do This" Diet is the only weight-loss program that puts together all of the factors that affect your weight—emotional, behavioral, mental, dietary, hormonal, chemical, and lifestyle factors—and teaches you how to incorporate these principles into your life. Finally, here's a plan that will help you say, "I can do this!"

Yes, *Dr. Colbert's "I Can Do This" Diet* is far more than a diet; it's a lifestyle. It will not offer you a quick-fix approach to anything. But more importantly, it offers you principles that are meant to last for life, principles that have been proven to work for thousands of individuals for more than a decade and counting.

Also different from diets you may have tried in the past, the "I Can Do This" diet offers an interactive online survey that will help you target hidden road-

blocks that often make dieting an endless cycle of losing and gaining weight. Have you tried a new diet only to stop losing weight after a few weeks? Learn why this plateau happens and how to get past it to your desired weight!

DROP THE DIET AND GET A LIFESTYLE

Most likely you picked up this book because you are on your last dieting straw. Maybe you have tried many of the diets out there, and, like my patients, you've seen temporary results once again turn into familiar flab. If you are one of the millions fed up with dieting, you have picked up the perfect solution, something that will put a stake in the heart of the dieter's approach to eating.

Unlike most hard-nosed diet creators, I adhere to the belief that food, like life, is to be enjoyed. Some foods take a needless toll on the body and should be avoided at all costs. Others have gotten lost in the fad-diet shuffle and ended up on the wrong side of the "eat/don't eat" lists. Still others can help you lose weight and even assist in keeping off those pounds.

The key, then, is finding a road map to help navigate through the often-treacherous territory of losing weight. And that is exactly what you hold in your hands. Every appliance and electronic gadget comes with an instruction manual. This book is your instruction manual for permanent weight loss. I wrote every chapter of this book with the phrase *long-term* foremost in my mind. As a result, this is an extremely practical guidebook that teaches you how to address your immediate issues while adopting a dietary lifestyle that is maintainable for years to come.

When you see the following symbols, you will find:

READ MORE ABOUT IT

Other books you can refer to for more information on topic being discussed

Other sections of this book where I address the same topic

My goal is not only to equip you with everyday tools for staying on course and avoiding detours but also to infuse you with the knowledge to overcome even bigger obstacles in the future.

That is why the first section of this book is all about explaining a few basic elements of weight gain and weight loss. And over the years, I have found that far too many people are illiterate when it comes to the basics of how our bodies process food—and how we can use that information to our advantage when managing our weight. Without getting too bogged down in scientific terms, we will explore several fundamental areas of weight loss.

After that comes a preparation for the actual program. It is one thing to educate people on what they must do to lose weight for life; it's another to count the cost and explain what that actually takes. In this second section, I will prepare you for this wonderful lifelong journey by helping you be honest with yourself and establish reachable goals, among other things.

That is followed by—you guessed it—the nuts and bolts of the "I Can Do This" program. Here I offer tips on designing a program catered just for you, including snacking, cooking, eating out, shopping, supplements, and many other issues. Though this is obviously the heart of this book, I strongly advise you to not skip ahead and only read that particular section. The reason is simple: that is exactly what a quick-fix, shortsighted dieter would do. I have written this third section so that anyone—even someone casually skimming through the book—can glean some helpful takeaways on how to lose weight for good. But without the heart and wisdom that are developed previous to those chapters, it might as well be just another eating plan to that person.

Finally, our road map ends with a self-test followed by my recommendations for what to do when you, for whatever reason, are stalled on the side of the road. There are very real physiological conditions (insulin resistance, hormone imbalance, neurotransmitter imbalance, and so on) that can prevent you from losing weight even if you are doing everything right. But there is hope. There are ways to overcome these conditions and find success. I have seen the results in my patients.

That's why, after taking the test, you will be encouraged to visit www .thecandodiet.com for the individualized, in-depth information I've provided there about conquering your particular roadblock to weight loss. The truth is, *everyone* will hit a plateau when it comes to losing weight and keeping it off. The key is being prepared to jump-start your body and your eating lifestyle.

I believe that by the end of this book you will have made an about-face in your approach to losing weight. Since you have picked up this book, I trust you realized the journey to controlling your weight does not include quick fixes. For making that decision, I congratulate you. The further you distance yourself from the old dieting mentality, the better off you will be. I cannot wait to see the new you...and I know you can't either.

SECTION I

UNDERSTANDING WEIGHT GAIN AND WEIGHT LOSS

1

THE OBESITY EPIDEMIC: WHAT WE'RE UP AGAINST

A FEW YEARS AGO a thirty-two-year-old man named Morgan Spurlock became Ronald McDonald's worst nightmare. Intent on correlating the rise of obesity in our nation with the fast-food giant, the independent filmmaker conducted a personal experiment—using himself as the guinea pig. For thirty days he ate nothing but McDonald's food. He downed three meals a day, sampling every item on the Golden Arches' menu. And whenever he was asked if he wanted his meal supersized, he accepted.

With cameras rolling the entire time, Spurlock transformed his body into a flab factory while consuming an average of 5,000 calories a day and gaining almost 25 pounds in a single month. He also turned his Academy Award–nominated documentary, *Super Size Me*, into a statement heard around the world.[1]

The jury is still out on whether Americans were actually paying attention. Though recent statistics indicate that the obesity rates in the United States may be stabilizing, they're still at unprecedented, staggering levels.[2] Since the 1960s, the proportion of obese Americans—now an astounding *34 percent*—has more than doubled.[3] Obesity currently kills an estimated four hundred thousand Americans each year and is the second-leading cause of preventable deaths in this country.[4] The number one avoidable killer? Cigarette smoking.[5] That means maintaining a healthy weight is up there with quitting smoking as the most crucial lifestyle change you could ever make. Because we're seeing a trend of people deciding to quit smoking, I predict that obesity will soon pass smoking as the number one avoidable killer of Americans.

Unfortunately, many doctors, nutritionists, and dietitians seem to completely miss or ignore this fact. They love to offer topical "Band-Aids" that alleviate patients' symptoms yet fail to tackle the root issues or consider the long-term ramifications of neglecting their patients' weight. One recent report from the Centers for Disease Control and Prevention (CDC) found that about a *third* of obese adults have never been told by a doctor or health-care provider

7

that they were obese.[6] Unbelievable! The results speak for themselves. In fact, they're screaming while most practitioners turn the other way.

As our nation faces the biggest health-care crisis in its history, it's time for us to realize that the answer isn't going to come from doctors, clinics, or the U.S. government. It's going to come from each person taking responsibility for their own health. And because obesity and overweight are at the root of so many health conditions, it only makes sense to start by getting yourself to a healthy weight.

Defining the Problem

Before we delve into what has so many people visiting the plus-size department, let's clarify the terms *overweight* and *obese*. Many people have a general sense as to how these words are different, yet in recent years the delineation has become clearer. Various health organizations, including the CDC and the National Institutes of Health (NIH), now officially define these terms using the body mass index (BMI), which factors in a person's weight relative to height. Most of these organizations define an overweight adult as having a BMI between 25 and 29.9, while an obese adult is anyone who has a BMI of 30 or higher.[7]

It's worth mentioning that a very small portion of individuals are overweight or obese according to their BMI (over 30) yet have a normal or low body fat percentage. Professional athletes, for instance, often have a high-muscle, low body fat makeup that causes them to weigh more than the average person, yet they are not truly obese (some football linemen and sumo wrestlers excluded, of course).

However, I have found that most of the people who come to me seeking help are not just overweight but technically obese, with a body fat percentage greater than 25

Calories Cost

Researchers have discovered that for every 100 extra calories a person eats each day, the additional costs beyond meals—such as health care and gasoline—add up to between 48 cents and $2.00. In fact, simply supersizing your meal for "only" 35 cents more can actually end up costing you between 82 cents to $6.64 in extra health-care costs.[9]

percent for males and greater than 33 percent for females.[8] Throughout this book when I discuss having a high BMI (over 30), I will be referring to obese people and not those few muscular types with high BMI but a normal or low body fat percentage.

THE FAT COST OF OBESITY

When all is considered, obesity comes with a fat price tag (pun intended) of nearly \$122.9 billion each year.[10] Recently William L. Weis, a management professor at Seattle University, calculated the total annual revenue from the "obesity industry"—which includes fast-food restaurants, obesity-related medical treatments, and diet books—as more than \$315 billion. That amounts to nearly 3 percent of the United States' overall economy![11] As shocking as that sounds, no dollar amount can do justice to the real damage being done.

If you are overweight or obese, you increase your risk of developing thirty-five major diseases, including (take a deep breath) heart disease, stroke, arthritis, type 2 diabetes, sleep apnea, gastroesophageal reflux disease, hypertension, high cholesterol, high triglycerides, Alzheimer's disease, infertility, erectile dysfunction, gallstones, gallbladder disease, adult-onset asthma, and depression. In fact, we now know that being overweight or obese increases your odds of developing more than a dozen forms of cancer. After reviewing more than seven thousand medical studies over the course of five years, a team of highly respected scientists from around the world concluded in 2007 that diet and weight have a direct effect on the chances of developing cancer. With help from the World Cancer Research Fund and the American Institute for Cancer, they listed the top ten recommendations for cancer prevention; *body fat* came in at number one. Their report also strongly recommended maintaining a normal range of body weight, which they identified as a body mass index between 18.5 and 24.9, to assist in cancer prevention.[12]

If you are an obese woman, you have a significantly higher risk of postmenopausal breast cancer—one and a half times more than a woman with an average healthy weight, to be exact. You also increase your chances of developing uterine cancer because of your weight. For pregnant mothers, the risk of delivering a baby with a serious birth defect is doubled if you are overweight and quadrupled if you are obese.[13] Men, your chances of developing prostate cancer are almost double if you are overweight, and even greater if you are obese.[14] (Prostate cancer is the second-most common cancer among men behind skin cancer.) A separate new study indicates that the greater a man's weight, the greater his chances of dying from a stroke.[15] Finally, for both men and women the odds of getting colon and kidney cancer increase with weight. And being obese triples your risk of developing Alzheimer's disease.

This is just a sampling of the physical implications of obesity. There are social and psychological ones too. Obese individuals generally contend with more rejection and prejudice than the average person. Often they are overlooked for

promotions or not even hired because of their physical appearance. Most obese people struggle daily with self-worth and self-image issues. They feel unattractive and unappreciated and are at an increased risk of depression. Many of us have experienced the humiliating experience of an obese person trying to fit in an airplane, stadium, or automobile seat that is too small. Maybe you have been that person. If you have, you are well acquainted with how obesity can affect the way others treat you, as well as how you treat yourself.

Globesity and a Culprit

Tragically, millions of others outside the United States struggle with the same issues. The World Health Organization calls obesity a worldwide epidemic. Obesity, along with its expanding list of health consequences, is now overtaking infection and malnutrition as the main cause of death and disability in many third-world countries. *Globesity*, as it has been termed, has officially arrived. And it seems Morgan Spurlock was on the right track in discovering a major reason why.

READ MORE ABOUT IT

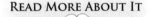

Learn more about fast food and obesity in *Fast Food Nation* by Eric Schlosser.

In *Fast Food Nation*, author Eric Schlosser reports that in 1970, Americans spent about $6 billion on fast food; in 2000, we spent more than $110 billion. Because corporate America is a global trendsetter, other countries have followed suit. Between 1984 and 1993, the number of fast-food restaurants in Great Britain doubled, as did the obesity rate among adults. Fast-forward fifteen years, and you will find the British currently eat more fast food than any other nation in Western Europe.

Meanwhile, the proportion of overweight teens in China has roughly tripled in the past decade. In Japan, the obesity rate among children doubled during the 1980s, which correlated with a 200 percent increase in fast-food sales. This generation of Japanese has gone on to become the first in the nation's history known for its bulging waistlines. Approximately one-third of all Japanese men in their thirties are now overweight.[16] Yes, the entire world

TRENDS IN CHILDHOOD OBESITY

Research shows that from 1980 to 2006, the prevalence of obesity has jumped from 5 percent to 12 percent in children ages two to five, from 6.5 percent to 17 percent in ages six to eleven, and from 5 percent to 17.6 percent in ages twelve to nineteen..[17]

is beginning to look more like Americans by adopting our fast-food eating habits.

A Child Shall Lead Them

How has an entire generation of hefty eaters changed the face of the world? By starting young. And once again, this unflattering trend originated in America. In the United States, one-fifth of our children are now reported to be overweight, and one out of ten (24 million adults) have diabetes. The CDC predicts that one out of three children born in the United States in 2000 will develop type 2 diabetes at some point in their life.[18]

As a result of childhood obesity, we are seeing a dramatic rise in children with type 2 diabetes throughout the country. And because of the connection obesity has with hypertension, hypercholesterolemia (high cholesterol), and heart disease, experts are predicting a dramatic rise in heart disease as our children become adults. The CDC reports that overweight teens stand a 70 percent chance of becoming overweight adults, and that is increased to 80 percent if at least one parent is overweight or obese. Because of that, heart disease and type 2 diabetes are expected to begin at a much earlier age in those who fail to beat the odds.[19] Overall, this is the first generation of children that is not expected to live as long as their parents, and they will be more likely to suffer from disease and illness at an earlier age.

If you do not lose weight for yourself, at least do it for your children. Children follow by example, by mirroring the behavior of their parents. Don't tell them to lose weight without doing it yourself. I'm sure most of you love your children and are good parents. But ask yourself: Do you love your children enough to lose weight? Do you love them enough to educate them on what foods to eat and what foods to

The Link to Illnesses

More than 90 percent of people who are newly diagnosed with type 2 diabetes are overweight or obese.[20]

Obesity also increases your risk of developing the following cancers: esophageal, thyroid, colon, kidney, prostate, endometrial, gallbladder, rectal, breast, pancreatic, leukemia, multiple myloma, malignant melanoma, and non-Hodgkin's lymphoma.[21]

Being overweight increases your risk of having GERD (acid reflux) symptoms by 50 percent; being obese doubles your chances.[22]

Excess weight is also commonly known to cause sleep apnea and hypertension (high blood pressure). In fact, 75 percent of all cases of hypertension in the United States are attributed to obesity.[23]

avoid? Do you love them enough to keep junk food out of your house and instead make healthy food more available? Do you love them enough to exercise regularly and lead by example?

If you answered yes to those questions, it is important that you not only take action for your children's sake but also that you make changes for them that last. I am ecstatic that you have picked up this book. I believe you now hold the key to truly changing your life. But let me be honest; this is not an easy fight when it involves your children's lives. The culture in which they are growing up is saturated with junk food that is void of nutrition but high in toxic fats, sugars, highly processed carbohydrates, and food additives. Consuming these foods has become part of childhood. For example, in 1978, the typical teenage boy in the United States drank seven ounces of soda a day; today he drinks approximately three times that much. Meanwhile, he gets about a quarter of his daily servings of vegetables from french fries and potato chips.[24]

If you're planning on taking a stand against this garbage-in, garbage-out culture, expect some opposition from every front. During the course of a year, the typical American child will watch more than thirty thousand television commercials, with many of these advertisements pitching fast food or junk food as delicious "must-eats." For years, fast-food franchises have enticed children into their restaurants with kids' meal toys, promotional giveaways, and elaborate playgrounds. It has obviously worked for McDonald's: about 90 percent of American children between the ages of three and nine set foot in one each month.[25] And when they can't visit the Golden Arches, it comes to them. Fast-food products—most of which are brought in by franchises—are sold in about 30 percent of public high school cafeterias and many elementary cafeterias.[26]

These fast-food establishments spend billions of dollars on research and marketing. They know exactly what they are doing and how to push your child's hot button. They understand the powerful impact certain foods can have on you at a young age. Have you ever thought of when you first started liking certain foods? For the majority of people, those preferences were formed during the first few years of life. That is why comfort foods often do more than just fill the stomach; they bring about memories of the fair, playgrounds, toys, backyard birthday bashes, Fourth of July parties, childhood

WORLD HUNGER

McDonald's feeds an astounding forty-seven million people a day around the world. That's more than the entire populations of Canada and Cambodia combined![27]

friends…the list goes on. The aroma of foods such as onion rings, doughnuts, or fried hamburgers can instantly trigger these memories, and as adults, we are often unconsciously drawn to these smells. Advertisers have keyed into this and learned to use the sight of food to stimulate the same fond childhood memories.

In the Genes or in the Water?

For every obese person, there is a story behind the excessive weight gain. Growing up, I would often hear it said of an obese person that "she was just born fat," or "he takes after his daddy." There's some truth in both of those. Genetics count when it comes to obesity.

In 1988, the *New England Journal of Medicine* published a Danish study that observed five hundred forty people who had been adopted during infancy. The research found that adopted individuals had a much greater tendency to end up in the weight class of their biological parents rather than their adoptive parents.[28] Separate studies have proven that twins raised apart also reveal that genes have a strong influence on gaining weight or becoming overweight.[29] There is a significant genetic predisposition to gaining weight.

Still, that does not fully explain the epidemic of obesity seen in the United States over the past thirty years. Although an individual may have a genetic predisposition to become obese, environment plays a major role as well. I like the way author, speaker, and noted women's physician Pamela Peeke said it: "Genetics may load the gun, but environment pulls the trigger."[30] Many patients I see come into my office thinking they have inherited their "fat genes," and therefore there is nothing they can do about it. After investigating a little, I usually find that they simply inherited their parents' propensity for bad choices of foods, large portion sizes, and poor eating habits.

If you have been overweight since childhood, you probably have an increased number of fat cells, which means you will have a tendency to gain weight if you choose the wrong types of foods, large portion sizes, and are inactive. But you should also realize that most people can override their genetic makeup for obesity by making the correct dietary and lifestyle choices. Unfortunately, many of us forget that to make these healthy choices, it helps to surround ourselves with a healthy environment.

That is becoming more difficult than ever as families give way to their hectic routines by grabbing breakfasts-on-the-go, ordering fast-food lunches, dining out for dinner, and skipping meals. After years of this, it is catching up to us. The average American adult gains between 1 to 3 pounds a year,

beginning at age twenty-five. That means a twenty-five-year-old, 120-pound female can expect to weigh anywhere from 150 to 210 pounds by the time she is fifty-five years of age. Is there any wonder why we have an epidemic of heart disease, type 2 diabetes, hypertension, high cholesterol, arthritis, cancer, and other degenerative diseases? We have to put the brakes on this obesity epidemic—and a lifestyle approach to eating is the answer!

ADDING CULTURE TO THE MIX

Just as environment often shapes your health habits, so does culture. The two walk hand in hand when it comes to causing obesity. As children, we develop our food preferences and habits based on our family environment. Yet every family is influenced by its surrounding culture, and culture often shapes the types of foods, recipes, and ingredients we choose on a regular basis.

I was raised in Mississippi. Ever since I was a child I remember how my mother's coffee cup always sat on the stove in the kitchen. But instead of coffee, it was filled with bacon grease. Whenever she cooked vegetables—any kind—she would add a few tablespoons of that bacon grease to add flavor. She fried almost everything: fried chicken, fried hamburgers, fried salmon, fried fish sticks, chicken fried steaks, fried chicken livers, fried ham, fried pork chops, fried bacon...you name it. Why did she do this? Because her mother had taught her to fry virtually any meat.

Mom also usually made gravies, all of which were grease-based. Most meals were served with corn bread or biscuits, either of which contained a hefty amount of Crisco shortening. We rarely ate grilled food, and when we did, it was a fatty cut of meat. I still remember my father making me eat all the fat on my steak. Since I was a skinny kid, he would say, "Son, that fat is good for you—it will help to fatten you up." I recall almost puking as I tried to get the fat down.

We were a typical Southern family. My brother, sister, and I were all raised to eat fried foods, greasy foods, biscuits, and corn bread—and top it all off with a large piece of cake or pie for dessert. Today, I see a similar thing happening in the southwestern part of the United States. This Southwest culture, which is in part defined by its Tex-Mex and Mexican eating habits, is helping to fuel the obesity epidemic. Most of these people are being raised on highly processed white breads or corn tortillas, white rice and fried white rice, corn chips, refried beans, fried tacos, enchiladas, nachos...the list goes on. Their diet typically contains a lot of fats, a lot of grease, a ton of highly processed carbohydrates, and a lot of sugar.

It is no coincidence that almost every year some Texas city has the unflattering distinction of having the largest number of obese individuals in the country. After Houston was named the "fattest city" multiple times in past years, 2008 saw Arlington, San Antonio, Fort Worth, El Paso, and Dallas all place among the top ten fattest cities of *Men's Fitness* magazine's "Annual Fattest and Fittest Cities in America Report." The year before, four of those cities made the dubious honor.[31] Not only do these overweight hot spots feature some of the country's best Tex-Mex and Mexican style foods, but they also offer extra large Texas portions with a blend of some of the most calorie-dense cultural foods around. Is there any wonder why Texans have a major obesity problem?

EATING WITH THE HEAD AND NOT THE HEART

We have discussed how genetics can sometimes, though rarely, prompt an individual's obese state. We have also talked about how the overwhelming majority of obesity cases are a direct result of environment and culture. These can be discouraging factors in light of the gloomy statistics and the ongoing epidemic. However, I want to end this chapter on a positive note by reminding you of a simple truth. In fact, it is what this book is all about.

> ### ENSALADA
> Just because a taco salad features the word *salad* doesn't mean it's healthy. With the massive fried tortilla shell, beef, cheese, sour cream, and additional items (plus the nutritionally useless iceberg lettuce), most taco salads add up to about 900 calories and 55 grams of fat.

Regardless of how difficult it sounds, your cultural tastes and foods can be changed over time with education, practice, and discipline. You can learn how to choose similar foods that have not been excessively processed as well as lower-fat alternatives. It's possible to discover—or rediscover—portion control and healthy cooking methods. Sure, you may still love your fried chicken, mashed potatoes and gravy, and chocolate cake. But soon you will be able to enjoy the same foods with just a fraction of the fat, sugars, and calories.

When I wrote the book *What Would Jesus Eat?* about the Mediterranean diet, I learned that most Middle Easterners ate differently than the typical American. That sounds obvious, but what distinguishes the two isn't. I found that those who are used to a Mediterranean diet typically would not leave the dinner table stuffed as most Americans do. Generally, they ate anything they wanted—but in moderation. They enjoyed their food and

socialized while eating. They had the uncanny ability to enjoy just a few bites of their favorite foods such as wine, dark chocolate, or even chocolate ice cream. Unlike most Americans, who scarf down a dessert as if they were inhaling it, those eating a Mediterranean diet actually savored just a few bites.

The real pleasure in most foods is in the first few bites. We will discuss this later, but for now, know that you can break out of your old cultural eating patterns. You do not have to follow a parent's poor food choices, and you can overcome your family's eating cultural patterns. (I certainly did!) And in the process, you will discover the true joy of eating.

"CAN DO" POINTS TO REMEMBER

1. Currently, one out of three Americans is obese.

2. An overweight adult is defined as having a BMI between 25 and 29.9, while an obese adult is anyone who has a BMI of 30 or higher.

3. Being overweight or obese increases your odds of getting more than a dozen forms of cancer.

4. The amount of overweight children has nearly doubled in the past twenty-five years, while the number of overweight adolescents has almost tripled.

5. Your children will model your eating habits and food choices. If you are not losing weight for yourself, at least do it for them!

6. As much as you may blame your family genes for your obesity, you must take responsibility for your own poor eating choices.

7. Though food choices are often shaped by your environment and culture, they can be changed.

2

The Seven Habits of Highly Effective Losers

T HE NATIONAL WEIGHT Control Registry (NWCR) at the Brown Medical School includes the names of more than five thousand individuals who have been successful at both losing and keeping off a significant amount of weight. Started in 1994 by Rena Wing, PhD, from Brown Medical School, and James Hill, PhD, from the University of Colorado, the NWCR was established to track and investigate why certain people succeed in controlling their weight long term while others do not. The requirements in being listed on the registry are clear: you must lose at least 30 pounds and keep it off for at least a year.[1]

While that may not sound like much to the person who has never struggled with weight issues, it is no small feat for those who are overweight or obese. It may surprise you to hear that only a measly 2 to 20 percent of dieters are able to maintain their weight loss. Those on the NWCR *are* able to maintain their weight loss—which should make you curious as to what sets them apart from the rest of overweight America. The NWCR provides some of these answers by the sheer nature of its enrollment process. The registry is open to anyone who meets the criteria, and unlike many studies, it involves detailed questionnaires that ask registrants about their diet history—both failures and successes—as well as what they are currently doing to maintain their weight-loss success.

The overwhelming majority of those who register with the NWCR are women (80 percent), and the range of weight lost is from 30 to 300 pounds, with the average loss being an impressive 66 pounds. Some members shed their pounds rapidly, while others did it slowly. (In fact, some registrants took as long as fourteen years to lose. Talk about perseverance!) The duration of successful weight loss and ongoing maintenance ranges from the minimum of one year to an incredible sixty-six years, with an average of five and a half years. The average female listed on the NWCR is forty-five years old and weighs 145 pounds, and the average male is forty-nine years old and weighs

190 pounds. Overall, 55 percent of the members lost weight with the assistance of some type of program, while 45 percent did so on their own. Both groups used a variety of diets, eating programs, exercises, and behavioral changes to get their lasting results.[2]

In other words, members of the NWCR are all over the place, as are their keys to success. There is no prototypical loser among them; neither is there a set method or magical diet. In fact, a 2003 *Consumer Reports* survey of more than thirty-two thousand dieters found similar results.[3] Most "successful" dieters tended to follow low-carb and high-protein diets rather than low-fat diets. (I use the term "successful" loosely because we must remember that statistics prove many of these respondents will regain their weight.) Numerous studies have given low-carb, high-protein diets the upper hand over low-fat diets because of diabetes prevention, metabolic syndrome improvement, and overall heart health.[4] Other findings indicate that low-fat diets are better for cardiovascular health.[5] Yet when it comes to sheer weight loss, a few hours researching online will prove not only that scientific studies vary widely on making a definitive assessment of which diet is best, but also that individuals respond differently to different diets.

> ### WORKING TWICE AS HARD
>
> The average woman has been on a diet ten times in her lifetime, compared to only five times for the average man.[6]

PICKING UP SOME HABITS

Years ago Stephen Covey wrote a monumental book titled *The Seven Habits of Highly Effective People*. It became such a megahit that it spawned a series of similar titles, courses, and seminars used around the world. The seven underlying principles, as you might guess, were simply drawn from observing successful models, people whom Covey considered worthy of imitating. I believe those listed as part of the NWCR deserve similar treatment. Although they run the gamut as to how they lost their weight and have kept it off, there are still some common threads

> ### CREATING NEW HABITS
>
> Many experts say that it takes twenty-one days to form a habit. Others say it takes forty days to form a new habit and ninety days to make that habit a natural part of your lifestyle. Regardless of the time frame, rest assured that whatever you continually practice will become a habit, so practice making healthy choices every day!

among all five-thousand-plus members. Before we go any further in this book, I think it would behoove us to take note of these common traits.

What really makes these losers different from all the gainers? By answering that question and understanding the characteristics of these successful eaters, you can then evaluate how you line up. I encourage you to consider each habit as a measuring stick. If you are weak in any of these habits, find the chapters in this book or the information online at www.thecandodiet.com that apply to those traits and take them to heart. Just as mimicking a professional basketball player's shooting form can often improve your shot, so can emulating these successful losers' habits help you lose your pounds—for good.

Habit #1: Modify your food intake.

In order to lose weight, 98 percent of registry members changed what they ate in some manner. Almost universally they consumed fewer calories; on average, they took in about 1,400 calories a day, which is considerably less than the average American. (I do not recommend consuming only 1,400 calories, especially for men who usually need at least 2,200 calories a day. Women, on the other hand, usually need at least 1,800 calories a day.) Most members switched to a low-fat diet, cutting their fat intake to an average of 24 percent of their total calorie consumption. The majority of registrants cut back on sugars and sweets, while also eating more fruits and vegetables.

Members also reported they went through a fast-food line less than once a week and ate out at restaurants no more than three times a week. And what may be the most interesting statistic of all: 88 percent practiced careful food selection rather than restricting the amount and types of foods they ate. In other words, they made healthy choices from a vast variety of foods.

> ### HERE TURKEY, TURKEY
>
> Not all turkey sandwiches are created equal. Rather than opting for a Sierra Turkey sandwich from Panera Bread, which has 840 calories and 40 grams of fat, choose a Subway six-inch Turkey Sub (330 calories, 8.5 grams of fat).[7]

As you continue through this book, you will find this last point to be one of the greatest assets of the "I Can Do This" program. After helping thousands of weight-loss patients, I have concluded that most people will not succeed unless things are kept simple. If you look at the most popular and instantly effective diets out there, you will notice they all have one thing in common: simplicity. I live by that rule of thumb, and as a result, my patients are always amazed at how easy the "I Can Do This" program is to implement—no calorie counting,

no keeping track of carb amounts or fat grams, no specialty foods. In fact, you will find there is an almost unlimited variety of foods from which you can choose, and it all comes down to being mindful of what's going in your mouth and eating the correct food combinations every three to three and a half hours.

Habit #2: Increase your activity level.

Being active is absolutely crucial for maintaining weight loss. More than 90 percent of NWCR members use physical activity as part of their ongoing lifestyle to control their weight. Along with changing their diet (only 1 percent relied solely on exercise to lose their weight), those individuals were physically active for approximately an hour a day and burned on average 400 calories each day. Ninety-four percent of registrants increased their physical activity mainly by walking—proving how simple and easy an active lifestyle can be. Most individuals stayed fit by engaging in such enjoyable activities as cycling, weightlifting, swimming, or jogging.

It's important that these people exercised more. Yet just as important to note is what they did less of—namely, being couch potatoes. Sixty-two percent of those registered watch fewer than ten hours of television each week. That is significantly less than the thirty-plus hours the average American spends glued to the tube.[8] Clearly, there is a direct correlation between losing weight and getting off the couch.

THINK AGAIN

Since the body burns calories during sleep, many dieters believe that skipping breakfast extends their fat-burning time. In fact, waiting more than ninety minutes after getting up to eat breakfast may increase your risk of becoming obese by almost 50 percent.[9]

Habit #3: Eat breakfast every day.

Nearly eight out of ten members ate breakfast every day during their weight-loss phase. We will touch on this throughout the book, but at this point just know that eating a healthy, well-balanced breakfast is instrumental in how successful your weight-loss efforts will be. Aside from setting the dietary tone for your day, eating a healthy breakfast boosts your metabolic rate, which enables you to continue burning a significant amount of calories and fat. It also helps to control your hunger, which in turn can ward off the temptation to binge eat later in the day. As you will learn, the effects of eating—or not eating—breakfast last long into the day. My most successful weight-loss patients understand this simple yet often-overlooked key.

Habit #4: Monitor your weight regularly.

A common trait of successful losers and maintainers is weighing themselves frequently. Many would weigh themselves on a daily basis. I do not recommend weighing yourself daily during the weight-loss portion of this program, mainly because pounds can easily become a source of discouragement. I have known many patients who became obsessed with each fraction of a pound, and when they hit any kind of plateau, they lost all momentum. Even though their bodies were in tune with the routine of losing weight, their emotions suddenly hit a fatigue point. And as we all know, you cannot lose weight without being both physically and emotionally connected to the process.

This is not to say you should not keep track of your weight at all. As you will discover, I recommend judging most of your initial performance by how your clothes fit and your body fat percentage—ultimately, how many inches you lose off your waist. Along with this, you will weigh yourself regularly (usually once a month). Once you've reached your goal weight, you are encouraged to weigh yourself daily during the maintenance portion of the program. Daily monitoring your weight once you have reached your goal will better enable you to maintain your goal weight.

The NWCR's research confirms that several years of successful weight maintenance increases the probability of future weight maintenance and that regularly keeping tabs on your weight helps this. In other words, if you have already maintained your weight loss for years and suddenly add a pound or two in one day, you are more likely to know how to respond to keep your progress intact. You would immediately know to either increase your activity level or adjust your diet to shed those pounds. The

I'll explain why I don't recommend daily weigh-ins in chapter 14.

NWCR found that, by simply monitoring their weight daily, most members were able to do this before a slight gain became a bigger problem. Remember, however, that this was during the *maintenance* phase, and not while these members were initially losing weight. Daily weighing helps you maintain your weight loss, but as I said, I do not recommend daily weighing while losing weight.

Habit #5: Stay consistent with your eating.

Registrants who successfully maintained their weight remained consistent with their eating patterns even during holidays, company parties, vacations, and cruises. Regardless of the special occasion, they kept their eating regimen

not because they were just following a diet but because it became a natural way of life. Obviously, there were exceptions to this: some NWCR members did cheat on occasion. But they did not let their cheating turn into bingeing or a habit. Instead, they were able to pick themselves up after their mistake and get back on track.

Understand that there will always be distractions, mistakes, and flubs. Most of these occur when you are confronted with the prospect of indulging in one of your favorite foods. The "I Can Do This" program isn't built to bar you from these favorite foods; it simply teaches you how to incorporate them into the bigger picture, which is the goal of losing those extra pounds and keeping them off.

Unfortunately, many people do not know how to handle the times when they fall off-track. For some, it starts with something as simple as deciding to "take a break" over a weekend or while on vacation. I will never forget a patient of mine who had successfully lost 100 pounds in eighteen months. He was on a regular exercise program and eating a healthy diet. He felt wonderful, so he rewarded himself by going on a cruise with his wife. When he returned from the cruise a week later, he had gained 20 pounds! Once on board, he had completely let loose, splurging on desserts, breads, multiple entrées with each meal, and, of course, the midnight buffets.

THE NEW 10 IS THE OLD 12

For years, high-end women's clothes manufacturers have practiced "vanity sizing," which is downsizing clothes to flatter consumers. Yet this practice is now a mainstream staple, with most clothes varying drastically not only from generations ago but also from retailer to retailer. As the average American woman has become larger, so have her clothes—yet the sizes have decreased, including recent additions of such misnomers as sizes "00" and "XXS."[10]

When I saw him, he assured me this would not be a problem and that he would simply get back on the program. That never happened. He continued to crave and eat these same types of foods, and he began coming up with more excuses each time he would indulge in them. Eventually he regained the hundred pounds he had lost; he simply could not get back on track.

I share that story to remind you of a key truth: the choice is up to you. Regardless of how much I pinpoint your lifelong struggle with weight in this book, ultimately I cannot save you. I can offer you advice and can describe a program that's been successful for thousands of others, but at the end of the day, *you* make the call. *You* have to learn these principles for yourself and believe in them enough to the extent that they become a natural part of your

everyday life. And unlike my patient who couldn't stay on track, *you* have to be aware of when you are losing ground. Which leads us to the next habit...

Habit #6: Control your portion sizes and your environment.

Yale researcher Diane Berry studied a group of women who maintained a weight loss of 15 to 144 pounds for at least a year. She found there were no fewer than three distinct behavioral characteristics consistent among these successful dieters. First, they were more aware of trigger foods and excessive portion sizes—two common traps for females. Second, they incorporated regular exercise into their lifestyle. And third, they recognized that to be successful, they would have to incorporate these behavioral changes into their lifestyles.[11]

Large portion sizes and comfort foods are two of the main reasons why obesity is an epidemic in this country. Those are common weak spots among dieters. So is the temptation to remain inactive and skip another workout. Both of these areas, however, can be easily managed by *doing* something. You have to actively manage your portion sizes and your food environment. Berry's final observation involves a changing mind-set. Behavioral changes have to be made for good, not just for a season of life. To be successful long term, you must habitually practice portion control, and you must habitually remove irresistible, tempting foods from your home and office.

I'll discuss more about irresistible foods and portion control in chapters 4 and 11 respectively.

Habit #7: Be accountable.

Being accountable has a twofold meaning. First, it involves being held accountable by others. Fifty-five percent of NWCR's members lost weight with the help of some outside force.[12] If it was a diet program, they most likely had someone holding them up to the diet's standards. Similarly, most of my patients will comment on how much more successful they are in losing weight when they meet with me on a regular basis than when they try to do it alone. Accountability has proven itself to

PERSON TO PERSON

When it comes to accountability, face-to-face meetings always win out. In one eighteen-month study that followed individuals who had successfully lost weight, those who kept in touch by newsletter had a 70 percent chance of regaining at least 5 pounds; those who kept tabs via the Internet had a 54 percent chance of gaining back the same amount, while only 38 percent of individuals who held each other accountable in person regained more than 5 pounds.[13]

be an incredible guiding force for losing weight, whether that comes through attending diet groups, meeting with another person, or keeping tabs through an online community. This is why weight-loss programs such as Weight Watchers have weathered the fad-diet phases throughout the years. They are built upon the idea that success comes with support.

Yet even the NWCR results prove that not every successful loser must be a part of a dieting group. I believe the key, then, lies in being accountable to yourself—and by that I mean coming to grips with the reality of your current situation. When you are overweight or obese, you know your condition. You are reminded daily by magazines, TV shows, billboard ads—even friends, families, and strangers—of how "unskinny" you are. Yet this does not necessarily lead to productive behavior.

One study found that individuals who were dissatisfied with their body shape used this as motivation to lose weight and met success.[14] These individuals were driven by a desire to feel attractive. Another study, however, revealed that individuals who were extremely dissatisfied with their physical appearance or who had a history of repeated weight loss were at a higher risk of failure.[15] Given these two extremes, we see that mild dissatisfaction can motivate you to lose weight, but extreme dissatisfaction may actually sabotage weight loss. So how do you avoid the latter?

We'll cover reprogramming your mind for weight loss in chapter 12.

Essentially, you must realize that psychological factors play a huge part in your overall success. Simply put, weight loss starts with the right thinking. I have found that most individuals who want to lose weight must first forgive themselves, then accept themselves, and eventually love themselves. I strongly recommend positive affirmations on a daily basis in order to reprogram your mind for weight loss.

At the same time, it's important to balance this positive, productive thinking with a reality that is first willing to admit to the present circumstances. You did not just wake up one day to find yourself overweight or obese. Either you repeatedly made poor eating choices that eventually developed into a lifestyle, or, as we'll cover in the last section of this book, you have become metabolically compromised—meaning you're unable to lose weight even when you follow an effective eating and exercise plan to a tee. Either way, the reality is that something has to change, or you'll keep getting the same results.

A recent study found that most individuals who maintained their weight loss reported less endorsement for medical causes of obesity. In other words, they did not blame their obesity on their genetics, thyroid dysfunction,

diabetes, or their increased fat cell number.[16] The successful maintainers of weight loss stopped making excuses and took responsibility for their obesity.

I have focused mainly on the NWCR's members during this chapter, but understand that they are not an isolated case. I have read hundreds, if not thousands, of scientific journals and research papers over the years, all trying to find the common traits among those who have managed to lose weight and keep it off. It is not a coincidence that the number of people registering with the NWCR continues to grow. People are catching on and taking note of the seven main habits of successful losers. I believe you will as well, in order to be successful at both losing weight and keeping it off for the remainder of your life.

"CAN DO" POINTS TO REMEMBER

1. Although those on the National Weight Control Registry (NWCR) differ in how they lost weight, many share certain habits from which we can glean.

2. Highly effective losers modify their food intake.

3. Just as important as increasing your activity level is not being a couch potato.

4. Eating a healthy, well-balanced breakfast is instrumental in how successful your weight-loss efforts will be.

5. Once they had reached their goal weight, most NWCR members monitored their weight so that a slight gain wouldn't become a bigger problem.

6. There will always be distractions, mistakes, and flubs; it's how you deal with those that determine your weight-loss success.

7. Effective losers practice portion control, and they identify and eliminate irresistible foods from their environment.

8. Being accountable means being held in check by others and being realistic with your current situation.

3

HUNGER VS. APPETITE

I F MOST PEOPLE would only eat the proper foods every three to three and a half hours, they would rarely be hungry and would probably never have a weight problem. You may think I'm oversimplifying, but after working with thousands of overweight and obese patients, I am still amazed how people seem to forget this simple truth. We Americans have grown accustomed to an all-you-can-eat lifestyle.

The truth is, there is a big difference between hunger and appetite, and we have confused the two. When it comes to weight loss, hunger is our friend and is easy to satisfy with the correct meal planning and timing of meals (every three to three and a half hours); appetite, on the other hand, can be our worst enemy. Hunger is defined as "a desire, need, or appetite for food." Appetite, meanwhile, is defined as "a desire to satisfy some craving of the body, specifically a desire for food or sometimes a desire for some specific food."[1] Appetite also usually deals with emotional eating.

The struggle most overweight and obese people have is not with hunger but with the appetite they have developed through years of poor dietary choices. In fact, many obese people no longer feel true hunger but instead are only tuned in to their appetites. Even when their stomachs are full, they remain unsatisfied and are preoccupied with food.

To understand why this happens, let's examine the science behind these two oft-misunderstood building blocks of weight loss. Although this will include a few terms you don't usually hear tossed around the office every day, my intent is not to bog you down with scientific terminology. Instead, I want to give you the tools to understand what's really going on behind your hunger and appetite—and, more importantly, how to tell them apart.

EVERYONE'S HUNGRY

Hunger is a purely physiological response that is triggered when your blood sugar falls below a certain level after a meal. An area of the brain called the hypothalamus controls both hunger and appetite, but it also controls your

metabolism, sex drive, temperature, and thirst. A certain part of the hypo-thalamus, called the ventromedial region, informs you when your stomach is satisfied—which is why it is also called the satiety center of the brain. Studies on lab rats have shown that those who have their ventromedial region of the hypothalamus destroyed literally eat themselves to death.[2]

The lateral hypothalamus is the hunger center of the brain, where the sensation of hunger actually originates. If this area of the brain is damaged, you lose your appetite and can become extremely thin. Additional studies on lab rats show that when this area of the hypothalamus is destroyed, the rats simply forget to eat and eventually starve to death.[3]

To avoid either of these situations, a fully functioning hypothalamus will detect whenever your blood sugar falls below a certain level and release a neurotransmitter called neuropeptide Y. This, in turn, activates the hunger center, which compels you to eat. At this point, the main foods you will natu-rally desire are carbohydrates and sugars, since they raise the blood sugar the fastest. (Interestingly enough, these foods also raise levels of serotonin, which is a neurotransmitter associated with feelings of satiety and well-being.) As your blood sugar increases, your pancreas releases insulin. Insulin then signals the cells to take in the sugar. It also tells the cells of the hypothalamus to absorb the sugar—and when this occurs, the hunger center is eventually turned off.

As you can see, low blood sugar is the main trigger for hunger. That is yet another reason why it is so important to not skip meals and to practice meal planning. Skipping meals is similar to driving your car on empty. Eventually you will run out of gas and get stuck on the side of the road. When you are running on food fumes, you set yourself up for a dietary disaster. Skipping meals not only triggers hunger by causing your blood sugar to plummet, but it also compels you to consume the very foods and drinks that can result in binge eating and, eventually, obesity. Think about it: What do sodas, cakes, pies, cookies, candy, and highly processed foods such as white bread have in common? They are high-glycemic and immediately raise your blood sugar. It generally takes about twenty minutes to get the signal to your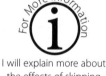

I will explain more about the effects of skipping meals in chapter 5.

brain's satiety center that you are full. Meanwhile, in those twenty minutes an out-of-control appetite can easily consume more than 2,000 calories. (Keep in mind that most men only need about 2,200 calories a day, and most women only need about 1,800 calories a day.)

It doesn't help that these processed foods are addictive by the very nature of what they contain. Sugar foods, fast foods, and the like all lack the proper

ratio of carbohydrates, proteins, fats, and fiber to ensure that the hunger center is turned off for many hours. Instead, as these foods are rapidly absorbed, they spike both the blood sugar and insulin levels. This often leads to a continual cycle of low blood sugar and frequent consumption of sugary, highly processed foods or drinks. Over time, it becomes harder to break this cycle as insulin levels become chronically elevated, causing fluctuations in blood sugar. And if the cycle continues, it's possible to become insulin resistant so that adequate blood sugar is never able to enter the cells—including those in the hypothalamus—and turn off the hunger center in the brain. The result is a ravenous appetite and eventually prediabetes or type 2 diabetes.

It should be obvious by now that controlling your *hunger* involves a purely physical solution. There are three keys to remember:

I explain more about the glycemic index in chapter 6.

1. Maintain a stable blood sugar by consuming regular, balanced meals and snacks (every three to three and a half hours).

2. Make healthy choices regarding foods that are low on the glycemic index.

3. Eat the proper proportions of carbohydrates, proteins, fats, and fiber—all of which we'll cover in upcoming chapters.

Controlling your *appetite*, however, is a different—and much more complex—story.

APPETITE FOR DESTRUCTION

Do you remember the first time you tasted ice cream? Probably not. Sure, your parents may have pictures of the messy birthday aftermaths from past cake and ice cream parties. But most likely, your penchant for the soft, heavenly substance came long before—as in the very first time some uncle or aunt decided to slip you a scoop without your parents knowing. In that moment, your brain instantly developed a love affair that has yet to end. In fact, you are reminded of it every time you finish your dinner and, regardless of how much you've eaten, think to yourself, "My, how a bowl of ice cream would hit the spot right about now."

What turns us into such Pavlovian eaters come dessert time? One word: *appetite*. It has often and fittingly been referred to as "hunger of the mind." Indeed, appetite involves the brain as much as the stomach. And some-

where between the two lies a complex process that includes taste, texture, sight, smell, memory, emotion, opinion, and judgment—all in addition to the equally intricate neurological and dietary reactions involved.

It can start with the simplest of things. The smell of freshly baked cookies. The sight of the Golden Arches. A co-worker's comment about visiting the state fair. The slightest nudge of your senses can spark an instant craving. It's how movie theaters have stayed in business for years, tempting movie-goers with preshow "reminders" of the buttery popcorn, gargantuan-sized soft drinks, and boxes of candy awaiting you at the concession stand. Other things can trigger your appetite as well. Social settings that involve some form of eating can cause you to consume certain foods to put you at ease. Your moods can determine what you reach for in the kitchen. When you are stressed, depressed, lonely, bored, anxious, angry, frustrated, irritated, or just plain moody, you can count on your appetite suggesting a few food-related remedies. Hormonal imbalance can prompt a similar physiological response. Women who are pregnant, menopausal, or premenstrual, and men with low testosterone levels, will often crave distinct flavors and foods.

Then there is the time factor. Ever wondered why people rarely crave ice cream, cookies, or cake for breakfast, yet these become instant after-dinner options? Or why is it that at four o'clock in the afternoon, no one at work reaches for a bag of broccoli, cauliflower, or cabbage? Instead, we roam the office to find something sweet or salty (and usually highly processed) to hold us over until the end of the workday. These are all direct results of a physiologically sparked craving, aka your appetite, that cannot be controlled without balancing brain and gut chemistry.

Whether it is through sight, smell, memory—whatever the trigger—the region of your brain that processes pleasure is stimulated. In response, your vagus nerve (the tenth cranial nerve) sends a signal to your stomach, which immediately releases digestive juices. At the same time, your pancreas secretes insulin, while your liver begins to adjust itself in preparation for whatever food it hopes to process in the near future. Yet behind every one of these bodily operations is a hormone that prompts the desire to eat: *ghrelin*.

HORMONES IN BALANCE

Fittingly known as the hunger hormone, ghrelin prompts you to want to eat. About every half hour the stomach secretes this substance when empty. Ghrelin, which wasn't identified until 1999, then makes its way to the brain, where it goes into three separate parts: the hypothalamus, which, as we

discussed earlier in this chapter, includes the hunger and satiety centers; the hindbrain, which controls the body's instinctive processes; and the part of the midbrain that produces feelings of pleasure and contentment. Once in the hypothalamus, ghrelin triggers the release of *neuropeptide Y*, which activates those familiar feelings of hunger.

When your stomach is filled, however, the ghrelin surges abate while another brain-gut process begins. An empty stomach is typically the size of your fist. As it fills with food, it stretches; when that occurs, three hormones are released from the gut and travel to the brain to relay the message that you are full and should stop eating. The first of these is *cholecystokinin* (CCK), which is released from the upper intestines. When it reaches the brain, it increases the feeling of satisfaction and encourages you to stop eating. This hormone signal does not last long, however, which is essentially why the other two are needed.

Think of these hormones, *glucagon-like peptide-1* (GLP-1) and *peptide tyrosine-tyrosine* (PYY), as the second line of fire. Released after CCK, they strongly inform the brain that you are full, while also telling the stomach to slow down its release of food into the intestines until any food still in the stomach has been adequately digested. This usually accounts for that extremely full feeling when you simply cannot eat another bite—and why you still feel that way two hours later.

What happens, however, when you refuse to listen to those first and second rounds of warnings sent by these gut hormones to tell you that you are full? Thankfully, the body comes prepared with the release of yet another hormone: *leptin*. Discovered in 1994, this appetite-suppressant is actually produced by your own body fat. Generally speaking, the higher your body fat, the more leptin you produce. Like the previous hormones mentioned, leptin travels to the hypothalamus—only it actually turns off hunger and stimulates the burning of calories.

The problem—you knew there had to be a catch—is that leptin does not always function the way it is supposed to. Although most overweight and obese individuals have elevated leptin levels, many times their bodies do not respond normally to it, or their leptin simply stops working. In other words, they develop leptin resistance because their bodies have produced so much that it has become numb to its effect. The good news for both obese and over-weight people is that when you do lose enough weight, your cells begin to respond normally to leptin, and it will once again suppress hunger.

IMBALANCED NEUROTRANSMITTERS

When gut hormones are out of balance, it is hard to determine when to stop eating. The same is true when neurotransmitters—those all-important chemical messengers—become imbalanced. There are three main neurotransmitter imbalances that can lead to a runaway appetite.

1. *Norepinephrine deficiency.* The most common of the three among obese patients, low levels of norepinephrine are often associated with depression. Norepinephrine is the key to keeping us alert and focused. When our norepinephrine levels are low, we can feel sluggish, tired, or exhausted, and often have trouble concentrating on one thing. This often propels an out-of-control eating lifestyle.

2. *Serotonin deficiency.* The second-most common, this is also associated with depression and anxiety. Since both these disorders are nearing epidemic levels in the United States, we can expect to see serotonin deficiency become even more common. Serotonin is the "feel good" neurotransmitter. It makes sense, then, that an imbalance of this neurotransmitter is associated with problems sleeping, cravings for sweets (especially chocolate) and carbohydrates, binge eating, panic attacks, compulsive eating, mental fixation on food, and obsessive-compulsive disorder (OCD). Your brain produces about 5 percent of your body's serotonin; the other 95 percent is produced in your digestive tract.[4] It's common to find individuals with serotonin deficiency displaying irrational behavior patterns over which they have little or no control. Interestingly, the female brain synthesizes 50 percent less serotonin than the male brain, which is why women usually crave sugars and starches more than men.[5]

3. *Dopamine deficiency.* Though serotonin is the "feel good" neurotransmitter, dopamine deals strictly with pleasure. Those sound almost identical, yet the brain processes them as two distinct things. When your dopamine levels are consistently low, you become prone to developing

For More Information

I will explain more about neurotransmitter imbalance in chapter 23. If you think you may be suffering from neurotransmitter imbalance, you can take the online test to find out. Visit www.thecandodiet.com for more information.

READ MORE ABOUT IT

For more information on neurotransmitters and how they affect your mood, refer to my book *The New Bible Cure for Depression and Anxiety*.

any kind of addiction—drugs, alcohol, cigarettes, gambling, sex. Among obese people, that addiction undoubtedly involves food. Like the other two deficiencies, an imbalance of dopamine can make you prone to depression, irritability, or moodiness. Most individuals who suffer from this find it hard to get excited about anything, which is why they often pacify their feelings with starchy, processed foods that deliver a "quick fix."

A REASON BEHIND EVERY CRAVING

I hope you are already getting a sense of how multilayered your appetite is. It is almost always associated with a mood, which is why it frequently leads you into emotional eating. This is important to realize the next time you have a sweet tooth. Your instant, supposedly overwhelming appetite is not just a sudden feeling; your body has gone through a series of complex processes to get to the point where you crave a chocolate chip cookie, a piece of key lime pie, or whatever food-of-the-moment it is. The same goes for starchy, salty, fat-filled, or high-carb foods. In every case, your gut and brain have been previously communicating via hormones and neurotransmitters and have arrived at a place where your mind has made a decision: *I'm craving something, and nothing else will appease my appetite.* If you eat consistently when you are not hungry and if you eat when you are depressed, lonely, stressed, and so forth, you may have a food addiction. Food addiction involves excessive craving and compulsive food consumption. I discuss more about food addiction in chapter 23.

> ### CRAMPS AND CHOCOLATE
>
> If you're a woman, you know what it's like to battle a craving for sweets, especially before your menstrual cycle. Although there are more factors at work, one of the reasons you may crave chocolate in particular is its high magnesium content. Magnesium deficiency exacerbates PMS, which can make chocolate a beloved "quick fix" as it helps to ease those cramps.

With that in mind, let's move on to the next chapter, where we'll tackle the question of why certain foods seem so irresistible—and what we can do to change that. Because the truth is, you *can* change it. In fact, by the end of this book you will know exactly how to control your hunger and tame your appetite whenever, wherever.

"CAN DO" POINTS TO REMEMBER

1. Hunger is triggered when the blood sugar falls below a certain level after a meal.

2. Appetite is much more complicated than hunger and may be triggered by the smell of food, sight of food, social settings, moods, and stress.

3. There are neurotransmitter mechanisms in the brain and hormonal mechanisms in the gut and brain that deal with hunger and appetite.

4. To control one's appetite, it is very important to balance neurotransmitters.

5. Your body goes through a series of complex processes to get to the point where you crave a certain food.

4

IRRESISTIBLE FOODS

VERY DAY IT hit her around three in the afternoon. Denise wanted a shake. Not just any shake—Denise always had a special craving for a mocha shake. And not just any mocha shake, mind you, but an Arby's large original Jamocha Shake.

Almost ten months ago, she had started running midafternoon errands for her boss that took her outside the office. Her five-minute drive down a few blocks to the local FedEx drop-off had turned into a ten-minute break that always included a pit stop at the nearby Arby's. At first, Denise's co-workers playfully ribbed her about leaving for her "afternoon sugar high." A few weeks in, however, they noticed the strange affect it had on her mood when she wasn't able to go at the usual time. She became cranky and easily irritated. Even Denise admitted the daily routine was taking a toll on her already over-weight frame.

By the time she walked into my office, Denise tipped the scales at more than 200 pounds. She was a tall woman, standing almost six feet, yet this thirty-two-year-old was obviously carrying far more weight than what was healthy for her body. Typically, when I take a weight-loss patient's history I ask her what foods she craves, how often she eats those foods, why and when she craves them, and similar questions. A yo-yo dieter in years past, Denise had the usual answers for why she craved an Arby's large original Jamocha Shake each day.

"I don't know," she said. "It relaxes me, I guess. I'm a personal assistant to my boss, so my schedule can get pretty stressful. I guess the shake is some-thing that unwinds me a bit during the day, makes me feel a little better in the midst of the craziness."

When I asked her if she ever could stop after just a couple of sips rather than downing an entire large shake each day, her answer was just as typical: "Are you kidding me? It's like I can't stop once that taste gets in my mouth."

CRAVINGS HAPPEN

In the last chapter we discussed the physical and psychological reasons behind a habitual craving like Denise's. We discovered the gut-brain chemistry that occurs whenever someone has developed such an appetite and been unable to ward off its demands. Though these cravings are perfectly normal, in this chapter I want to dig deeper and ultimately debunk the notion that certain foods cannot be avoided once an appetite is awakened.

Almost every overweight and obese person has a particular food that brings about a temptation at specific times of the day. Most of these people give in and end up devouring the whole bag, box, container, or serving of whatever food they're craving. Before we go any further, let me remind you: regardless of how bad or often your cravings are, you are not a slave to this kind of eating pattern. Cravings are bound to happen; the key is learning what to do when they come and to reduce hunger and stabilize the blood sugar by eating the correct foods every three to three and a half hours. Once you understand the reasons behind your cravings and make adjustments to your environment and your schedule, you will be able to control the temptation of seemingly "irresistible" foods.

It's true: the deck is already stacked against you regarding these foods—mainly because of the culture in which we live. People most often crave dense, high-calorie foods—which are exactly what fast-food restaurants and all-you-can-eat establishments offer.

During a yearlong study called the Comprehensive Assessment of the Long-Term Effects of Restricting Intake of

FOOD ADDICTION: WHEN CRAVINGS ARE OUT OF CONTROL

Food addiction is a very real and debilitating eating disorder for many people. If your cravings are impossible for you to control, you may need professional help to overcome this disorder. Food addicts abuse food similarly to the way drug and alcohol addicts abuse those substances. This unhealthy obsession with food affects men and women of every age and race and can accompany other eating disorders such as anorexia, bulimia, and compulsive overeating. If you think you may be suffering from food addiction or any eating disorder, there is hope. I encourage you to call the eating disorder helpline at 1-800-941-5313.

I'll discuss food addiction further in chapter 23. If you think you may be suffering from a food addiction, you can take the online test and find out. Visit www .thecandodiet.com for more information.

Energy (CALERIE) trial, researchers at Tufts University discovered the most commonly craved foods were those high in calories. Participants did not just crave carbohydrates (as is usually believed), but they specifically craved high-calorie foods. These included foods high in both sugar and fat, such as chocolate, as well as salty snacks such as chips and french fries.[1]

A separate study from the Food and Brand Lab at the University of Illinois went a step further in identifying these specific foods. According to this survey of more than one thousand individuals, Americans' favorite comfort foods are: potato chips (23 percent), ice cream (14 percent), cookies (12 percent), chocolate (11 percent), and pizza or pasta (11 percent). Interestingly enough, the study also revealed that these comfort foods are not limited to snacks and that gender plays a part in what kinds of foods are consumed. While women do prefer more convenient foods that involve less preparation (i.e., snacks), men lean more toward meal-related foods such as steak, burgers, and casseroles.[2]

STOP—IT'S TRIGGER TIME

To eventually conquer food cravings, it is essential to know the specific times of day we are most susceptible to them. Not only do we have to identify these appetite trigger times, but we must also modify our behavior, food selection, and eating times to combat our natural tendency to give in. Part of this adjustment includes knowing how to recognize stress cues and potential signs of brain chemistry imbalance. Remember, you are not alone in this; virtually every overweight person encounters daily cravings for high-calorie "irresistible" foods.

The most common appetite trigger times are between 3:00 p.m. and 6:00 p.m. and from 8:00 p.m. to 11:00 p.m. Although the precise time varies from individual to individual and may alter slightly depending on such factors as mood or environment, most people will notice they have a consistent time of day when their appetite seems to come to life with a vengeance. Unfortunately, this is often compounded with one of the most common mistakes I find overweight and obese patients making: they skip meals instead of eating every three to three and a half hours to reduce their hunger.

I cannot stress enough how important it is to keep both an adequate amount of fuel in your body *and* the right type of fuel. Both are key in keeping your blood sugar and insulin levels normal in order to prevent a runaway appetite. This starts by having a healthy breakfast, a healthy lunch, and a healthy dinner, as well as a healthy midmorning, midafternoon, and evening snack. Skipping meals is the absolute worst thing you can do when battling your craving for irresistible foods.

If you're like most people, when you skip a meal, you probably end up compounding the situation by heading to the nearest vending machine, convenience store, fast-food restaurant, or candy dish. In an effort to quickly feel better and pacify your hunger, you down chips, bagels, or doughnuts—anything with lots of calories (and sugars and fats). Remember, the majority of those who lose weight and keep it off are the ones who do not skip meals, especially breakfast. In fact, a study from the University of Colorado found that 78 percent of those who lost weight and maintained their weight loss ate breakfast every day.[3]

I discuss the importance of combining the right fuel mixture for each of your meals as well as your snacks in more detail in chapters 16 and 17.

Without overstating the obvious, you must realize that when your trigger time hits, you will probably not be craving broccoli, lettuce, asparagus, or okra. Instead, you will be reaching for the most calorie-dense foods available to quickly raise your blood sugar and fuel your body in order to turn off the craving. And even if you begin eating three meals a day of the correct types of food and healthy snacks, your appetite trigger time may continue. For instance, you may be driving to an important appointment at two thirty in the afternoon when all of a sudden your appetite is triggered. Without preparation, you would likely pull into the nearest McDonald's and scarf down a Quarter Pounder with cheese, a large order of french fries, and a soda. While your stomach might feel much better, we all know how quickly the guilt would come on.

Instead, you can be prepared and overcome the craving with something that not only satisfies your hunger but also keeps you on the path toward weight loss. This is why it is important to keep in your purse, automobile, or office desk healthy snacks, supplements that raise serotonin or norepinephrine levels, and fiber supplements such as PGX fiber that can actually prevent appetite trigger times. A healthy energy bar is a great example of a healthy snack that can be kept at the office, as are nuts, seeds, and fruits

I discuss the supplements that raise serotonin and norepinephrine online. You can access this important information after taking the test at www.thecandodiet.com.

such as an apple, pear, orange, or grapefruit, along with a protein drink. Another great snack is a slice of whole-grain bread (approximately 5 grams of fiber per slice) and a protein such as 4 to 8 ounces of low-fat cottage cheese, low-fat plain yogurt, low-fat plain kefir, or sliced turkey or roast beef and a handful of nuts or seeds. Just be sure to eat slowly and chew every bite about thirty times to allow your brain to receive the message that you are satisfied. You are actually providing the ideal fuel mixture to turn off the appetite. If

your appetite trigger time is in the late evening, you can do the same thing then. You can also take two to three PGX fiber capsules with 16 ounces of water to fill your stomach before consuming your snack.

Taming the Environment

Part of combating a potential trigger-time pitfall is taming your food environment. Remove junk foods such as chips, cookies, crackers, cakes, pies, candies, and other treats from your cabinets, pantry, and refrigerator. And, of course, remember to get rid of the high-fat, high-sugar ice cream from the freezer. By removing temptation, it is much easier to stand strong when the irresistible urge hits. Stock your pantry and refrigerator with healthy food alternatives rather than bags of chips or cans of soda. The latter will only leave you feeling guilty and defeated. If you were an alcoholic trying to be sober, you surely would not keep your refrigerator and cabinets stocked with beer, wine, or whiskey. In the same way, if you are changing your lifestyle to involve healthier, more beneficial foods, then get the unhealthy, detrimental ones out of the house. Although "out of sight, out of mind" isn't a surefire bet when it comes to certain foods, it does increase your odds of being able to resist them when you don't have a home full of temptations.

Of course, there are plenty of excuses against this idea of taming the environment. Probably the most popular I hear among weight-loss patients is, "I can't get rid of these snacks because my kids enjoy them." If your kids habitually eat these foods, they will likely become overweight or obese as well. Do you really want that? I doubt it. If your kids truly desire these foods and you don't want to completely deny them, treat them once or twice a week at the mall or a restaurant—but not in the home. The main point is to keep the irresistible foods out of your house. Also, make sure that you never go shopping when you are hungry, and avoid eating at buffet-style restaurants.

Fill Up Before

Various studies have shown that grocery shopping on an empty stomach can lead to a 15 to 40 percent higher tab.

Mindless Eating

One of the most harmful yet subtle ways people fall prey to a lifestyle that leads to obesity is through mindless eating. This is simply eating when you are channel surfing, watching a movie, working on the computer, or talking on the phone. During these types of activities you usually don't realize that you have

eaten an entire bag of popcorn, bag of chips, box of crackers, or container of ice cream. To avoid this, you need to have designated eating areas in the home, such as the kitchen and dining room; all other areas should be off-limits to eating. When you allow yourself to eat in your bed or on the couch while watching TV—or anywhere you want for that matter—you will probably fall prey to mindless eating. You are also more likely to be influenced by food or beverage commercials on TV. Again, it is no coincidence that after a soda commercial, you're likely to walk over to the refrigerator and get a soda—all without realizing that you have just been reeled in like a fish on a line by crafty advertisers.

> **READ MORE ABOUT IT**
>
> Learn more about this dangerous trap of eating mindlessly in *Mindless Eating* by Brian Wansink, PhD.

Instead of eating mind*lessly*, we must be mind*ful*. Understand that the true pleasure of most foods is in the first few bites as you savor the flavor of that food. Your taste buds are engaged in a pleasurable experience as you enjoy the present moment. By eating consciously, you become more aware of the type of food you choose as well as the amount that you consume. You are also more prone to ask yourself if you really are hungry and if you truly desire the food you are eating. Most people never go to the mall and buy a suit or a dress without asking for the price. Yet most overweight individuals sit down and unconsciously consume thousands of calories in a single meal without even realizing the price they are paying with their health. And then they wonder why those clothes they bought at the mall don't fit anymore!

TRAINING THE TASTE BUDS

I have found that one of the simplest things we can do to overcome irresistible food urges is to train our taste buds to enjoy a lower-calorie, lower-fat, and lower-sugar alternative for whatever food we are craving. For example, instead of high-fat, high-sugar Häagen-Dazs chocolate ice cream, find a low-fat, low-sugar alternative such as a piece of Dagoba premium organic dark chocolate, which has only 4 grams of sugar. And instead of occasionally consuming a huge bowl or a half-gallon carton of ice cream in one sitting, try one scoop of low-fat, low-sugar ice cream or frozen yogurt one or two times a week. (But don't keep the ice cream at home.) By savoring each bite and practicing mindfulness, you can literally retrain your taste buds to enjoy many alternative foods.

Remember, whatever you continually practice will eventually become a habit. It is not difficult to learn how to enjoy foods with significantly fewer calories

and to savor just a few bites instead of bingeing on massive quantities of a particular food. Instead of choosing junk chocolates—which the majority of candy bars are with their blend of inferior chocolate, corn syrup, artificial flavors, and colorings—try a small amount of fine dark chocolate. By slowly eating, enjoying, and savoring a small amount of the "real stuff," your senses become engaged, and usually you end up satisfied after a few bites.

> ### ANOTHER REASON TO LIKE CHOCOLATE
>
> Reason No. 253 why chocolate is so good: it contains *tryptophan*, an essential amino acid that affects how much serotonin is released into your brain. And "feel good" serotonin, as we learned in the last chapter, typically diminishes cravings for sweets and carbohydrates.

JUST SAY NO

One of the keys to mindful eating is mentally visualizing yourself saying no to tempting foods. When my wife, Mary, and I fly on American Airlines, a flight attendant will typically come by after a meal with these massive, warm, freshly baked, *very tempting* chocolate chip cookies. Mary absolutely loves those cookies, but in years past she was trying to lose weight, and every flight presented an incredible challenge for her. She couldn't resist the temptation of those heavenly smelling and tasting cookies, which caused her to become more frustrated with herself.

It was not as if she would one day instantly be freed from the temptation or that she would suddenly be empowered on the spot to say no. She had to visualize herself saying no. In fact, she had to *practice* this visualization often in her head to train herself for when the moment actually arrived. And she did just that, imagining herself boarding the plane, eating her meal, waiting for the flight attendant to pose the question, and then responding with a firm, "No, thank you."

I will never forget the time we were flying to California and it happened. After finishing our lunch, the flight attendant politely leaned over with a batch of warm, moist, incredibly alluring chocolate chip cookies and asked Mary if she wanted one. "No, thank you," she said. I turned and looked at Mary, shocked. "Are you sure?" I asked. She smiled and reaffirmed her decision. You see, she had already mentally rehearsed refusing those cookies, visualizing herself saying those words hundreds of times—and this time she had actually succeeded in saying them! Since then, she has done this repeatedly. And the good news (especially for many of you who have a similar craving) is that now on some occasions she actually accepts the cookie and is able to control her appetite by only eating

one or two bites. She has also since done this with other foods that used to be irresistible to her, including bread, chocolate, and desserts.

Mary is now able to practice mindful eating by taking just a few bites of her former weakness and putting down the rest. The wonderful result is that she savors those bites and does not crave the foods afterward. Again, this is not some magical ability that she just woke up with one morning and decided to use; she repeatedly practiced and visualized this. First, she learned to say no to her comfort foods and overcame the overwhelming temptation. Then she reduced her hunger by meal and snack planning. Finally, she was able to reintroduce small amounts of those favorite foods and, by practicing mindful eating, not binge on the food but remain in control of her eating. I believe you can do the exact same thing.

HOOKING THE CUSTOMER

One of the ways restaurants enhance the flavors of their foods and get you to come back is by adding lots of monosodium glutamate (MSG) to their dishes. Besides making you hungry again only hours after eating, MSG has several other negative side effects, including severe headaches and shortness of breath. Although Chinese restaurants get the worst rap for using the salt-like powder, many fast-food chains and sit-down establishments use it as well.

SIMPLY IRRESISTIBLE

The reality is that depriving yourself of your favorite foods will almost always ultimately end in bingeing on those foods—which, as we all know, leads to guilt and condemnation. If you really love chocolate, for instance, there is no way that you are going to stop eating chocolate for the remainder of your life. Again, this is one of the main reasons most diets do not work in the long run. Instead, you can implement the principles in this chapter and throughout this book so you can have the ability to control your irresistible urges for these foods.

One final note: it is important that you accept the fact that there are some irresistible foods you simply cannot resist. Manufacturers of foods such as specially flavored chips, crackers, cookies, candies, and pastries have carefully crafted these products so that the majority of consumers cannot eat just one. They are also highly aware that they essentially make a substance that, at least for overweight and obese people, can have the same effect as a drug. Most people who are hooked on irresistible foods are stress eaters or emotional eaters; many may have a food addiction. Those foods are doing more than just raising their blood sugar and turning off their hunger signal in the brain; they are literally giving them comfort. Like getting Valium or a

shot of morphine, comfort foods or companion foods start a reaction in the brain and throughout the rest of the body that causes a release of powerful neurotransmitters and brain chemicals such as endorphins. These have a tremendous calming and numbing effect on the mind and the body, which is why so many people experience a high when they eat these irresistible foods.

Instead of reintroducing junk foods that are actually designed to stimulate your appetite and get you hooked, learn to choose and savor natural foods such as natural, high-quality, low-sugar dark chocolates. Unlike artificial foods that literally program you to consume the whole package, a few bites of quality natural foods will generally satisfy your craving for that food.

Until you have mastered the principles of the "I Can Do This" program, I strongly urge you to not keep any irresistible foods in your house. Easy access to these foods sabotages any weight-loss efforts. Rally the support of your family and friends to do this, since you may not be able to follow through with this difficult move alone. With their help, you can overcome your cravings and control your appetite. You can identify your irresistible foods, as well as your appetite trigger times, and eliminate those foods from your home, office, car, closet, purse, or wherever you are the most tempted. You can also choose healthy snacks and eat ever three to three and a half hours.

Now that we have tackled the issues of controlling hunger and appetite, along with the cravings that come with them, let's move on to discover exactly how your body processes the foods you consume—good or bad.

"Can Do" Points to Remember

1. Identifying your appetite trigger times is important. (The most common ones are between 2:00 p.m. and 5:00 p.m. and from 8:00 p.m. to 11:00 p.m.)

2. When you skip a meal, you set yourself up for cravings for irresistible foods that are typically high in sugar or refined carbohydrates.

3. Tame your food environment by removing junk foods and sweets from your house.

4. Mindless eating is simply eating unconsciously—while watching TV, a movie, a ball game, while working on the computer, etc.

5. Practice training your taste buds to enjoy natural foods instead of man-made artificial foods.

5

HOW METABOLISM WORKS

I LOVE WATCHING TIME-LAPSE videos. Whether it's a nightly weather report showing the day's cloudscape or a montage of a busy street corner's ebb and flow of people, there is something fascinating about getting to see months, weeks, days, or hours of time condensed into mere seconds.

My interest in this began years ago when I saw a documentary using time-lapse filming to capture the effects of the ocean on the coastline. I sat mesmerized as I watched waves pound away at the rocks, day after day, tide in and tide out. After first glance, it appeared the water was not doing anything special. Even after several months and years, the coast essentially looked the same. Yet the documenters proved that had their video been able to track thousands of years—or even billions of years as some geologists claim—I would have been able to see an entirely different landscape formed. By repeatedly and ceaselessly beating down the shoreline, the ocean was actually wearing down the rocks. Eventually, even these seemingly immovable structures could be molded into completely different forms through the power of erosion.

Repeat dieting, or what is often referred to as yo-yo dieting, has a similar effect on our bodies. More specifically, it wears down our metabolism. Generally, when you yo-yo diet, your muscle mass decreases and your body fat increases. Even without dieting, the average person loses between 5 and 7 pounds of muscle mass every ten years after age thirty-five.[1] When you are a repeat dieter, however, you usually lose even more of this muscle mass. Even on many diets that result in weight loss, approximately half of the pounds you lose are fat, and the remainder is usually metabolically active muscle and water. It's hard to stress enough how detrimental this is to gaining sustained control over your weight. Muscle is extremely valuable! In fact, muscle cells burn about seventy times more calories than fat cells, which is why they are so crucial for maintaining weight loss.

Unfortunately, each time you hop on and off another diet, you typically lose valuable muscle and regain extra fat. Worse still, you are gradually becoming fatter by dramatically lowering your metabolic rate. Studies show that with every decade of muscle loss, your metabolism also decreases by

about 5 percent.[2] In essence, every time you drop out of another diet attempt, you make the next one even more difficult.

To find out how you can stop this cycle and restore your metabolic system, let's first take a look at how metabolism works.

Burn While You Rest

Metabolism is defined as the chemical processes continuously going on in living cells or organisms that are essential for the maintenance of life.[3] It is actually the sum total of all chemical reactions in the body. Keep in mind that your tissues and organs never take a break. Your heart always pumps, your lungs always take in a breath, your liver never stops with its five hundred different functions—including filtering the blood; removing toxins; processing fats, proteins, and carbohydrates; producing bile; and detoxifying chemicals, toxins, and metabolic waste. Your brain and nervous system, digestive system, immune system, hormones, bones, joints, muscles, every tissue of your body—these all require energy and never stop performing their functions, which all contribute to the metabolic rate. Since it takes energy for your heart to beat, your lungs to breathe, and all your organs to function properly, the metabolic rate is simply the rate at which you burn calories in a nonactive state. When considered over a twenty-four-hour period, this is called the basal metabolic rate (BMR) or resting metabolic rate. You typically burn about 75 percent of your calories during a state of rest. As I will discuss later in this chapter, there are several things that influence your metabolic rate, including your stress level, muscle mass, eating behaviors, food choices, and activity level.

One of the biggest factors that affect the metabolic rate is skipping meals, which I've already mentioned. When you do not eat for more than twelve hours, your metabolic rate goes down by about 40 percent. This sets you up for weight gain, which is compounded when you consume high-carbohydrate, high-fat foods since your body will not burn as many calories in this lowered metabolic state. This is also why eating a healthy breakfast (literally breaking a "fast" through the night as you sleep) is so essential. Individuals who eat breakfast are typically leaner than those who skip breakfast because their metabolic rate is generally higher.

As you might guess, body fat is not metabolically active tissue. Muscle tissue, on the other hand, is extremely metabolically active. The more muscle you have, the higher your metabolic rate will be. The more fat you have, the slower your metabolic rate will be. Think of this another way if it helps: it takes far more energy to maintain a pound of muscle than a pound of fat. A good way to

increase your metabolic rate is to increase your muscle mass and decrease your body fat.

ALL IN THE CALCULATIONS

Figuring out a ballpark BMR is easy.* There are more specific formulas for calculating your BMR, but I want to keep our discussion simple, so I'm going to share a general formula instead. There are three easy steps: First, simply multiply your weight in pounds by ten. Second, determine the number of calories you burn in a day by multiplying the number of minutes you exercise each day by four. Third, add this total to the first number.

For example, if you weigh 200 pounds and exercise thirty minutes a day, you would calculate your calories burned per day as follows:

Body weight in pounds x 10
  (200 lbs. x 10 = 2,000)

Number of minutes exercised x 4
  (30 minutes x 4= 120)

2,000 + 120 = 2,120 calories burned per day

Using this formula, you would burn approximately 2,120 calories a day. Keep in mind that this is only a rough estimate of the metabolic rate; it does not apply to people who are metabolically compromised or have a depressed metabolic rate.

EASIER SAID THAN DONE

"Losing weight isn't rocket science. All it takes is eating less and exercising more." How many of us have heard that oversimplified solution for most of our overweight years? I've had plenty of obese patients who wanted to wring the necks of all the well-meaning but insensitive people who offered this as a word of "advice." As if these patients had never tried!

* When calculating BMR, it's important to realize that the typical male has significantly more muscle mass than a typical female, while women usually have a significantly higher amount of body fat than men. Therefore, a one-size-fits-all BMR is not entirely accurate or realistic. The formula I discuss here is a very crude way to measure your BMR.

Other BMR Formulas[4]

The Harris Benedict formula

The Harris Benedict formula factors your height, weight, age, and sex into your BMR. This makes it more accurate than the simple formula I showed you on the previous page, which is based on weight alone. (When looking at the following formula, keep in mind that 1 inch equals 2.54 centimeters and 1 kilogram equals 2.2 pounds.)

Men: BMR = 66 + (13.7 x weight in kg) + (5 x height in cm) - (6.8 x age in years)
Women: BMR = 655 + (9.6 x weight in kg) + (1.8 x height in cm) - (4.7 x age in years)

For example, a thirty-year-old woman who is 5 feet 6 inches tall (167.6 cm) and weighs 120 pounds (54.5 kilos) would formulate her BMR like this:

655 + 523 + 302 - 141 = **1,339 calories/day**

The Katch-McArdle formula

The Katch-McArdle formula can provide the most accurate BMR estimate of all because it takes your body fat percentage and lean mass into account. You have to know what your body fat percentage is in order to use this formula, which looks like this:

BMR (men and women) = 370 + (21.6 x lean mass in kg)

Using our same example of a thirty-year-old woman who is 5 feet 6 inches tall (167.6 cm) and weighs 120 pounds (54.5 kilos), we now add that she knows her body fat percentage is 20 percent (24 pounds), which means her lean mass is 96 pounds (43.6 kilos), and her BMR formula looks like this:

BMR = 370 + (21.6 x 43.6) = **1,312 calories/day**

Factoring your activity level

After calculating your BMR with either the Harris Benedict formula or the Katch-McArdle formula, you still need to factor in your activity level before you know exactly how many calories you need to consume each day. Here's a breakdown of several activity levels:

Sedentary = BMR x 1.2 (little or no exercise, desk job)
Lightly active = BMR x 1.375 (light exercise/sports one to three days a week)
Moderately active = BMR x 1.55 (moderate exercise/sports three to five days a week)
Very active = BMR x 1.725 (hard exercise/sports six to seven days a week)
Extremely active = BMR x 1.9 (hard daily exercise/sports and physical job or two times a day training; i.e., marathon, contest, etc.)

Let's say our thirty-year-old woman is moderately active, so going by the Harris Benedict formula, her daily calorie needs are:

1.55 x 1,339 = **2,075 calories/day**

Going by the Katch-McArdle formula, her daily calorie needs are:

1.55 x 1,312 = **2,033 calories/day**

In our example, the difference in the daily calorie needs between the two formulas is minimal (2,075 calories vs. 2,033 calories) because the person we used as an example is average in body size and body composition. The benefit of factoring lean body mass into the Katch-McArdle BMR formula increases for people whose body composition is closer to either end of the spectrum (very muscular or very obese).

The truth is, that formula for weight loss is spot-on. To shed pounds, usually we do need to eat less and exercise more. But what happens when doing these things doesn't work? What do you do when you have followed every diet and exercise program to the tee and still haven't seen any results?

If this describes you, first let me remind you that you are not alone. As we explore the various reasons why people get stuck in their efforts to lose weight, you will see that many of these factors are reaching epidemic proportions. If you suffer from one or more of these factors, you're accompanied by millions of others—and the club is growing. Second, know that you may be metabolically compromised. All that means is that your metabolism is sluggish and has yet to recover. Somehow—usually through chronic dieting and binge eating—it has been worn down to the point of barely working, which means your body isn't burning fuel the way it should be.

I explain more about overcoming the challenges of losing weight when you are metabolically challenged in chapter 22.

BREATHING TEST: THE BEST WAY TO MEASURE YOUR BMR

A routine pulmonary lab test, called indirect calorimetry, can measure oxygen consumption, carbon dioxide production, and respiratory exchange rate. This provides accurate and useful information in providing a detailed picture of the body's metabolic processes at rest.[5]

This can happen for a myriad of reasons, several of which are covered in the last chapter of this book and at www.thecandodiet.com. But the overall result is that your body gets locked into *storing* fat rather than *burning* it. Sadly, many obese and metabolically compromised Americans are unaware of the everyday factors that have contributed to their condition. With that in mind, let's examine some of the major factors that can severely affect your metabolic rate.

AVOID STARVATION MODE

The World Health Organization classifies any diet containing fewer than 2,200 calories a day for the average man and 1,800 calories a day for the average woman as a starvation diet. When you excessively restrict calories and your caloric intake drops below your BMR, you have just entered the starvation zone. Simply put, all your organs and tissues must get their daily calories. When they do not, your brain thinks you are starving and begins to lower your metabolism to conserve energy so you can survive. This is a normal physiologic response.

Unfortunately, many diets fail to recognize this and instead go against nature—and we all know who wins that matchup. When you intentionally starve yourself, you not only disrupt your body's natural eating cycle, but you also significantly lower your metabolic rate. I have had many patients complain to me how they have spent entire days eating nothing but 2 ounces of chicken and a dry salad, yet they still cannot lose weight. Then, after eating just a single baked potato, they suddenly gain a pound. Sound familiar?

This can be frustrating if you have strictly adhered to the latest fad diet, but what must be understood is the real harm of skipping meals. When you do not eat, your brain interprets your actions as a famine. It simply does the natural thing and locks into self-protection mode by signaling your metabolism to slow down in order to conserve energy. Without knowing it, you have then turned on the starvation response. You can imagine, then, what effect repeatedly doing this has on your body. Many dieters have reset their metabolic rate time and time again, and the result has been like a stove that no longer functions on high settings but instead only simmers. Though these dieters' internal fires burn, they cannot burn hot enough for them to lose weight.

DON'T SKIP OUT!

When you don't eat sugar or starches for more than twenty hours, the glycogen (stored sugar) supply in your liver and muscles eventually becomes depleted, causing the liver to break down proteins from muscles and other tissues in a replenishment effort. Because the liver is unable to provide adequate amounts of sugar using this method, you end up feeling fatigued, lethargic, forgetful, spacey, shaky, and light-headed. This can also trigger the tremendous sugar and starch cravings many people experience in the mid to late afternoon.

CHRONIC STRESS

Chronic stress also lowers the metabolic rate. Our bodies are designed to secrete two stress hormones when we are stressed: epinephrine and cortisol. A "fight-or-flight" hormone, epinephrine works immediately by racing through our bodies when triggered by such stressors as an emergency, running late for an appointment, or an argument with a spouse. When our bodies are unable to fight or flee, we become like rush-hour commuters stuck in bumper-to-bumper traffic on the interstate—we are left literally stewing in our own stress juices. Epinephrine revs up the stress response by raising our blood pressure and increasing both our heart rate and our breathing. When the perceived stress is over, the epinephrine level typically drops back to normal.

Cortisol, on the other hand, works more slowly, giving us stamina to cope

with long-term stress. However, when the stress response becomes stuck as a result of long-term stress, the ongoing elevation of cortisol causes the body to continually release sugar into the bloodstream from glycogen. Glycogen is simply stored sugar, generally held in the liver and muscles. When glycogen is released into the bloodstream, it causes insulin levels to rise, which in turn lowers the blood sugar. Low blood sugar causes more cortisol to be released, leading to weight gain. Excessive insulin also causes the body to store fat in adipose tissue, while also preventing the body from releasing fat from the tissues, even during exercise. In other words, stress programs us for fat storage and contributes significantly to insulin resistance.

Elevated cortisol levels can also cause the body to burn muscle tissue as fuel. Cortisol is a catabolic hormone, which means it causes the body to break down muscle to produce energy, leading to an even lower metabolic rate. As any weightlifter knows, muscle tissue is pricey fuel; we sacrifice our metabolic rate when we burn muscle tissue as fuel. Cortisol is the only hormone that increases as we age.

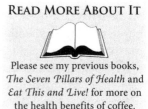

READ MORE ABOUT IT

Please see my previous books, *The Seven Pillars of Health* and *Eat This and Live!* for more on the health benefits of coffee.

Certain foods and beverages will raise cortisol levels, including everyday items such as caffeinated beverages and coffee. In fact, drinking two cups of coffee raises your cortisol levels by approximately 30 percent within a single hour. I am not recommending that you stop drinking coffee—it does have health benefits—however, I do recommend that you not drink more than two cups a day.

Eating excessive amounts of sugar, white bread, and other high-glycemic foods without the proper ratio of protein, fats, and fiber can cause hypoglycemic episodes, which are bouts with low blood sugar that also raise cortisol levels. Whenever your blood sugar drops, your body is naturally signaled to increase cortisol production. Another way this can happen is through food allergies and sensitivities and by skipping meals and snack times.

AGE ·

Getting older ushers in many health changes, including losing muscle and gaining fat. As we age, not only do we lose muscle mass, but also most people experience decreased levels of hormones—particularly anabolic hormones, which help build muscle and include testosterone, dehydroepiandrosterone (DHEA), and growth hormone. This hormone imbalance can severely stunt any weight-loss efforts.

Among women, this is often seen when they produce either too much or too little estrogen. Both can cause weight gain, particularly in the abdomen, hips, and thighs. Estrogen in the form of birth control pills or hormone replacement therapy commonly causes weight gain. At the same time, many postmenopausal women often chalk up their "menopots" to a lack of estrogen, when in fact it may be due to too much estrogen. In general, the more body fat you have, the more estrogen you make. And the more estrogen you make, the more body fat you have; it's a vicious cycle.

This is also the reason why so many obese men have enlarged breasts—their fat cells are simply making too much estrogen. Yes, men have estrogen, just as women have testosterone. In fact, both men and women can struggle with weight gain as a result of low testosterone. Understand that hormones need to be balanced to correct the metabolic rate, build muscle, and burn fat—all of which, of course, affect your weight.

BELLY FAT AND ESTROGEN

Did you know that belly fat actually produces estrogen? It's true. High levels of estrogen may lead to gynecomastia (enlarged breast tissue in men) and continual weight gain, especially in the hips, waist, and thighs.

GENDER

Women typically have a higher percentage of body fat and lower metabolic rate than men. Although there is currently no consensus on a specific "healthy" range of body fat percentage, and ranges vary according to age, most studies indicate a good goal for women is to keep your body fat under 30 percent (for women, obese is defined as a body fat percentage—not BMI—greater than 33 percent; 31–33 percent is borderline). For men, that goal is less than 20 percent (for men, obese is defined as greater than 25 percent; 21–25 percent is borderline).[6] By design, women have a lower metabolic rate than men because they typically carry an extra 7 percent to 8 percent of fat on them, even at a healthy weight. Add to this that a woman's metabolic rate declines at the rate of approximately 5 percent per decade of life, beginning at age twenty.

SIT OR GET FIT?

Obese people sit down an average of 152 minutes more each day than more slender individuals.[7]

INACTIVITY

Sedentary individuals have a significant loss of muscle mass with aging. I stated earlier that adults naturally lose 5 to 7 pounds of muscle every ten years after age thirty-five

just by aging, and, as you might guess, inactivity further accelerates this process. The less active we are, the more body fat we keep—and, naturally, the more muscle we lose. By age sixty, most people have lost about 28 pounds of muscle and replaced most of that with much more fat.

I have found this to be especially true among women. I check body fat measurements on all my weight-loss patients and have commonly encountered women with 50 percent body fat or more. It is extremely rare to find this among male patients. Most of these cases have been a result of combining gender with a lack of exercise and metabolic compromise. Obviously, women have the disadvantage of carrying a higher percentage of body fat and generally will not lose weight as fast as men. Because of this, it is even more important that they be educated about the effects exercise has on metabolism, as well as understanding the unique challenges they face. Remaining sedentary simply compounds the situation and increases their chances of obesity.

GENETICS

MYSTERY GENE

Although many are quick to dispute the existence of a "fat gene," several independent population-based studies have identified a gene that may be responsible for up to 22 percent of all cases of obesity and may be associated with diabetes. It should be noted, however, that research is still in its early stages.[8]

Though it can easily become an excuse for being overweight, your genetic blueprint greatly influences your metabolic rate. As I mentioned in chapter 1, numerous studies have shown that adopted children rarely resemble the weights of their adoptive parents, but instead they mimic their biological parents' weight. Too often, however, these individuals use this "genetic card" to account for their obesity and become resigned to being obese for the remainder of their life. I have found that not to be the case and have seen many of these individuals boost their metabolic rate and lose weight by following this program.

MEDICATIONS

Certain medications can lower your metabolic rate and cause weight gain. These include birth control pills, hormone replacement therapy, prednisone and other steroids, various antidepressants, antipsychotic medications, lithium, insulin and insulin-stimulating medications, cholesterol-lowering medications, some anticonvulsant medications, some antihistamines, and certain blood pressure pills, such as beta-blockers. Ironically, many physicians treat diseases caused by

obesity such as hypertension, diabetes, depression, and elevated cholesterol with the very medications that lower the metabolic rate and result in more weight gain. That is why I typically use vitamins, supplements, and other nutrients alongside the "I Can Do This" program to treat obesity-associated problems rather than just medications. I discuss this more in chapter 23.

Online I discuss thyroid solutions that won't interfere with your weight-loss goals. You can access this information after you take the test at www.thecandodiet.com.

Thyroid Problems

A low or sluggish thyroid can also cause a decreased metabolic rate, though this is often an overlooked problem to the weight-loss equation. I have seen hundreds of cases in which patients reached the end of their rope after adhering to every diet under the sun but never losing weight, only to discover their thyroid was prohibiting them from making progress. Thyroid blood tests should be checked on a regular basis to ensure that the thyroid is functioning normally.

Although men can develop thyroid disease as well, the overwhelming majority of those suffering from thyroid issues are women. An estimated thirteen million American women have some kind of thyroid dysfunction.[9] The sad part is that many of them do not even know it and struggle with weight loss (along with other issues) their entire lives. Researchers say that about 10 percent of younger women and 20 percent of women over age fifty regularly experience mild thyroid problems that impact their weight, attitude, and overall health.[10] You can find more about this in chapter 23.

Half the Equation

Every overweight individual has a reason for his overweight condition. Yet sadly, most who have been unsuccessful with diets over the long haul never find out the underlying reason for their inability to lose pounds for good. In this chapter, we have touched on many of these various causes as they relate to metabolic rate, ranging from skipping meals to chronic dieting to chronic stress to aging to medications. In doing so, I have tried to help you understand the many ways your metabolic rate can be affected—which you now know directly influences maintaining weight loss.

This is only half the equation, however. Revealing how metabolism works is essential for understanding how to lose pounds and keep them off. Just as important is knowing the solution: developing a low-glycemic lifestyle. With

that in mind, let's now look at how we can raise our metabolic rate and keep off those pounds for good.

"CAN DO" POINTS TO REMEMBER

1. Muscle cells burn about seventy times more calories than fat cells, which is why they are so crucial for maintaining weight loss.

2. Your BMR is simply the rate at which you burn calories during a twenty-four-hour period in a nonactive state.

3. Skipping meals or going for more than twelve hours without eating lowers your metabolic rate by about 40 percent.

4. The more muscle you have, the higher your metabolic rate.

5. A sluggish metabolic rate is usually caused by crash diets, yo-yo diets, overeating, skipping meals, and choosing the wrong foods.

6. Chronic stress lowers the metabolic rate and programs the body to store fat.

7. Aging usually is associated with hormonal imbalance, muscle loss, and a lower metabolic rate.

8. Many medications lower the metabolic rate.

THE GLYCEMIC INDEX AND GLYCEMIC LOAD

THIRTY-FIVE-YEAR-OLD BARBARA HAD battled obesity since her first pregnancy ten years earlier. After having three children, she was 80 pounds overweight and extremely frustrated. Sure, she had tried numerous diets and had lost the usual 5 or 10 pounds. But after stopping these diets, she always gained her weight back, and sometimes even more. The main problem, Barbara figured, was her hectic schedule. She worked full-time, in addition to carpooling children to and from school and activities, preparing dinner, cleaning house, and being a wife and a mother.

Her hectic pace left Barbara little time to prepare food for her family, eat for herself, and clean up. So instead of depriving her family, she decided to cut back on her own meals. She usually either skipped breakfast entirely or grabbed a cup of coffee (with cream and sugar) and a bagel or doughnut at work. For lunch, she ate out—usually a

MOST LIKELY TO BE CONSUMED?

Did you know that besides water, carbohydrates are the most consumed substance in the world?

hamburger, french fries, and a Diet Coke. And almost every afternoon, she wandered into the office break room for a snack. Fellow employees were always bringing in doughnuts, cookies, bagels, cake, or chips.

After work, Barbara would prepare dinner for the family each night, which almost always consisted of a bread (such as rolls or biscuits), meat, starch (including potatoes, rice, and pasta), and a vegetable. She believed she was preparing a well-balanced meal, and since her children were a healthy weight and her husband was not overweight, she figured she was doing something right. Still, it was hard for her to understand why she was 80 pounds over-weight if she ate the same dinners as the rest of her family each night.

CONTROLLING BLOOD SUGAR AND INSULIN

Barbara was unknowingly choosing foods that raised her blood sugar, spiked her insulin levels, and programmed her for weight gain. Among her core problems was that she was consuming way too many processed carbohydrates, as is the case with most Americans. Unfortunately, most of the carbohydrates we eat in our country are extremely refined and convert to sugar very rapidly.

Take white bread, for example. The wheat in white bread is highly processed and refined. During the milling process, the wheat grains are cracked and then pulverized by a series of rollers. The starchy endosperm portion of the grain, which is high in carbohydrates, is separated from the bran, which contains fiber, magnesium, and vitamins. It is also separated from the wheat germ, which contains polyunsaturated fats and vitamins. The wheat germ and fiber are then sold to health food stores, while the general public gets the rest. After processing the starchy endosperm, machines then grind it more, bleach it white, and eventually turn it into flour. This flour is then used to make bagels, breads, buns, cereals, crackers, cookies, muffins, pasta, cakes, and so on. Unfortunately, this commonly used but highly refined flour usually raises the blood sugar and stimulates the release of insulin, which sets people up for weight gain.

That is exactly what was happening with Barbara. When she actually ate breakfast rather than skipping it (a move that was equally as bad, in her case), she drank coffee with sugar and ate a bagel. The sugar in the coffee and the highly processed carbohydrates in the bagel caused Barbara's blood sugar to rise rapidly. Once eaten, processed carbohydrates behave similarly to sugars in the GI tract and are absorbed rapidly, causing a sugar spike in the bloodstream. To lower the blood sugar, the pancreas secretes insulin to drive the sugar into the tissues of the body. However, when we consume sugar or highly processed carbohydrates and fail to complement them with sufficient quantities of proteins, fats, and fiber, this poor fuel mixture often causes too much insulin to be secreted by the pancreas.

When your blood sugar rises rapidly after consuming sugary foods and refined carbohydrates, you usually feel happy, good, energetic, full, and satisfied. However, if the pancreas secretes excessive amounts of insulin, your blood sugar eventually comes crashing down. This, in turn, can cause you to feel spacey, sweaty, lethargic, sluggish, irritable, hungry, light-headed, jittery, anxious, and shaky. In addition, your heart may race, or you may develop a headache. I have already discussed how the brain's hunger center immediately detects when the blood sugar falls and how it sends out hunger signals.

Whenever this occurred for Barbara, she would systematically look for a snack in her break room such as a Snickers bar or a leftover doughnut so her symptoms would go away. Unfortunately, this would start the vicious cycle all over again, raising her blood sugar once again. As a result, Barbara's body was programmed for weight gain.

For her, the culprits were skipping meals, high-glycemic snacks, and excessive insulin. This hormone is a double-edged sword; although it is needed for health, too much insulin sets us up for weight gain, obesity, and a host of deadly diseases. Excessive insulin in the bloodstream is called hyperinsulinemia, and when we elevate our insulin levels we program our bodies to actually store fat. If these levels remain elevated for too long, we can develop insulin resistance, in which the body's tissues no longer respond normally to insulin. When this occurs, insulin sends blood sugar into the muscles and liver to be stored as glycogen, but it also causes fat to accumulate in the liver, in the blood (in the form of elevated triglycerides), in the muscle cells, and especially in the abdomen, causing an ever-expanding waistline. This also prevents the body from releasing stored fat even with exercise. Elevated insulin levels and insulin resistance are associated with many diseases, including type 2 diabetes, elevated triglycerides and cholesterol, heart disease, hypertension, polycystic ovary syndrome, autoimmune disease, Alzheimer's disease, and even some cancers.

YOUNG AND SWEET

Sugary cereals weren't introduced until the early 1950s, when companies began to target kids. Among the first cereals was Kellogg's aptly named Sugar Smacks, which contained an astounding 56 percent sugar.[1] The product was later renamed Honey Smacks, but don't let that fool you; sugar is still the number one ingredient on its label.

GLYCEMIC INDEX 101

To get a better feel for how quickly insulin levels shot up in individuals after they consumed carbohydrates, doctors and scientists created the glycemic index. This was first identified in the early 1980s by Drs. David Jenkins and Thomas Wolever, who were professors of nutrition at the University of Toronto in Canada. In their studies at the time, they focused on individuals with type 2 diabetes and found that certain carbohydrates increased blood sugar levels and insulin levels, while other carbohydrates did not. They followed this up by testing hundreds of different foods to determine their glycemic index values.

Because their methods and findings have proven to be so reliable, they are the standard by which we measure the internal processing of foods.

In essence, the glycemic index gives an indication of the rate at which different carbs and foods break down to release sugar into the bloodstream. More precisely, it assesses a numeric value to how rapidly the blood sugar rises after consuming a food that contains carbohydrates. Keep in mind the glycemic index is only for carbohydrates and not for fats or proteins. Sugars and carbohydrates that are digested rapidly, such as white bread, white rice, and instant potatoes, raise the blood sugar rapidly. These are high-glycemic foods and have a glycemic index of 70 or higher.

On the other hand, if foods containing carbohydrates are digested slowly and therefore release sugars gradually into the bloodstream, they have a glycemic index value of 55 or lower. These foods include most vegetables and fruits, beans, peas, lentils, sweet potatoes, and the like. Because these foods cause the blood sugar to rise more slowly, the blood sugar levels are stabilized for a longer period of time. Low-glycemic foods also cause satiety hormones to be released in the small intestines, which keeps you satisfied longer.

As an example of the various glycemic index values for different foods, glucose has a value of 100, while broccoli and cabbage, both of which contain little or no carbohydrates, have a value of 0 to 1. In truth, there is nothing fancy about the glycemic index. One of the most important factors that can determine the food's glycemic index value is simply how much the food has been processed. Generally speaking, the more highly processed a food, the higher its glycemic index value; the more natural a food, the lower its glycemic index value.

> ### RULE OF THUMB: THE GLYCEMIC INDEX
> Low-glycemic foods: 55 or less
> Medium-glycemic foods: 56–69
> High-glycemic foods: 70 or above

THE GLYCEMIC LOAD

Almost twenty years after Drs. Jenkins and Wolever came up with their measurement, researchers at Harvard University developed a new way of classifying foods that took into account not only the glycemic index value of a food but also the quantity of carbohydrates that food contains. This is called the glycemic load (GL). It gives us a guide as to how much quantity of a particular carbohydrate or food we should eat.

For a while, nutritionists scratched their heads as patients desiring to lose weight were eating low-glycemic foods yet were not losing weight. In fact,

some were actually gaining weight. The problem, they discovered through the GL, was that overconsuming many types of low-glycemic foods can actually lead to weight gain. And these patients were eating as many low-glycemic foods as they wanted, simply because they had been told that foods with a low glycemic index value were better for weight loss.

A food's GL is determined by multiplying the glycemic index value by the quantity of carbohydrates a serving contains (in grams), and then dividing that number by 100. The actual formula looks like this:

(Glycemic Index Value x Carb Grams Per Serving) ÷ 100 = Glycemic Load

To show you how important the GL is, let me offer some examples. Some wheat pastas have a low glycemic index value, which makes many dieters think they're an automatic key to losing weight. However, if a serving size of that wheat pasta is too large, it may sabotage your weight-loss efforts because, despite a low glycemic index value, the GL is high. On the other extreme, watermelon has a high glycemic index value but a very low GL, which makes it OK to eat in a larger quantity. As another example, white potatoes have a GL that is double that of yams.

I will teach you a simple method to calculate portion sizes of foods in chapter 15.

Don't worry. You will not have to calculate the GL for every item at every meal you eat. Instead, I will teach you a simple method to calculate portion sizes of foods. The main point is that by understanding the GL, you can identify which low-glycemic foods can cause trouble if you eat too much of them. These include low-glycemic breads, low-glycemic rice, sweet potatoes, yams, low-glycemic pasta, low-glycemic cereals, and so forth. As a general rule, any large quantity of a low-glycemic "starchy" food will usually have a high GL.

Keep in mind also that if you use the GL without considering the glycemic index, you will probably be eating more of an Atkins-type diet with lots of fats and proteins and very few carbohydrates—which is not a healthy way to eat in the long run and can cause insulin resistance.

GLYCEMIC INDEX VALUES OF COMMON FOODS[2]

To look up the glycemic index values of other foods not listed here, go to www.thecandodiet.com.

Food	Glycemic Index Value
Asparagus	<15
Broccoli	<15
Celery	<15
Cucumber	<15
Green beans	<15
Lettuce (all varieties)	<15
Low-fat yogurt (artificially sweetened)	<15
Peppers (all varieties)	<15
Spinach	<15
Zucchini	<15
Tomatoes	15
Cherries	22
Milk (skim)	32
Spaghetti (whole wheat)	37
Apples	36
All-Bran cereal	42
Lentil soup (canned)	44
Orange juice	52
Bananas	53
Potato (sweet)	54
Rice (brown)	55
Popcorn	55
Muesli	56
Whole-wheat bread	69
Watermelon	72
Doughnut	75
Rice cakes	82
Corn flakes	84
Potato (baked)	85
Baguette (French bread)	95
Parsnips	97
Dates	103

TOO GOOD TO BE TRUE?

When I first met Barbara, she was ready to throw in the towel as far as losing weight. Yet within a matter of weeks, we discovered the two core issues holding her back. First, she began eating three good meals each day, along with a healthy midafternoon snack. Second, she made a basic switch from

high-glycemic carbs to delicious low-glycemic carbs with a low GL. In her words, the transformation was "simply amazing." She no longer had cravings for sugars and starches, and she felt satisfied and energetic. By following the "I Can Do This" program, Barbara lost 80 pounds in less than a year—all without dieting or starving herself.

Pending your current condition, it's possible you could have the same results in the same amount of time. This program incorporates both low-glycemic-index foods as well as low-glycemic-load foods, which is why the information in this chapter is crucial to understand. Though you don't necessarily have to know the details or history behind every glycemic term, it helps to have a basic understanding of the glycemic index and glycemic load—and how they can affect your weight loss success.

Often people will tell me after being on the "I Can Do This" program for a few months that they find it hard to believe it can be this easy. I don't mean to sugarcoat (pardon my word choice) the journey; at times it is tough for individuals having to overcome multiple obstacles. Yet even these people are amazed at how unrestrictive this program is. It does not have diet phases as so many diets do. Instead, you will be eating the same types of foods to lose weight as you do to maintain your weight loss. The only difference is that portion sizes will change. You won't have to deprive yourself, but instead you will be eating delicious, healthy foods that will significantly reduce hunger cravings and help control your appetite. And most people find the best aspect of this program is that, after the first month, you are also allowed treat foods from time to time—even ones that are moderate or high glycemic. The key is to make sure they are eaten in modest portions and with the correct fuel mixture of good proteins, good fats, and adequate fiber.

My goal when I established the "I Can Do This" program was to emphasize moderation so that people could still enjoy their favorite foods while being able to live on it for the rest of their lives. Remember, as I said in the introduction of this book, one of the main reasons diets don't work for the long haul is because they can't be maintained. In

DON'T FORGET

Always check with your doctor before beginning this program.

other words, they're not practical. On this eating program, you will not be starving or eating diet foods. Instead, you will notice an increased energy level, you will sleep better, and you will actually feel better. You won't have to cook different foods for the rest of your family. This program is healthy for children, the elderly, and patients with diabetes, heart disease, cancer, or any other disease—whatever your condition. In fact, you will be consuming

plenty of fiber, vitamins, minerals, healthy fats, antioxidants, and phytonu-trients that significantly reduce your risk of such diseases as heart disease, type 2 diabetes, hypertension, high cholesterol, cancer, Alzheimer's disease, polycystic ovary syndrome, and autoimmune disease.

The "I Can Do This" program also helps your body preferentially lose weight in the abdominal area, therefore reducing your waist size. You will also improve your bowel regularity due to the high-fiber content of this program. Many patients even say it slows down the aging process, as they claim to look younger and have more energy.

If all those reasons are not enough to follow this program, here is another one that should catch your attention: *your children will be healthier.* I have seen countless families have their lives turned around when Mom or Dad began the eating program and, for sheer convenience's sake, included everyone else in the meals. In every case where there was a concerted effort to include the children, they became healthier, lost weight if they were overweight or obese, and were more resistant to disease. They usually had more energy and typically were better behaved. That, in turn, often resulted in better grades at school.

Too good to be true? Keep reading, and you can judge for yourself.

"CAN DO" POINTS TO REMEMBER

1. Most of the carbohydrates we eat in our country are extremely refined and convert to sugar very rapidly.

2. When we eat sugar or highly processed carbohydrates and fail to complement them with sufficient quantities of proteins, fats, and fiber, our pancreas secretes excessive insulin.

3. Too much insulin sets us up for weight gain, obesity, and a host of deadly diseases.

4. The glycemic index measures how rapidly the blood sugar rises after consuming a food that contains carbohydrates.

5. Generally speaking, the more highly processed a food, the higher its glycemic index value; the more natural a food, the lower its glycemic index value.

6. The glycemic load (GL) provides a guide as to how much quantity of a particular carbohydrate or food we should eat.

7

CARBOHYDRATES: A CASE OF THE TORTOISE AND THE HARE

WE HAVE ALL heard the story of the tortoise and the hare. The hare races ahead but fails to reach the finish line, while the slow but steady tortoise eventually passes him and wins the race. When it comes to how your body processes carbohydrates, the race that takes place within you is reminiscent of this classic fable. In this chapter, we will take a look at two main types of carbohydrates: "tortoise carbs" and "hare carbs."

Before we get started, I want to explain that I am *not* talking about simple carbs vs. complex carbs, which are two common categories for carbs. Instead, I'm calling low-glycemic carbs "tortoise carbs" and high-glycemic carbs "hare carbs." I'll explain why in the paragraphs to come.

Unfortunately, carbohydrates have received a bad rap over the past few years. I have met countless individuals who in their initial appointments with me preached the detriments of all carbs because that's what they had been taught from past diet experiences. They had climbed on board the high-protein diet train and weren't about to get off—even though their health was suffering as a result. At times it was downright funny how adamantly they swore off carbs, as if touching them would instantly add a pound or two. The problem was, they couldn't sustain the no-carb approach for long, which is why they were in my office weighing more than they did before.

The truth is carbohydrates are critical for good health. When combined with the correct portion of fats and proteins, good carbs give you energy, calm your mood, keep you full and satisfied by turning off hunger, and actually assist in losing weight. They also help you to enjoy meals and snacks, enable you to handle stress better, allow you to sleep more soundly, improve your bowel functions, and give you an overall feeling of well-being. The National Institutes of Health (NIH) actually recommends that 45 to 65 percent of our daily energy intake come from carbohydrates, with 25 to 35 percent of energy coming from fats and only 15 to 35 percent from proteins.[1] I typically recommend about 40 percent of our calories come from low-glycemic carbohydrates,

30 percent from lean proteins, and 25 to 30 percent from healthy fats. As you can tell, carbohydrates are crucial for a healthy lifestyle—which means they are crucial for maintaining weight loss.

HARE CARBS

Unfortunately, most of the carbohydrates overweight and obese people consume are not the kinds that assist with weight loss. Instead, they are the "hare carbs," or high-glycemic carbs, ones that cause the blood sugar to rapidly rise. As I have already alluded to, this starts a chain of events that, over time, traps people in a fat-storage mode and prevents them from finishing the weight-loss race. The underlying cycle of hare carbs is obvious enough: the faster you absorb the carbs, the higher your insulin level rises, the more weight you gain, and the more diseases you develop.

AMERICA'S WORST FOOD

Is it any wonder that the worst restaurant dish in the United States, as selected by *Men's Health* editor in chief David Zinczenko, is bursting with carbs, calories, and fats? Outback Steakhouse's Aussie Cheese Fries with Ranch Dressing has a staggering 2,900 calories—more than most dieters' daily limit—240 grams of carbohydrates, and a mind-blowing 182 grams of fat. This for a dish that's supposed to be a preamble to the main course![2]

The problem is, it's easy to find these bad carbs—they're everywhere! Food manufacturers have taken nature's fruits, vegetables, potatoes, sugarcane, corn, wheat, rice, and other grains and processed and refined them by milling, pressing, squeezing, cooking, and separating the whole foods into parts. Their procedures turn natural foods into man-made ones. Instead of fruit, we get processed, pasteurized juice, jams, pastries, and the like. Instead of sugarcane and corn, we end up with white sugar and sodas containing high-fructose corn syrup. Instead of whole-wheat bread, we receive white bread, crackers, pasta, highly processed cereals, buns, bagels, pretzels, cakes, or muffins. And instead of brown rice or wild rice, we are given white rice and rice cakes.

Have you ever wondered why there aren't more restaurants and fast-food chains touting natural carbs such as whole-grain breads, steel-cut oatmeal, whole fruits, broccoli, asparagus, beans, peas, or legumes? First, because these carbs are actually more filling—which means customers rarely overeat them and are less likely to purchase other items from the menu. Second, it is because these types of carbs do not preserve as well—which should make you wonder what exactly is being put in the bad carbs to make them last so long.

Finally, the majority of the food industry does not pitch these natural carbs because they do not sell as well. And why would that be? Because that's the culture they have created!

Welcome to the dark side of carbohydrates, where restaurant menus, grocery-store shelves, and home pantries overflow with highly processed high-glycemic carbs such as white bread, white rice, crackers, chips, cakes, pies, sodas, cookies, candy, and doughnuts. Is it any wonder why our country is hooked on these addictive foods?

THE CARBOHYDRATE AND THE SUGAR ADDICT

When people crave highly processed carbohydrates, they are actually craving sugars. And more often than not, they are hooked on sugar. The digestive system quickly turns those highly processed carbohydrates into sugar, which is rapidly absorbed into the bloodstream. This, in turn, spikes insulin levels, which drives the sugar into the cells and tissues. In only a few hours, when the cells in the hypothalamus sense inadequate sugar, the appetite is again triggered. Meanwhile, the brain communicates that it needs a new "fix."

RULE OF THUMB: BREADS

The more processed and refined bread is, the less fiber it contains—and ultimately, the less filling. Look for brands that carry at least 3 grams of fiber per slice. I also recommend double-fiber breads and sprouted breads.

If you think I am going overboard with the continuous drug addiction analogy, here's proof that I am not: Sugar and highly processed carbs release natural opioids in the brain. Your brain actually has opioid receptors. Ever heard of a "runner's high"? This euphoric sensation occurs when exercise stimulates the brain to form endorphins. These neurotransmitters are similar in molecular structure to morphine but are much milder. They activate the brain's pleasure center.

Like exercise, sugars and highly processed carbohydrates are also able to trigger the release of such endorphins—which is why we call the result a "sugar high" or "sugar rush." Most people are unconsciously stimulating the pleasure centers in their brains, creating a sugar high, by having a hit of sugar, white bread, muffin, bagel, doughnut, soda, or something similar. Yet again, this is proof of how easy it is to become a sugar or carbohydrate addict; we are naturally programmed this way.

This opioid effect—and our natural inclination for it—has even been studied in infants. At Johns Hopkins University, researchers studied one- to

three-day-old infants to observe their response to sugar. These babies were each placed in a bassinet for five minutes, and when they began to whimper or cry, they were given either a small amount of sugar in water or just plain water. Researchers discovered that the sugar water stopped the crying, while plain water did nothing.[3]

In addition to activating opioid receptors, sugar and highly processed carbs also have a physiologically calming affect because of the release of serotonin in the brain. When the brain's serotonin level is increased after you have eaten sweets or a refined starch, you typically experience within twenty to thirty minutes a significant emotional relief. This also suppresses your appetite, improves your mood, helps you relax, makes you sleep better, and contributes to an overall feeling of well-being. Meanwhile, your body is programmed to store fat, all the while craving the next intake of feel-good but highly processed carbs.

TORTOISE CARBS

Over the years, I have attended a few financial seminars on investing money. At almost every one, the financial expert would use the tortoise-and-hare analogy to show how long-term investing always wins out in the end. Though some investors manage to beat the odds by playing the market for short-term gains, it is undoubtedly the slow and steady, "in it for the long haul" investors who wind up with greater earnings. Because of this, these instructors would hardly spend any time talking about next year's hottest stocks but instead would offer plenty of advice on how to find those stocks or mutual funds that were consistent winners.

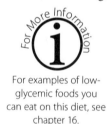

For examples of low-glycemic foods you can eat on this diet, see chapter 16.

When it comes to weight-loss success, "tortoise carbs" are like those long-term investment champs. These are the carbohydrates that slowly raise the blood sugar and enable you to lose weight, prevent diseases, and complete your race toward the finish line. We have spent the first part of this chapter discussing the lousy effects of "hare carbs"; now let's spend the rest of the chapter on these natural, unprocessed carbs that can keep you healthy.

For starters, low-glycemic tortoise carbs can be broken down into the following groups:

1. Vegetables
2. Fruits

3. Starches such as whole-grain breads, whole-grain pasta, corn, oatmeal, unprocessed cereals, and sweet potatoes

4. Dairy products such as milk, yogurt, kefir, butter, and cheese

5. Legumes such as beans, peas, lentils, and peanuts

6. Nuts and seeds

Even though most of these tortoise carbohydrates are healthy, it's still possible to choose the wrong types of starches and dairy or overeat low-glycemic starches such as whole-grain bread and pasta, thereby sabotaging your weight-loss efforts. For this reason, and because there are other ways carbohydrates stall weight-loss efforts, it's important to incorporate the glycemic index and glycemic load principles we discussed in the last chapter.

IS IT A HARE OR A TORTOISE?

The faster your body digests a carbohydrate, the faster it raises your blood sugar—and therefore the higher its glycemic index value will be. This is what makes a carb a hare rather than a tortoise. Yet how exactly can you differentiate between the two? Here are a few traits that will help distinguish between a tortoise and a hare:

1. *Fat content.* With the exception of seeds, nuts, and dairy, most tortoise carbohydrates are low in fat. As we will learn later, fats are not an inherent evil as some diets make them out to be. In fact, adequate amounts of fats in a meal are absolutely essential for both keeping you satisfied longer and slowing the rate in which carbohydrates are broken down and released in the bloodstream—which is why most low-fat diets fail. This doesn't give you the license to down a bag of Doritos or other highly processed, high-fat carbohydrates just

STAMP OF APPROVAL

To help make shopping for whole-grain products easier, look for the "100% Whole Grain" stamp with a golden-yellow background and black border. Foods bearing this stamp contain an entire servings' worth of whole grain (16 grams), as opposed to those bearing the basic stamp, which only have half a serving's worth of grain and are mixed with refined grains.[4] The 100% Whole Grain Stamp indicates that all of the grain in a product is whole grain; the basic Whole Grain Stamp is for products that may also contain some refined grain.

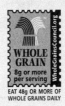 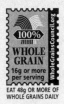

to get your fat content. Obviously, you sabotage your weight-loss efforts when you do this.

2. *Fiber content.* Generally, a higher fiber content of a food slows down the absorption of sugar, making the carb a tortoise.

3. *Form of starch.* Certain starches such as potatoes, white bread, and white rice contain amylopectin, which is a complex carbohydrate that the body rapidly absorbs. However, whole grains, beans, peas, legumes, and sweet potatoes contain another complex carb called amylose, which is digested more slowly and raises the blood sugar in a slower fashion as well. Many corn products such as corn meal, corn pasta, and corn flakes are digested fairly rapidly and therefore are considered hare carbohydrates (with a high glycemic index value). However, corn on the cob or frozen corn is digested more slowly and only gradually raises the blood sugar.

For More Information

In chapter 9, I will show you the difference between good fats and bad fats. There are also several examples of balanced snacks and meals provided in Appendix F.

4. *Ripeness.* The riper the fruit, the faster it is absorbed. An example of this is the difference between yellow bananas and brown, spotted bananas. The latter raise the blood sugar much faster than regular yellow bananas since they are riper and have a higher sugar content.

5. *Cooking.* Most pasta can be either a tortoise carbohydrate or a hare carbohydrate, depending on how you cook it. If you cook pasta al dente, which means only about five or six minutes and leaving it firm, it is typically a tortoise carbohydrate and has a low glycemic index value. If the pasta is cooked for a longer period of time and is very soft, it is a hare carbohydrate and has a high glycemic index value. Also, thicker pasta generally has a lower glycemic index value than thinner types of pasta, while whole-grain pasta is lower glycemic than refined white pastas.

6. *Milling type.* A finely ground grain is a hare carbohydrate and has a higher glycemic index value than coarsely ground grain, which has a higher fiber content and thus is a tortoise.

7. *Protein content.* The higher the protein content of a food, the more it helps prevent a rapid rise in blood sugar and makes the food more likely to be lower glycemic—and thus a tortoise carbohydrate.

Fiber

Fiber is one of the most important carbohydrates for weight control. It lowers the glycemic index value of food, creating a tortoise-type carbohydrate, and

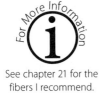

See chapter 21 for the fibers I recommend.

prevents the sugar spike and elevated insulin levels that occur with high-glycemic foods. Even high-glycemic foods such as sugars, cakes, pies, and cookies can be turned into medium-glycemic foods by eating sufficient fiber. For years I have been telling patients, "Fiber covers a multitude of dietary sins!"

Fiber also keeps you full and satisfied for longer periods of time. It significantly reduces your appetite by filling your stomach and by slowing down the rate at which sugars are absorbed into the bloodstream. Eating high-fiber foods also takes longer to chew and dramatically slows down the very act of eating, which helps to prevent you from consuming excessive calories before the satiety center in your brain realizes it.

Unfortunately, most Americans do not eat enough fiber. Though the numbers vary with age, the Institute of Medicine recommends that men consume about 38 grams of fiber a day and women consume around 25 grams of fiber daily. According to the institute, however, the average man and woman in the United States each currently consumes less than half that amount.[5]

To get the full benefit of fiber, it helps to know the difference between two major types of fiber: soluble and insoluble. Most dietary fiber is indigestible and is excreted in the stool. Although both types of fibers slow down the rate at which carbohydrates are digested and enter the bloodstream, there are some noticeable differences.

> ## It's All About Fiber
>
> Since only 5 percent of Americans consume an adequate amount of daily fiber, women hoping to lose weight should concentrate more on getting enough fiber rather than following through with low-carb, low-fat, or high-protein diets. This was confirmed by a study of more than forty-five hundred people, which also discovered that women on a low-fiber, high-fat diet have an increased risk of being overweight or obese.[6]

Soluble fiber. This type of fiber dissolves in the intestines, while insoluble fiber does not. Foods high in soluble fiber include legumes, beans, peas, lentils, apples, citrus food, oats, barley, flaxseeds, and psyllium seeds and husks. Soluble fiber forms a sticky, gummy substance as it passes through the intestines. Acting like a sponge, it soaks up and traps excessive cholesterol, sugar, and toxins and excretes them in the stool. Soluble fiber not only helps

you lose weight and decrease your appetite, but it also lowers your cholesterol and blood sugar, which reduces your risk of heart disease.

Insoluble fiber. Derived from the cell walls of plants, this type of fiber consists mainly of cellulose, which is indigestible. It is found mainly in whole grains, wheat bran, and in lower amounts of fruits and vegetables. Insoluble fiber adds bulk to the stool, relieves constipation, and helps to sweep the colon clean. It not only aids in controlling the appetite, but it also prevents constipation and diverticular disease.

Both soluble and insoluble fiber will help control your appetite, lower cholesterol levels, stabilize blood sugar, decrease your risk of chronic disease, improve bowel function, and assist you in losing weight.

SUGAR

We have already talked about the different types of carbohydrates; now let's briefly discuss sugar. Unfortunately, statistics show that Americans have become a little too familiar with this elemental substance. The average American consumes about 158 pounds of sugar a year—about 50 teaspoons a day![7] Let's put that into perspective: A single 12-ounce can of carbonated soda typically contains around 8 to 10 teaspoons of sugar.[8] If you drink soft drinks throughout the day, you can see how this added sugar intake quickly adds up. And it's even worse for teenagers, who often consume almost twice that amount.[9]

> **NATIONAL SUGAR HIGH**
>
> Overall sugar consumption for the average American has increased 30 percent since 1983.[10]

Most everyone knows the foods that are high in sugar—desserts, sodas, candy, cookies, cakes, pies, doughnuts, and the like. The general public is a little less knowledgeable about those starchy foods that, while not touted as high-sugar items, are usually high glycemic. I cannot stress enough how important this is in losing weight and keeping it off. As we discussed earlier, sugar usually triggers the release of endorphins that give us a sugar high. It acts more like a drug and leads to cravings for more and more sugar. Eating sugar programs the body for weight gain. It also makes us more susceptible to insulin resistance, metabolic syndrome, type 2 diabetes, and heart disease. Excess sugar also triggers free-radical reactions in our bodies, leading to chronic disease, accelerated aging, and plaque formation in our arteries. In some cases, excess sugar can cause glycation, where sugar molecules react with protein molecules to cause wrinkled skin and damaged tissues. The

bottom line is that too much sugar does not produce a pretty face or body but instead a fat and flabby body and a wrinkly face.

Sweeteners

For several years the dieting gimmick was—and to a degree still is—simply to replace these excess sugars with artificial sweeteners. There are plenty of sweeteners available, with the most widely known being aspartame and sucralose. I do not recommend either one of these. (For detailed reasons on why neither of these work, see my book *The Seven Pillars of Health*.) There are, however, three natural sweeteners that are safe and low glycemic.

Stevia

This is an herbal sweetener with no calories and a glycemic index value of 0. It is my favorite natural sweetener, and I use the liquid form of stevia in my coffee and tea. In this form, it is very sweet—approximately 200 times sweeter than sugar, in fact. Because of this, you only need to use a tiny amount of it. Stevia is also available in granulated form. Products such as Truvia contain granulated stevia in convenient single-serving packets and can be found in most grocery stores. If powdered or liquid stevia is too sweet for you, I suggest you try the granulated form, which is more like the consistency and sweetness of sugar.

Xylitol

A sugar alcohol, xylitol also has a very low glycemic index value. It also kills bacteria and prevents dental cavities. I have used xylitol as a nose drop to treat patients with sinus infections. It tastes just like sugar with no aftertaste and is a good substitute for sugar for cooking or baking. Because

Unnaturally Sweet

Splenda, which is made by turning sugar into a chlorocarbon, is approximately 600 times sweeter than sugar.[11]

Agave Nectar and High-Fructose Corn Syrup

In spite of what you may have heard, agave nectar is not made from the sap of the agave plant but from the starch of the agave root bulb. The agave root contains starch—similar to the starch in corn or rice—and a complex carbohydrate called inulin, which is made up of fructose.

Similar to the way cornstarch is converted into high-fructose corn syrup (HFCS), agave starch is put through a chemical process that converts the starch into a fructose-rich syrup—anywhere from 70 percent fructose and higher, according to several agave nectar Web sites.

That means that the refined fructose in agave nectar is even more concentrated than the fructose in HFCS. For comparison, the HFCS used in sodas is 55 percent refined fructose. For this reason, I do not recommend using agave as an alternative to sugar, syrup, or other sweeteners.[12]

it is a sugar alcohol, however, some individuals may experience bloating, gas, diarrhea, or other gastrointestinal issues when using xylitol in larger quantities. Because it is a natural sweetener and our bodies do produce it, I still recommend using it in very low doses initially to avoid any GI disturbance.

Just Like Sugar (chicory)

Just Like Sugar is a natural sweetener made up of four ingredients: chicory root, which is a probiotic food that helps improve your GI function; calcium, which helps lower blood pressure and helps to prevent heart attack, osteoporosis, and dental problems; vitamin C from organic orange juice; and the zest of orange peel (this is what flavors it to taste sweet). In addition to supporting your weight-loss efforts, Just Like Sugar does not promote tooth decay. It's available at retail stores like Whole Foods and many health food stores, and I find it's a wonderful natural alternative to sugar and harmful artificial sweeteners without the intense sweet aftertaste that deters some people from using stevia. (See Appendix H.)

Every carbohydrate—whether tortoise or hare, good or bad—needs a digestive companion, so to speak. And one of the most important factors of losing weight is what is being combined with the carbs you eat. With that in mind, let's see what types of healthy proteins we can choose to lose weight and feel great.

"Can Do" Points to Remember

1. Good carbohydrates are typically low-glycemic, nonrefined, nonprocessed grains, vegetables, fruits, and legumes. When combined with the correct portion of fats and proteins, these "tortoise" carbs give you energy, calm your mood, keep you full and satisfied by turning off hunger, and actually assist in losing weight.

2. Bad carbohydrates ("hare" carbs) include sugars and highly processed or refined foods such as white bread, white rice, most processed cereals, bagels, pretzels, most crackers, muffins, and so forth.

3. Sugars and processed carbohydrates exert an opiate-like effect on the body and may create a sugar or carbohydrate addiction.

4. The riper the fruit, generally the higher the glycemic index and the faster it is absorbed.

5. Adequate fiber on a daily basis helps control the appetite, balance the blood sugar, and prevent disease.

6. Excessive sugar and processed carbohydrate intake may age you prematurely.

7. There are wonderful natural sweeteners, including stevia, xylitol, and Just Like Sugar.

8

The Power of Protein

MANY PEOPLE BELIEVE that a high-protein diet is healthy and the best way to lose weight. However, we have seen that excessive protein may actually damage the body by decreasing kidney function and setting you up for osteoporosis. Many meats and protein sources are also high in saturated fats, which can increase the risk of high cholesterol and heart disease. A high intake of saturated fats may also predispose you to develop insulin resistance, which is usually associated with weight gain and increases your chances of developing type 2 diabetes and hypertension (high blood pressure).

I do not recommend either a high-protein diet or a low-protein diet, but a moderate intake of protein foods on a daily basis. High-protein diets are generally considered diets in which more than 30 percent of the calorie intake comes from proteins. Many of these diets, however, recommend more than 50 percent of the calorie intake as protein. Compare that to the average American diet, which contains approximately 15 percent of calories from protein, or the Asian diet, which runs close to the 12 percent mark.[1]

According to the Institute of Medicine, the recommended dietary allowance (RDA) for protein is 0.8 grams per kilogram (or 2.2 pounds) of body weight.[2] Based on this recommendation, a 154-pound man would need approximately 56 grams of protein a day. However, that number also varies with activity level. A marathoner, for instance, needs 1.2 to 1.4 grams of protein per kilogram of body weight, while a bodybuilder aims for 1.4 to 1.8 grams of protein for each kilogram of body weight.[3] When factoring in both extremes of the activity scale, the average recommended daily requirement for protein is approximately 50 to 75 grams per day for adult females and 70 to 100 grams daily for adult males, depending on their activity levels.

The truth is, however, that it is extremely rare in the United States for an adult or child to have a protein deficiency. Our meat-and-potatoes approach to eating has created a culture known for its beef and chicken obsession. We like hearty meat, and we like lots of it. I venture to say that has had a direct effect on the success of these high-protein diets, regardless of how unhealthy

some are. The key, as always, is moderation. Studies have shown that men with diets high in red meat have an increased risk of prostate cancer, and it is typically a more aggressive form of prostate cancer. However, men who eat fish three times a week have approximately half the risk of developing prostate cancer compared to men who rarely eat fish.[4] Also, frying or grilling meat, chicken, or fish so that it is charred or well done is also associated with an increased risk of cancer.

Generally speaking, the more protein you eat, the more calcium you excrete. Calcium neutralizes the acids that are produced when proteins are digested and absorbed into the body. With a moderate intake of protein, your blood contains enough calcium to neutralize these acids. When you consume too much protein, however, your body may have to cannibalize the bones and teeth in order to get enough calcium to buffer the onslaught of acids produced from excessive proteins. In fact, an oft-cited Nurses' Health Study found that women who consumed more than 95 grams of protein a day were 20 percent more likely to fracture a wrist than those eating less than 68 grams of protein a day.[5] I am in no way indicating that protein is your enemy. Instead, we simply need to practice moderation by consuming smaller portions of healthy protein sources.

In 2002, the NIH advised ranges of carbohydrates, fats, and proteins. Among their recommendations was that protein should make up 15 to 35 percent of a person's daily consumption of energy or total calories. I believe that anything more than 35 percent of our daily calories as protein is simply too much. I tell my patients to get approximately 30 percent of their daily calories from lean protein, 40 percent from high-fiber, low-glycemic carbohydrates, and 25 to 30 percent from healthy fats. I also strongly believe in consuming some protein with each meal and snack. As you will see, it helps to create the correct fuel mixture that keeps your appetite controlled, your energy up, and your blood sugar and insulin levels in check—all while your metabolism continues to burn off those extra pounds.

NO PROTEIN DEFICIENCY HERE

At the Big Texan Steak Ranch in Amarillo, Texas, steak lovers can down a 72-ounce steak for free—as long as they finish it. For those who don't, it's a seventy-two-dollar bill. Of the forty-thousand-plus who have taken up the challenge, more than thirty-three thousand have failed—and undoubtedly left with indigestion.[6]

THE FUNCTION OF PROTEIN

Most of us can remember seeing a picture of proteins from a high school or college biology class. Proteins are composed of amino acids and often illustrated to look like a string of beads, with each bead being one of twenty different amino acids. The body is able to manufacture twelve amino acids, which are known as nonessential amino acids. The remaining eight amino acids, however, are essential and must be supplied by the food we eat. Because our bodies are unable to store proteins in the same way they store fats and sugars, we constantly need new proteins, and we need these on a daily basis. Overall, there are at least ten thousand different proteins throughout your body. These make up the main component of digestive and metabolic enzymes, hormones, antibodies, and lipoproteins that carry cholesterol.

Essentially, proteins and amino acids are the building blocks for the body. They are used to repair and maintain tissues such as muscles, connective tissue, our skin, our hair, our bone matrix, and even our nails. If you do not have adequate protein, you will not be able to adequately maintain these tissues I just listed, as well as enzymes, hormones, and your immune system. As a result, you will age faster and eventually develop disease.

PROTEIN AND WEIGHT LOSS

Though protein is not the main piece of the dietary puzzle for weight loss—I argue that there can never be just a single component—it plays a key role. Your body is able to lose weight and keep it off when you eat balanced meals and snacks that contain an adequate amount of healthy proteins, carbohydrates, and fats in the correct ratios. That means the correct choices of protein are extremely important in helping you achieve permanent weight loss.

HOLD THE SALAMI

Regardless of brand name, salami (with 6 grams of fat and 323 milligrams of sodium per ounce) remains one of the most unhealthy deli meats on the market. This high-sodium, fat-laden mixture of processed meats should be avoided at all costs and replaced by low-sodium turkey or chicken breast.

Including protein in a balanced meal actually makes you feel more satisfied after eating and helps to decrease hunger between meals. High-protein foods slow down gastric emptying, which is simply the movement of food from the stomach to the intestinal tract. This, in turn, keeps you fuller longer. As you might guess, this also helps to stabilize blood sugar. Protein, like fat, helps to prevent the rapid

rise in blood sugar after eating refined carbohydrates and sugars. Protein also helps to raise the metabolic rate for one to three hours after eating.

With the understanding that eating protein with your meal is vital for weight loss, let's look at some of the healthiest sources of protein. As we'll see in the remainder of this chapter, these include fish, poultry, lean meats, eggs, low-fat dairy, legumes, whole grains, nuts, and seeds.

ANIMAL PROTEIN

READ MORE ABOUT IT

For my recommendations for grilling meat, poultry, and fish, refer to *The Seven Pillars of Health* and *Eat This and Live!*

Animal proteins are typically a higher-quality protein than plant proteins and contain all the essential amino acids. This category includes dairy, eggs, meat, poultry, and fish, all of which have all the essential amino acids needed and thus are a higher-quality protein. I strongly recommend certified free-range meats and chicken or organically fed beef, chicken, or turkey. These meats are free of antibiotics and hormones.

Why do I have such a big beef (sorry, I couldn't resist) with the average mass-produced package of meat? Because of sloppy slaughterhouse practices and slack regulations, meat can at times be contaminated with deadly *E. coli* O157:H7 bacteria. Their feed and water may also be contaminated with various toxins. You may not realize it, but any toxins the animal consumes are typically stored in the fatty tissues of the animal.

Feedlot animals are typically grain-fed and are fattened considerably since they are sold by weight. This results in cuts of meat that are quite high in saturated fat. That is why it is so

FROM FARM TO FORK

TIME magazine ran an article in August 2009 that included a comparison of organic, free-range cattle and conventionally raised cattle. Here's a recap:[7]

	Organic Cows	Conventional Cows
Prevalence	1 percent of all cattle	99 percent of all cattle
Diet	Grass	Grass and corn
Supplements Given	None	Chemicals: antibiotics and sometimes growth hormones, bloods, and fats
Human Impact	Omega Effect: Higher in beta-carotene, vitamin E, and omega-3 fatty acids	Fat Attack: Higher in fat, helping to fuel the obesity epidemic

important to choose the leanest cuts of meat and trim away any visible fat. That includes peeling off the skin of the chicken and the turkey.

Instead of frying meat, which boosts its fat content, try grilling, baking, broiling, or even stir-frying at low temperatures. Again, be careful with grilling since charred or well-done meats (yes, even chicken and fish) usually contain heterocyclic amines that are associated with cancer.

Finally, it should be obvious that you need to avoid high-fat junk meats that are loaded with salt, nitrates, and nitrites—and are also associated with an increased risk of certain cancers. These meats include hot dogs, bologna, salami, pepperoni, sausage, bacon, and other highly processed items. I realize you may on some occasion want bacon or sausage. If you choose to eat these, choose Canadian bacon or the leanest cuts of bacon and sausage, and please squeeze the pieces between two napkins to remove as much fat as you can. In addition, choose nitrite- and nitrate-free bacon, turkey bacon, or turkey sausage.

Those are the renowned fatty meats. On the other side of the spectrum, lean meats can include lean beef, lean pork (such as pork chops), ham, tenderloin, veal, lamb, buffalo, elk, pheasant, duck, chicken, turkey, and fish and shellfish (canned or frozen). After reading through that list, many of you may be thinking, "You mean I can eat red meat or pork or shellfish every day and lose weight?" Not exactly. I strongly recommend that you limit these foods to once or twice a week, and limit portions to 2 to 6 ounces for women and 3 to 8 ounces for men of the leanest cuts (and preferably free-range). I strongly believe that chicken, turkey, fish, eggs, and low-fat dairy are much healthier choices of protein. However, lean pork and shellfish are not fueling the obesity epidemic.

LOW-MERCURY FISH

Anchovies
Butterfish
Catfish
Clam
Crab (domestic)
Crawfish/crayfish
Croaker (Atlantic)
Flounder
Haddock (Atlantic)
Hake
Herring
Mackerel (N. Atlantic, chub)
Mullet
Oyster
Perch (ocean)
Plaice
Pollock
Salmon (canned or fresh)
Sardine
Scallop
Shad (American)
Shrimp
Sole (Pacific)
Squid (calamari)
Tilapia
Trout (freshwater)
Whitefish
Whiting

Fish

For selecting the best fish for your protein, I strongly recommend ocean fish instead of farm-raised fish. The latter typically contain much higher levels of polychlorinated biphenyls (PCBs), which are carcinogens, as well as other contaminants. Larger predatory fish are typically higher in mercury content and include swordfish, shark, king mackerel, and large tuna. The small tuna or tongol tuna found in most health food stores is typically very low in mercury. Alaskan wild salmon is another favorite of mine because of its lower mercury content.

If you are consuming fish low in mercury, you can eat fish a few times a week. However, the American College of Obstetricians and Gynecologists recommends only two 6-ounce servings of fish a week for pregnant women,[8] and the American Academy of Pediatrics recommends no more than 7 ounces of fish a week for children.[9]

Eggs

Eggs had a bad reputation for many years of raising cholesterol due to the supposedly high cholesterol content of the yolk. We now know that this is not exactly true. Eggs actually have little effect on the LDL cholesterol for many people, which is the bad cholesterol. In fact, I have had many patients who ate three eggs every day and had very low cholesterol levels. There are now omega-3-enriched eggs and organic eggs that help to provide your body beneficial fats while lowering cholesterol and serving as good sources of protein. Therefore, the majority of people can eat up and enjoy organic or omega-3 eggs. However, if you are being treated for high cholesterol, consult your physician regarding this. If you do not know your cholesterol levels, ask your doctor to check your lipid panel.

Also, remember that poached or hard-boiled eggs are generally healthier and lower in calories; however, you can still fry and scramble your eggs on low heat in a small amount of healthy oil such as extra-virgin olive oil, macadamia nut oil, coconut oil, a small amount of organic butter or Smart Balance, Pam Olive Oil spray, or Smart Balance Butter Burst spray.

Dairy

Like eggs, there are forms of dairy that have been given a bad reputation for years because of their high fat content. Items such as whole milk, sour cream, cream, butter, cheese, and ice cream have all been declared bad because they are typically high in saturated fat and associated with elevated cholesterol and heart disease. As a result, most doctors have recommended that their patients

avoid these foods. Unfortunately, most Americans consume too much of these high-fat sources of dairy.

However, there are now plenty of healthy low-fat sources of dairy, including skim milk, low-fat cheeses, low-fat sour cream, low-fat yogurt, and low-fat kefir. These are good sources of protein and are high in calcium. Research has shown that the more calcium-rich food you consume, the more likely you are to lose weight and, in particular, lose fat.

I would again recommend organic products to avoid the pesticides, antibiotics, and hormones, as well as other toxins that dairy animals are given. There's another benefit to organic products: for many people with food allergies or sensitivities to dairy, organic may be better tolerated. These people may normally experience eczema, rashes, congestion, recurrent infections, or excessive mucus production from eating dairy foods. Many times, however, these symptoms can be avoided by switching to organic, low-fat yogurt or kefir, or to low-fat goat milk products. (Of course, those who are severely allergic to all dairy would be wise to simply stay away from these products, organic or not.)

ALLERGIC OR INTOLERANT?

Lactose intolerance is not the same thing as food allergies or sensitivities to dairy. If you are lactose intolerant, your body's digestive tract does not produce enough lactase enzyme for proper digestion of the lactose (milk sugar) in dairy products. The symptoms of lactose intolerance—gas, bloating, and diarrhea—can be alleviated by consuming lactose-free dairy products or taking lactase supplements such as Lactaid.

If you are not familiar with kefir, I recommend you try it out. Kefir is a cousin of yogurt and is simply fermented milk that is rich in beneficial bacteria. With both kefir and yogurt, however, avoid the premixed fruit blends, which are usually high in sugars and can sabotage your weight-loss efforts. It is best to choose organic, low-fat, plain yogurt and kefir products and add your own fresh fruit to it.

Also, many dieters complain about not being able to eat cheese. On the "I Can Do This" program, you will still be able to enjoy small amounts of your favorite low-fat or skim-milk cheese lightly sprinkled over your food. Just do not eat it by the slice, as this generally leads to mindless eating.

Plant proteins

Plant proteins are typically lower-quality proteins since most are low in at least one of the essential amino acids. Legumes and beans have less of the amino acid methionine, and grains have less of the amino acid lysine. Vegetarians are

able to combine plant proteins with their regular meals to have a high-quality protein. For example, by combining corn and beans, whole wheat and peanut butter, or rice and beans you can form complete proteins. Soy, however, is an exception and is already considered a complete protein.

The potential problem with combining two starches to make a complete protein is that it is easy to slow down or entirely stop your weight loss if your portions are too big. If you can keep this in mind, however, there is no reason you should not enjoy the added benefits and flavors of these proteins. For instance, whole grains and legumes are excellent sources of fiber and are also loaded with nutrients. Black bean soup and a small amount of wild rice is a complete protein and very filling—and yes, you will most likely start losing weight if you regularly consume it.

A word of caution about beans: As we learn from a young age, beans can cause excessive gas and bloating. This can easily be avoided by soaking the beans, peas, or lentils in a pan with three times their volume of cold water in the refrigerator overnight. The next day, discard the water they were soaked in and cook your beans. Most of the substances in the beans that cause flatulence are removed in the soaking process. And in case you are eating out, you can take a couple of the over-the-counter product Beano before eating beans. This provides the enzyme that enables you to digest the beans and thus prevent flatulence.

FIVE BEANS FOR LIFE

1. Red beans—gram for gram, these contain more antioxidants than blueberries and are a great source of iron.

2. Kidney beans—the second-best bean source of antioxidants, these are also a solid choice for providing fiber.

3. Black beans—along with providing plenty of antioxidants, black beans contain the most magnesium among beans.

4. Black-eyed beans—the top bean source of calcium, they also are great for providing both magnesium and folate.

5. Pinto beans—like red beans, they rank higher than blueberries in antioxidants and are also the best source of selenium.[10]

Soy

I mentioned soy earlier as a complete protein that can stand on its own. This is because, despite being considered a legume or bean, it contains all the essential amino acids to make it a complete protein. Fermented soy such as tofu, miso soup, tempeh, and natto are easily digested and assimilated. Soy has been

proven to lower cholesterol, diminish the risk of myocardial infarction (MI) and heart disease, decrease hot flashes in menopausal women, and may prevent both memory loss and breast cancer.

Unfortunately, there is a potential dark side of soy, as recent and somewhat controversial research indicates. Many scientists now believe that overconsuming soy may do more harm than good. High consumption of isoflavones, which are the estrogen-like plant chemicals contained in soy, may stimulate the production of breast cancer cells. It may also increase the chances of developing serious reproductive, thyroid, and liver problems.[11]

Besides this, most soy products are processed and have a low biological value compared to other proteins—meaning the body doesn't use them very efficiently. This includes two of the most commonly consumed soy products, soy milk and soy protein. These products can interfere with thyroid functioning and lower the metabolic rate, making it more difficult to lose weight. In general, there are many adults and children on soy milk or soy protein powder, and it may be doing them more harm than good, especially if they are trying to lose weight.

If you enjoy soy, I recommend cutting back or eliminating soy products altogether if you desire to lose weight. And let me emphasize this: the final word on soy is not yet in. Even the soy skeptics say the bottom line is to opt for natural forms of soy rather than chemically altered or genetically modified (GM). Because it remains a somewhat controversial protein, my advice is to proceed with caution; do not eat or drink soy products every day, but if you must consume soy, do it only a couple times a week.

DIABETES AND SOY

For the last few years I have been warning people about the use of soy because I've seen many people have adverse reactions to consuming it. Others in the medical community are beginning to speak out as well.

Gabriel Cousens, MD, calls soy a *diabetogenic*, meaning it produces diabetes. Cousens explains that 90 percent of all soy is genetically modified (GM). Soy is also one of the top seven allergens. The isoflavones in soy can make a person estrogenic, contributing to cancer and breast and uterine fibroids. Cousens also links soy to decreased thyroid production, stunted growth in children, lowering of good (HDL) cholesterol, insulin resistance, heart disease, and Alzheimer's disease.[12]

Nuts

Nuts are a fair source of protein and a good source of fiber. They contain beneficial fats, including polyunsaturated and monounsaturated fats. A small handful of almonds, walnuts, or pecans several times a week or as a snack is

extremely beneficial for weight loss. Be careful, however, to limit the nuts to a small handful since they do contain many calories.

Protein powders

Whey protein is a complete protein that is high in quality and easy to digest and absorb into the body. This is an excellent way to add protein to your meals and snacks. Whey protein contains the amino acid leucine, as well as the other branch chain amino acids that help maintain muscle tissue and promote fat loss. By stimulating the release of two hormones, CCK and GLP-1, whey suppresses the appetite. It is also crucial for the immune system and increases the levels of glutathione, which is one of the most important antioxidants in the body.

Unfortunately, most whey protein sold over the counter in health food stores is low-quality whey. I strongly recommend undenatured whey protein, which is a superior quality, or whey protein isolate. Also, there are some excellent vegetarian protein powders such as Life's Basics Plant Protein and PureLean Protein, which contains pea, hemp, and rice protein with chia seed. However, I do not recommend lower-quality protein powder such as soy, caseine, or egg proteins.

CHILL…FOR PROTEIN'S SAKE

Did you know that stress can affect how much protein you absorb? Chronic stress is associated with a decreased output of pancreatic enzymes as blood is shunted away from the digestive tract. This, in turn, can impair your ability to digest proteins.

THE WORD ON DIGESTION

Most Americans do not have a problem *eating* protein. The problem is in *digesting* protein. Despite eating adequate amounts, many people are unable to sufficiently process and absorb protein. Most of us eat rapidly and do not chew our food enough, which makes it difficult to adequately digest proteins. This is especially true with many meat lovers. I've seen countless people scarf down a steak by chewing the meat only a couple of times and washing each bite down with big gulps of iced tea. If these steak fans are older, they are most likely missing out on the protein's value because they lack the enzymes and hydrochloric acid to properly digest it.

READ MORE ABOUT IT

Please see *The Seven Pillars of Health* and *Eat This and Live!* for more information regarding the digestive benefits of proper chewing and other eating habits.

By simply slowing down, relaxing, and chewing every bite thirty times, we can help with the digestion and absorption of the protein we consume. Some individuals—particularly those over the age of fifty—will still need a digestive enzyme and/or hydrochloric acid supplements to help them adequately digest and absorb protein foods.

"CAN DO" POINTS TO REMEMBER

1. The average recommended daily requirement for protein is approximately 50–75 grams per day for adult females and 70–100 grams daily for adult males.

2. The more protein you eat, the more calcium is needed to buffer the onslaught of acids produced from excessive proteins—which can lead to your body possibly even cannibalizing the calcium from your bones and teeth.

3. Adequate amounts of protein eaten with each meal and snack will decrease hunger and help you lose weight.

4. If you do not have adequate protein, you may ultimately age faster and be prone to develop disease.

5. Free-range or organic lean chicken and turkey, organic or omega-3 eggs, wild-caught fish, and organic low-fat dairy are the best choices of animal proteins.

6. Organic legumes, whole grains, and nuts are the best plant proteins.

7. Proceed with caution with soy products.

8. Protein powder such as undenatured whey protein is a good way to add protein to your meals and snacks.

9

FATS THAT MAKE YOU FAT AND
FATS THAT MAKE YOU LEAN

A S A KID, I remember there was no feeling worse than getting blamed
for something you didn't do. Coloring on the wall. Breaking an appliance. Letting the cat out of the house. Hitting a baseball through the
next-door neighbor's window. We have all watched as someone did something wrong, only to turn around and find others pointing the finger at us.
It's not fun being guilty when you're not.

For decades, physicians, nutritionists, dietitians, and other health authori-
ties have blamed fats for every diet-related problem under the sun. The obesity
epidemic. Elevated cholesterol. Heart disease. It seems someone, years ago,
came up with a masterful plan to indoctrinate a single "truth" and transform
an entire country's dietary mind-set. The premise: *fats will make you fat.*

As a result, a whole country flocked to anything labeled "low-fat" or, better
yet, "*no* fat." Anyone and everyone started going on low-fat diets, cooking
from low-fat cookbooks, and eating low-fat crackers, low-fat chips, low-fat ice
cream, and even low-fat cookies. Since the 1960s, Americans have decreased
their consumption of fat from 40 percent of their daily caloric intake to 38
percent of their total calories in the 1980s to a current level of approximately
33 percent of their calories.[1] There is one big problem, though.

We're still gaining weight.

In fact, obesity has skyrocketed in this country to unparalleled proportions, while the average weight of Americans has steadily increased during
this same forty-year stretch. If fats are supposed to make you fat, then why
has cutting back on them made Americans fatter? Clearly, something doesn't
add up.

THE FAT TRUTH

First things first: fats will not necessarily make you fat. The truth of the matter
is there are good fats that enable you to lose weight and bad fats that cause

you to gain weight. The good fats are, in fact, very good; they help prevent heart disease, lower cholesterol, decrease inflammation, and ward off a multitude of diseases. The bad fats...not so much. These are the ones that deserve the finger pointed at them, and we will talk about them a bit. The bottom line that needs to be understood, however, is that too much of any fat—whether good or bad—will make you fat.

Overall, fats are critically important for our health. Among their many roles, their main purpose in the body is to provide fuel for cells. Each of the trillions of cells in your body is surrounded by a fatty cell membrane composed primarily of polyunsaturated and saturated fats. The saturated fats provide a rigid support for the cell membrane. The polyunsaturated fats, meanwhile, add flexibility to the cell membranes and allow the transfer of nutrients inside the cells and waste products to be passed outside the cells. These cell membranes need a proper balance of both saturated and polyunsaturated fats.

Likewise, we need a proper balance of fats in our diet to help with the absorption of fat-soluble vitamins, including vitamins A, D, E, and K. We also need fats to produce hormones that regulate inflammation, blood clotting, and muscle contraction. Approximately 60 percent of your brain is composed of fat. You need cholesterol to make brain cells, and most of your cholesterol comes from saturated fats. Fats make up the coverings that surround and protect nerves. They help to satisfy hunger for extended periods. And they even cook dinner for you.

OK, so that last one was a stretch. But as you can see, fats are not the villains we have made them out to be. In this chapter, we will find that good fats actually have tremendous health benefits.

TYPES OF FATS

Fats can be broken down into two main types: saturated and unsaturated. Within the unsaturated fats category are three smaller groupings.

1. Omega-6 fats
2. Omega-9 fats
3. Omega-3 fats

Omega-3 and omega-6 fats are polyunsaturated fats, while omega-9 fats are monounsaturated fats. And actually, only two of the fats within these subcategories are absolutely required for health: linoleic acid, which is an

omega-6 fatty acid, and alpha-linolenic acid, which is an omega-3 fatty acid. Our bodies are capable of producing all other types of fats by consuming these two fatty acids. That leaves omega-9 fats left out in the rain, as they are considered nonessential fatty acids.

Got it? Of course not. I don't expect you to understand the terms and details of fats, especially when many biology students have a hard time remembering them. The subject of fats and fatty acids can get extremely confusing to most people. So for simplicity's sake, I have decided to categorize fats into three main categories: bad fats, good fats, and fats that can be good or bad depending on the amount that is ingested.

Bad Fats

Trans fats
Trans fats are simply man-made fats that we have already alluded to throughout the early chapters of this book. These fats are present in margarine; shortenings; most commercially baked foods; many deep-fried foods; many commercial peanut butters; and many processed foods such as crackers, cookies, cakes, pies, and breads. The problem with trans fats is that they are synthetic toxic fats that raise the cholesterol level, form plaque in the arteries, and increase a person's risk of obesity, heart disease, type 2 diabetes, and even cancer.

Trans fats are also associated with inflammation in the body. Many diseases are associated with inflammation, including heart disease, Alzheimer's disease, arthritis, and autoimmune diseases, to name a few. Inflammation is also associated with truncal obesity.

How bad are trans fats? Open up a tub of margarine and set it outside in your garage. Typically, no insects will even go near it. So how in the world did we wind up putting this substance in the majority of our foods today? Good question. After being developed in Germany and mass-produced in England, trans fats came on the scene here in America in 1911 with the introduction of Crisco. To boost sales, free cookbooks were given away— cookbooks in which every recipe required the hydrogenated shortening.[2] By the time World War II came around, butter was in short supply, and trans fats became ingrained into our culture. Processed food companies had the perfect fat for profits. It would not spoil or turn rancid. Better yet, it was cheap and had an extremely long shelf life.

My, how the times have changed. In January 2007, the U.S. Food and Drug Administration (FDA) almost entirely banned Crisco. Rather than completely

fold shop, however, the product's maker agreed to reformulate its shortening to contain zero trans fats per serving.[3] This fell more in line with the NIH's general recommendation to either not eat trans fats at all or to eat them in only very small quantities. The reasons go beyond adding a few pounds. By consuming trans fats, your cells and cell membranes actually become hydrogenated or partially hydrogenated as they stiffen and grow rigid. This, then, affects the transport of nutrients into the cells and waste products out of the cells and leads to inflammation.

FOODS THAT OFTEN HAVE TRANS FATS

1. Fast foods
2. Packaged foods
3. Frozen foods
4. Candy and cookies
5. Baked goods
6. Chips and crackers
7. Toppings, dips, and condiments
8. Soups
9. Margarine and butter
10. Breakfast foods

In the same Nurses' Health Study I referred to in the last chapter, researchers found that the women who consumed the most trans fats—about 3 percent of their daily energy, or about 7 grams of fat—were twice as likely to develop heart disease over a fourteen-year period than those who ate the least amount of trans fats.[4] Overall, experts agree that each gram of trans fat consumed increases your risk of heart disease by approximately 20 percent. In addition, trans fats further your risk of becoming obese by increasing insulin resistance and by increasing the size of fat cells, which in turn enables them to store more fat than regular fat cells. Trans fats literally program your body for fat storage.

With all these detriments, you would think the general public might catch on. And the good news is that we are— slowly. Beginning in January 2006, the FDA mandated the labeling of all foods containing trans fats. Fortunately, many fast-food restaurants, as well as many processed food companies, no longer use these toxic fats. But that does not mean they aren't still out there. As of this book's writing, a typical store-bought doughnut still contained 3.2 grams of trans fat and a large order of french fries from the average fast-food restaurant typically contained 6.8 grams of trans fats. Though these amounts certainly vary according to where they come from, the point is that we must still beware of these trans fats. Learn to read labels and avoid any foods that contain hydrogenated, partially hydrogenated, or trans fats.

Refined polyunsaturated fats

This is another type of bad fat that causes weight gain. There are actually good polyunsaturated fats (including omega-3 fats), as well as unrefined polyunsaturated fats such as cold-pressed vegetable oils, seeds, and nuts. The majority of Americans, however, consume excessive amounts of refined polyunsaturated fats. These fats are included in most salad dressings and most commercial vegetable oils such as sunflower oil, safflower oil, corn oil, soybean oil, or most any other type of commercial vegetable oil. These omega-6 fats have been refined and heated to high temperatures and thus are typically high in dangerous lipid peroxides, which trigger inflammation in the body. These fats are also associated with weight gain, again because of their tendency to increase insulin resistance, which sets the stage for obesity.

Deep-fried foods

Deep-fried foods such as french fries, onion rings, fried chicken, deep fried fish, hush puppies, and any other item that is deep-fried is loaded with fats. Simply imagine taking a sponge, dropping it in water, and then wringing all the water out of the sponge. That is similar to what you are doing when you take french fries, onion rings, chicken, or any other type of food and throw it into a deep fryer. That food is literally soaking up all the grease and all the fat—only you are not wringing it out like the sponge but instead putting in your mouth. And in the process, your body is being programmed (by eating fried foods) to store the fat.

Many of the oils that restaurants use in their deep-fat fryers actually create inflammation in the body. We now know that truncal obesity, heart disease, Alzheimer's disease, arthritis, and autoimmune diseases are associated with inflammation. Parents who regularly feed their children french fries, deep-fried chicken, and fried chicken strips are unknowingly setting up their children for a lifelong struggle with obesity.

> **MISLEADING LABELS**
>
> On January 1, 2006, all packaged foods sold in the United States began to list trans fat content on their nutrition labels. But under FDA regulations, "if the serving contains less than 0.5 gram [of trans fat], the content, when declared, shall be expressed as zero."[5] That means you could eat several cookies, each with 0.4 grams of trans fat, and end up eating several grams of trans fats even though the label says zero!

FATS THAT MAY BE GOOD OR MAY BE BAD

Some fats can be good or bad, depending on the amount ingested. These include saturated fats and unrefined omega-6 fats, which are polyunsaturated fats. First, let's take a look at saturated fats.

THINKING GREEN

Canola oil, which is used by many restaurants for deep-frying, actually releases twice the amount of an air pollutant called acetaldehyde than extra-virgin olive oil when heated to 350 degrees Fahrenheit. At 475 degrees Fahrenheit, two and half times as much acetaldehyde is released.[6]

Saturated fats

Whether a saturated fat is good or bad depends on the type and amount consumed. Saturated fats are found primarily in animal products, including meat such as beef, pork, lamb, and poultry. More precisely, they are found in animal fat, as in the visible fat that typically surrounds a piece of steak. They are also found in marbled fat, which is the fat inter-mixed with the meat that makes prime rib and rib eye steak so juicy. Finally, satu-rated fats are also found in the skins of poultry; dairy products, including butter, cream, half-and-half, milk, and cheese; as well as a few vegetable oils, including palm oil, palm kernel oil, and coconut oil.

Thousands of studies prove that excessive intake of saturated fats is associated with an increase of LDL cholesterol, which is the bad form of cholesterol, and with an increased risk of atherosclerosis. Many people are unaware of all the different types of saturated fats. Short-chain saturated fats are present in coconut oil and palm kernel oil, both of which are excel-lent sources of fuel for the body and easily digestible. These fatty acids are healthier saturated fats and less likely to elevate cholesterol levels, unless consumed in excess. Coconut oil also contains lauric acid, which is a satu-rated fat that helps the immune system function and is even present in breast milk.

The next type of saturated fats includes the medium-chain triglycerides (MCTs). These are also found in coconut oil and palm kernel oil, with coconut oil being the most concentrated source of MCTs. These fats are also digested and utilized differently from other saturated fats. They are first sent to the liver and rapidly converted to energy, much as carbohydrates are. Athletes use these fats quite frequently because they produce immediate energy and typi-cally are not stored as fat. MCTs also help to increase the metabolic rate. Even

though it is not efficient, MCTs can be stored as fat, especially if you consume too many calories and do not exercise enough.

The worse types of saturated fats are the long-chain saturated fats, especially fatty cuts of meat such as most regular hamburger meat, ribs, rib eye, prime rib, sausage, and bacon—all of which are associated with raising LDL cholesterol. Long-chain saturated fats are present in all meats, especially fatty and high-fat dairy products such as butter and cheese.

Approximately 5 to 10 percent of your food intake should be made up of saturated fats. However, if you have elevated levels of cholesterol, the National Cholesterol Education Program (NCEP) recommends that no more than 7 percent of your daily calories should come from saturated fat.[7] When you consistently consume more than 10 percent of your total calories as saturated fat, you increase your risk of high cholesterol, atherosclerosis, insulin resistance, and weight gain.

Bad fat cutback

So how do you lower your intake of saturated fats? It's not complicated. Choose extra-lean cuts of meat, low-fat or nonfat dairy products, peel the skins off poultry, trim off all visible fats, and limit eating red meat to two or three times a week (no more than 18 ounces total per week). I recommend choosing more turkey, chicken, and fish, which are typically low in saturated fats provided they are free-range, organic, and not farm-raised fish. I also urge you to limit your portion sizes of meat to 2 to 6 ounces for women and 3 to 8 ounces for men per meal. This is equivalent to 21 to 42 grams of protein per meal, which is plenty of protein for anyone.

For some, this may seem like a small amount of meat. Men especially like to eat huge steaks. But did you ever consider that an 8-ounce steak is half a pound? No matter how much you love steak, realize that it is loaded with saturated fats (especially if it's rib-eye steak) that are locking you into obesity, often via insulin resistance. And as you recall, insulin resistance is when the body's tissues do not respond normally to insulin. This programs the body for fat storage and weight gain, which is why it is so important to choose extra-lean sources of meat and low-fat or nonfat dairy and watch your portion sizes. Realize also that free-range, grass-fed, or organically fed animals typically have significantly less saturated fat than grain-fed animals. Buffalo, bison, and elk, as well as other wild game, are all good choices for low-saturated-fat meats.

Omega-6 fats

We all need small amounts of unrefined omega-6 fats on a daily basis for good health. The omega-6 fatty acid, linoleic acid, is an essential fatty acid that everyone requires. However, the majority of Americans take in excessive amounts of this, often in the form of salad dressings and other refined oils such as corn oil, sunflower oil, and safflower oil. Many processed foods, as well as fast foods and restaurant foods, are extremely high in refined omega-6 fatty acids. The recommended ratio of omega-6 fatty acids to omega-3 fatty acids should be approximately 4:1. Currently, most Americans consume about a 20:1 ratio![8] Omega-3 fats suppress inflammation whereas excessive omega-6 fats promote inflammation. Remember, inflammation is associated with truncal obesity and disease.

> **READ THE LABEL**
>
> Since foods can still contain up to 0.5 grams of trans fats per serving while being labeled as having zero trans fats, the best way to avoid consuming trans fats unawares is to look for the words *partially hydrogenated* or *shortening* on the label. If either of these words is on the label, don't eat the product!

Instead of refined omega-6 fats, choose expeller- or cold-pressed oils in very small amounts. These oils include grape seed oil, walnut oil, and sesame seed oil. Other healthy sources of omega-6 fats include practically all seeds and nuts. Although seeds and nuts are high in fat, they are also high in fiber, which is filling, satisfying, and actually prevents the absorption of some of the fat. Keep in mind, however, that an excessive consumption of even good omega-6 fats can cause weight gain and may be associated with insulin resistance, which triggers fat storage. As always, the key is moderation. Any kind of fat—even healthy fats if taken in excess—can lead to weight gain.

HEALTHY FATS

GLA

Gamma linolenic acid (GLA) is produced in the body from linoleic acid (LA). Think of GLA as a "super LA." It is an extremely beneficial fatty acid that helps to decrease inflammation in the body. Oils that contain GLA include borage oil, evening primrose oil, and black currant seed oil. Unfortunately, GLA is not found in most foods. Even though LA is the essential fatty acid, many individuals are unable to convert LA to GLA and are thus at a higher risk of developing inflammation, an impaired immune response, allergies, and insulin resistance. This also means, of course, that the risk of

weight gain and fat storage increases due to their bodies' inability to produce adequate amounts of GLA.

Most people who naturally produce the extremely beneficial GLA are young and healthy. That is because the body's ability to convert LA to GLA is impaired by excessive stress, an excessive intake of trans fats or saturated fats, an excessive intake of omega-6 fats, and even older age.

Omega-3 fats

Without getting into too many details and confusing you, I think it is important to go a little deeper in explaining omega-3 fats, since they are mentioned frequently and are often automatically associated with fish. There are actually three types of omega-3 fats: alpha-linolenic acid (ALA), which is found in flaxseeds and flaxseed oil; eicosapentaenoic acid (EPA), found in cold-water fish; and docosahexaenoic acid (DHA), which is also found in cold-water fish as well as some algae. Approximately 99 percent of Americans are deficient in these healthy fats.

Unfortunately, many individuals are unable to produce EPA and DHA from ALA because the enzyme that makes this conversion is often impaired. Again, this is usually due to stress, older age, and excessive intake of trans fats, saturated fats, and omega-6 fats. Therefore, even if you are eating a lot of omega-3 fats in the form of flaxseed oil and flaxseeds, you still may not have adequate amounts of EPA and DHA since your body is unable to convert ALA to the most powerful omega-3 fats, EPA and DHA.

Omega-3 fats—particularly EPA and DHA—have many benefits. They decrease inflammation in the body, lower cholesterol and triglycerides, assist in preventing and treating heart disease, help neurotransmitters in the brain function optimally, support the immune system, and prompt the body to release stored fat. The best sources of omega-3 fats are fatty fish such as salmon, mackerel, herring, and sardines. Quality fish oil supplements are also good alternatives. (See Appendix H.)

A diet with sufficient amounts of omega-3 fats will usually prevent and eventually reverse insulin resistance. These fats help the body to start *losing* weight in the abdominal area, making it less likely that weight will be stored there. In fact, good fats in the form of fatty fish or quality fish oil capsules are a must for anyone wanting to lose weight in the abdominal area. Belly fat is associated with inflammation, and fish oil decreases inflammation in the body. Individuals who consume plenty of omega-3 fats also decrease their risk of developing diabetes. I strongly recommend that in choosing

fish, select wild salmon or wild-caught ocean fish instead of farm-raised fish.

I mentioned earlier the benefits of choosing free-range, grass-fed, or organically fed animals. Animals that are typically grain fed include cows, pigs, and even chickens. Their meat usually contains a very low concentration of omega-3 fatty acids and significantly higher amounts of omega-6 fatty acids. Grain-fed meat is also typically high in saturated fats. Together these fats increase the risk of insulin resistance and inflammation, and thus promote weight gain, usually in the belly. However, free-range or grass-fed animals, on the other hand, typically have much higher concentrations of omega-3 fats in their tissues and lower levels of omega-6 fats, as well as lower levels of saturated fats.

THE REALITY OF AMERICA'S FARMS

The sad state of America's food industry isn't new, but a recent article in *TIME* magazine sheds light on some surprising statistics:

- The number of US farms today is less than 2 million, compared to 6.8 million in 1935.

- In 1940, the average farmer fed 19 Americans; today he feeds 129 people.

- By 2015, worldwide demand for meat and poultry is predicted to rise by 25 percent.

American farms are becoming more efficient, but at what cost? You might like to picture your bacon and eggs coming from animals raised on a serene hillside farm by Old MacDonald. But it is much more likely that they came from a "factory farm" or concentrated-animal feeding operation (CAFO), where a thousand or more animals are cramped into prison-like living conditions, making it necessary to pump them with antibiotics while they are fed corn instead of grass to fatten them for slaughter as quickly as possible.[9]

Monounsaturated fats

The last group of good fats that I would like to talk about are monounsaturated fats. Certain Mediterranean diets consume up to 40 percent of their daily calories from monounsaturated fats, primarily in the form of olive oil. In what became known as the Seven Countries Study, Ancel Keys, PhD, and other researchers studied more than twelve thousand men between the ages of forty and fifty from 1958 to 1964. Keys discovered that those in the Mediterranean groups had the lowest mortality rates from all causes. Greek men had the lowest mortality rate overall, as well as the lowest rate of heart disease. The Finnish men, on the other hand, had the highest rate of heart disease and consumed almost 40 percent of their calories from

fats—with more than 50 percent of this coming from saturated fats. Though the Greek men consumed about the same amount of calories from fat, the majority of the fat they consumed was monounsaturated fat in the form of olive oil. Among other things, the study proved that olive oil and other monounsaturated fats are extremely healthy fats.[10]

Monounsaturated fats are in the omega-9 category and are considered nonessential fats since the body can make them from other fats. Regardless of this, monounsaturated fats are extremely healthy, as they help lower LDL cholesterol without decreasing HDL cholesterol (the good kind). They also help to support the immune system and aid in weight loss by decreasing insulin resistance. Foods high in monounsaturated fats include olives, olive oil, almonds, avocados, macadamia nuts, peanuts, peanut butter, cashews, hazelnuts, sesame seeds, Brazilian nuts, and canola oil. These fats are liquid at room temperature but solidify when refrigerated.

Along with the other benefits I have mentioned, monounsaturated fats such as extra-virgin olive oil help to decrease insulin resistance, which, as you know by now, enables you to lose weight if consumed in moderation. This is particularly key for individuals trying to lose weight who are eating salads often. Many people sabotage their weight-loss efforts on salad dressings alone. A simple solution that I always strongly recommend to my patients is to switch from commercial-type salad dressings to extra-virgin olive oil with balsamic vinegar or any other type of vinegar (four parts vinegar to one part oil) and use a salad spritzer.

FATS THAT MAKE YOU LESS FAT

A study from Brigham and Women's Hospital in Boston reveals why a Mediterranean-style diet using olive oil trumps a traditional low-fat diet when it comes to losing weight. Those on the traditional low-fat diet limited their fat intake to 20 percent of their total calories, while those on the Mediterranean diet were allowed to consume 35 percent of their calories from olive oil, nuts, and other monounsaturated fats. After six months, both groups lost weight—not surprising since both were consuming significantly fewer calories than the average American diet. Yet after eighteen months, only 20 percent of those on the low-fat diet stuck with their diet, and most began to regain their lost weight. Meanwhile, the majority of those on the Mediterranean diet not only remained on it, but they also kept their pounds off.[11]

THE FAT PROBLEM

As mentioned at the beginning of this chapter, the majority of Americans consume approximately one-third of their total calories from fats. Even though this is a fairly safe amount of fat, Americans continue to gain weight and suffer from an epidemic of being overweight and obese. For this reason, I recommend approximately 25 to 30 percent of your total calorie intake as fats (making sure to choose *good* fats) in order to lose weight. I cannot stress enough the importance of both the *type* of fats and the *ratio* of fats consumed.

I typically suggest about 10 percent of your fat intake to be monounsaturated fats and 10 percent as polyunsaturated fats in a 4:1 ratio of omega-6 to omega-3 fats. In other words, if 2.5 grams of your fats are omega-3 fats, then you would be looking to consume 7.5 grams of omega-6 fats.

Finally, I believe no more than 5 to 10 percent of your fat intake should be saturated fats. I strongly recommend that you avoid all trans fats, fried foods, and refined omega-6 fats, such as most regular salad dressings. Consuming modest amounts of omega-3 fats, monounsaturated fats, GLA omega-6 fats, and cold-pressed omega 6 oils will help decrease insulin resistance, which in turn enables you to lose weight.

Whenever I explain fats to patients, they seem to understand it best when I tell them that they simply need an oil change. You would not dare think of driving your car year after year and never change your car's oil because eventually you would ruin the engine. Our bodies are no different. We need the proper balance of good healthy oils in

CHEAP FOOD AT A HIGH PRICE

Americans today are paying less per calorie for our food than in the past, but these cheap foods are feeding some very unhealthy eating habits and contributing to an obesity epidemic that is now affecting two-thirds of the population. According to a recent *TIME* magazine article, Americans spend less than 10 percent of their incomes on food today; this is down from 18 percent in 1966. Surprised? Wondering how this is possible? It's because the federal government has given more than $50 billion to the corn industry, and many other grains receive similar government subsidies to keep the prices of these foods artificially low.

However, fruits and vegetables don't receive the same price support as corn and other grains; that's why one dollar can buy you 875 calories of soda but only 250 calories of vegetables or 170 calories of fruit. That's also why McDonald's can offer you such a bargain—only $5 for a Big Mac, fries, and a Coke—but that "bargain" contains more than half of the calories you should consume in an entire day (almost 1,200), not to mention all of the bad fats and other unhealthy ingredients.[12]

our body for all our cells, tissues, and organs to function properly. Fats are not evil; they're essential. Remember, even your brain is made up of 60 percent fat. You can use the right proportion and the right amount of good fats to actually help you lose weight—and fat. Now go get an oil change!

"CAN DO" POINTS TO REMEMBER

1. Among their many roles, the main purpose of fat is to provide fuel for cells.

2. Too much consumption of any fat, whether good or bad, can make you fat.

3. Bad fats include trans fats and refined omega-6 fats such as most commercial oils, salad dressings, and deep-fried foods.

4. Fats that are good in moderation and fats that are bad in excess include saturated fats and unrefined omega-6 fats such as seeds, nuts, and cold-pressed vegetable oils.

5. Good fats include omega-3 fats such as fish oils and flaxseed oils; monounsaturated fats such as extra-virgin olive oil, avocados, almonds, and other nuts and seeds; cold-pressed omega-6 oils; and GLA omega-6 fatty acids such as borage oil, evening primrose oil, and black currant seed oil.

10

BEVERAGES: ARE YOU DRINKING YOURSELF OBESE?

F RESH-FACED YOUTHS FROM all over the world standing on a hilltop singing about the world in perfect harmony. Sportscasters analyzing "Bud Bowl" highlights from a gridiron showdown between helmet-clad bottles of Bud Light and Budweiser. A partying bull terrier named Spuds Mackenzie. Polar bears watching the aurora borealis while sipping from Coke bottles.

These are some of the beverage industry's ingenious ways to change perception. You have to hand it to them: they certainly know how to market a drink. From hilarious beer commercials to ridiculous—but always memorable—soft-drink ads, marketers have brilliantly taught America that instant fun comes in a can. And as is usually the case, they are more interested in distracting you with a fond memory or good feeling about their product than informing you about its actual content and potential health hazards. Like the fact that a 12-ounce can of Coke Classic contains 140 calories and 39 grams of sugars. Or that a "healthy" bottle of Dole's Ruby Red grapefruit juice packs in 63 grams of carbs (55 of which are sugars) and 260 calories for every 15 ounces. Or even that a supposedly "diet" carbonated drink can possibly lead to greater weight gain than a regular soda.

Meanwhile, we continue to guzzle their drinks.

It's taking its toll on our waistlines too. According to the Beverage Marketing Corporation, the average person (adult or child) ingests approximately 192 gallons of liquid a year. That amounts to approximately 3.7 gallons a week, or half a gallon a day.[1] That's a decent amount. The problem, however, doesn't lie so much in *how much* we are drinking but *what* we are drinking. For years I have taught that we need to consume about two quarts or half a gallon of *water* each day. Let's take a look at the percentages of types of beverages people consume to see just how far off we are from this mark.

WHAT THE AVERAGE AMERICAN DRINKS[2]

Type of Beverage	Percent of Total Beverage Consumption
Carbonated soft drinks	28.3 percent
Beer	11.7 percent (total alcohol consumption was 13 percent, with wine at 1.2 percent and distilled spirits at 0.7 percent)
Milk	10.9 percent
Bottled water	10.7 percent
Coffee	9.0 percent
Fruit beverages	4.7 percent
Tea	3.8 percent

According to the chart above, 40 percent of all beverages consumed were carbonated soft drinks and alcoholic beverages, while more than two-thirds of drinks consumed were high-calorie beverages. We are literally drinking ourselves fat.

FEELING THIRSTY?

Why do we continue to guzzle down the extra calories and sugars with apparently no thought for change? Beyond the fruity flavors and "great taste/less filling" arguments, it starts with a basic driving force: thirst. Your thirst center is located in the hypothalamus of the brain. Thirst is the main way that your body signals you that you need to ingest more fluids. This is actually triggered by a decrease in blood volume or an increase of sodium in the blood. Drinking a beverage increases the blood volume and dilutes the sodium in the blood, and thirst then abates.

This isn't necessarily the case among elderly people. Because they often suffer from an impaired sense of thirst, they are more prone to dehydration; essentially, the sodium in their blood rises too high. To prevent this and quench thirst, we usually gulp down water or a host of other beverages. The problem for those trying to control their weight, however, is that many of these drinks do not effectively curb the appetite or satisfy hunger.

It's all part of beverage makers' plans. Their concern is how their drink can most effectively appeal to your need to quench your thirst. As a result, near any grocery store or convenience store you will almost always find a massive billboard or poster showing a cool, refreshing drink. It's why there is usually a refrigerated container full of ice-cold drinks near every checkout line. The

truth is, any cool beverage that is low in sodium will quench your thirst. But do you realize that when you gulp these down you are also ingesting about 10 teaspoons of sugar with each 12-ounce can of soda? This does absolutely nothing to turn off or turn down your hunger or appetite. On the contrary, it actually stimulates your appetite.

When you absorb the sugar or high-fructose corn syrup from a soda into your bloodstream—usually a rapid process—it spikes your blood sugar, causing a surge of insulin to be released from the pancreas, which in turn eventually triggers the appetite. In reality, the soda is simultaneously quenching thirst *and* triggering appetite—yet that soda cannot effectively curb hunger. So what usually happens next? If you are like the average American, usually within an hour or two you find yourself reaching for a high-calorie snack to raise your blood sugar. Many of us are caught in this soda snare.

BIG GULPS

The National Soft Drink Association now reports that the average person consumes more than six hundred 12-ounce servings of soft drinks a year. Young males age twelve to twenty-nine are the biggest consumers, gulping down an astounding 160-plus gallons a year, which amounts to almost 2 quarts each day.[3]

THE SODA SNARE

Anne was one of those stuck in the trap. A forty-two-year-old accountant, her days typically began by eating a small bagel with cream cheese and drinking a glass of orange juice. Around midmorning she drank a soda, and for lunch she usually had a healthy soup along with another soda. She would add a "pick me up" soda around 3:00 p.m., and then ate a healthy dinner and drank iced tea at night. Even though she worked out five days a week, always passed on desserts, and did not consume excessive calories, she could not understand why she never lost weight. It was even more frustrating when she looked around at many of her slender co-workers, most of whom ate more than she did—including desserts—but never seemed to gain a pound.

After a while, she noticed that instead of drinking sodas, her slender co-workers were drinking water and unsweetened tea. She could not bring herself to go cold turkey, so she compromised and switched from drinking regular soda to diet soda. Within a few months of doing this, she had actually gained 5 more pounds. Talk about frustrating! By the time she scheduled an appointment at my office, she was 35 pounds overweight and about to give up.

Upon taking her dietary and beverage history, it did not take long to figure

out the source of her problems. Her sodas and diet sodas were killing any efforts she made at losing weight. When I switched Anne over to water with lemon and unsweetened green tea and adjusted her food intake, she began to lose weight. Within six months, she had lost the 35 pounds, and she felt and looked great.

Diet sodas

Anne's case is more common than you might think. I have met with hundreds of exasperated patients who thought their solution was changing from regular sodas to diet ones. "After all, there's barely anything in them, right?" they usually ask. Because of labeling alone, diet sodas have often been associated with diets. Somewhere between the first reduced-calorie drink and emergence of artificial sweeteners, we believed we could lose weight merely by making the switch to diet sodas.

A handful of studies have shown the exact opposite. These reports indicate that drinking diet sodas can actually cause weight gain—more weight than regular sodas, in fact. One study covering eight years' worth of data found that drinking one or two cans of soda each day led to a 32.8 percent greater chance of becoming overweight. When diet sodas were consumed in place of regular ones at the same rate, the risk increased to a whopping 54.5 percent.[4]

I'll be honest; the exact reasons for this are not yet fully known. Researchers have yet to understand what the direct connection is between the contents of diet drinks and weight gain. What we do know is that somehow diet sodas trigger the body to store fat. Some researchers believe that the tremendous sweetness of many of these artificial sweeteners, which are typically 200 to 2,000 times sweeter than sugar, causes us to crave more sweets. The sweet taste literally primes the taste buds for more sweets.

Soda drinkers, and especially diet soda drinkers, are also less likely to enjoy the sweetness of fruit, instead leaning toward stronger flavors and greater sweetness to make foods taste good. Their taste buds become hooked on super-sweetness. In addition, even thinking about sweets can cause the body to release more insulin. Higher insulin levels, in turn, lower the blood sugar in the body, which triggers hunger and puts us in fat-storage mode. These diet sodas are most likely increasing

DIET DRINKS AND METABOLIC SYNDROME

A recent study of more than ninety-five hundred people found those who consumed at least one can of diet soda a day had a 34 percent higher chance of developing metabolic syndrome than those who did not drink diet sodas.[5]

insulin levels and setting up people for increased hunger and fat storage—which was exactly what happened with Anne.

As the soda grows (so goes the waistline)

There is another factor to the connection between growing waistlines and sodas—both regular and diet. In the 1950s, Coke was only sold in a 6½-ounce bottle. Now cans of soda are 12 ounces and the standard bottle is 20 ounces. The Center for Science in the Public Interest says the average daily soda consumption for every adult American is about 18 ounces of soda. We now drink more than twice the amount of soda consumed in early 1970s.[6]

It obviously does not help that most fast-food restaurants and convenience stores offer supersized drinks. From Burger King's 42-ounce "king" offering to 7-Eleven's infamous *Super* Big Gulp, which weighs in at an astounding 44 ounces (as if it wasn't big enough before), Americans are free to guzzle down as much as they want, whenever they want—and with free refills too! Do we realize that by doing this we're not only loading up on more than 400 calories for most of these drinks, but we're also consuming more than *100 grams* of sugar (not counting refills)?

There is no denying this mega-expansion on how we view beverage sizes has affected our younger generation. The average teenager now drinks approximately two 12-ounce cans of carbonated soft drinks a day, which correlates to approximately 20 teaspoons of sugar and makes up 13 percent of their caloric intake. (This does not include the recent rise in consumption of high-sugar energy drinks.) In 1950, Americans drank four times as much milk as soda; yet today, according to the USDA, that has been reversed, with Americans drinking four times as much soda as milk.[7] Since soda consumption has replaced milk in teens' diet, they will probably be at an increased risk of developing osteoporosis. Is it any wonder the CDC reports that over the past thirty years the national obesity rate has more than tripled in teenagers?[8] Soda consumption is a huge contributing factor to this. (In fact, Michael Jacobson, cofounder and executive director of the Center for Science in the Public Interest, believes so strongly in this that he is lobbying to require obesity warning labels on soda cans similar to the Surgeon General's warning on cigarettes.)

The health risks of drinking sodas are obvious. A recent study published in the journal *Circulation* suggests that drinking one or more sodas a day—including diet sodas—is associated with an increase of other risk factors for heart disease. Among those evaluated, those who drank a soda or more each day increased their risk of becoming obese by 31 percent, had a 30 percent

higher chance of increasing their waistline, a 25 percent increase in the likelihood of developing elevated blood sugar levels, and were 32 percent more prone to developing lower HDL (good) cholesterol levels. The interesting point was that it made no difference whether the soda was diet or regular soda.[9]

As the connection between sodas and obesity continues to solidify, we know one thing for certain: this "liquid candy," which comprises approximately 10 percent of the calories in the American diet, is certainly not all it's cracked up to be.[10]

ALCOHOL

After sodas, the most common beverage consumed in the United States is alcohol. Like carbonated soft drinks, alcohol has some drawbacks when it comes to losing weight. While carbohydrates and proteins have 4 calories per gram, and fat has 9 calories per gram, alcohol comes in around 7 calories per gram. In other words, alcohol is closer in calories to fat than to carbohydrates.

Alcohol increases blood sugar levels, leading to elevated insulin levels, which as we know programs the body for weight gain and fat storage. Your body will preferentially use the alcoholic fuel at the expense of not burning fat stored until the alcohol is utilized. Not only does alcohol increase insulin levels, but it also raises cortisol levels. These two are a dynamic duo for weight gain, especially for increasing abdominal fat. One of the main reasons alcoholic beverages cause weight gain is that they decrease our ability to control our eating, while also decreasing our inhibitions. So at the same time alcohol stimulates our appetite, it's also causing us to lose our ability to say no to tempting high-calorie foods.

By far the most widely consumed alcohol in America is beer, which is notoriously high in carbohydrates. A typical 12-ounce can of beer comes packed with 148 calories and 13 grams of carbohydrates. And although we have somewhat turned the beer-guzzling, pot-bellied football fan into a cultural icon, a belly born out of six-packs gulped down in front of the television is no laughing matter. In fact, that beer belly is actually the belly becoming "bubble wrapped" with an ever-expanding omentum. The omentum is a fatty drape of tissue that literally hangs beneath the muscles inside your abdomen. This is toxic fat associated with high cholesterol, hypertension, type 2 diabetes, and heart disease. Typically the more alcohol you drink, the larger your omentum becomes, and the more difficult it is for you to lose weight.

Alcohol by itself causes weight gain, but when combined with sugars and

stress, your body literally becomes a belly-fat-forming machine. Some of the worst examples of this can be found in bars across America during "happy hour." After a stress-filled day, workers pour into a bar to relieve their tension with a social drink. But how many of them realize the pint-size margarita they just ordered has more than 670 calories and 43 grams of carbohydrates? Coupled with their stress levels, empty stomachs, and a handful of sweet-and-salty bar snacks, they are creating a metabolic disaster that is rapidly bubble-wrapping their abdomens in fat.

COFFEE AND OTHER CAFFEINATED BEVERAGES

Both alcohol and caffeine act as mild diuretics in the body, which increases urination and water loss. Therefore, some people may notice some mild weight loss when consuming alcoholic and caffeinated beverages. In fact, what they are usually only losing is temporary water weight. Many Americans are unknowingly already mildly dehydrated, and instead of drinking water that hydrates them, they turn to coffee and other caffeinated beverages. As a result, they become stuck in the caffeine trap.

SHOT TO THE HEART

According to the coffee connoisseurs at Italian manufacturer Illy Coffee, a shot of espresso has 35 percent less caffeine than a cup of brewed coffee.[12]

I am not against drinking coffee, since it is a good source of antioxidants. Consuming high-calorie coffee drinks such as lattes and cappuccinos, however, is helping to fuel the obesity epidemic by raising both insulin and cortisol levels in the body. With a Starbucks on nearly every city corner and its coffee offered at almost every supermarket and restaurant, these drinks are becoming as problematic as sodas. And the problem, just as it is for carbonated drinks, is in the ever-increasing sizes. The three drink sizes at Starbucks are the venti (24 ounces), grande (16 ounces), and tall (12 ounces). When you combine this with the "extras" that often go in a drink, it's easy to see how the line between sodas and coffees is diminishing. A grande Caffè Mocha with whipped cream (and using 2 percent milk), for instance, contains 330 calories, 175 milligrams of caffeine, and 33 grams of sugar. A venti Caffè Vanilla Frappuccino Blended Coffee with whipped cream, meanwhile, contains 560 calories, 160 milligrams of caffeine, and 84 grams of sugar.[11]

For years many nutritionists have recommended caffeine for weight loss. It's true: caffeine is able to increase the metabolic rate mildly for a short period of

time. It makes you more alert, more energetic, and more productive—which usually translates to a more active, calorie-burning lifestyle. Nine out of ten Americans consume some type of caffeine on a regular basis and in moderate doses of approximately 150 to 300 milligrams a day, which is equivalent to about one to two cups of coffee a day.[13] This is not harmful and does not cause weight gain. *It is what you add to your coffee that sets you up for weight gain,* especially the sugar, artificial sweeteners, or cream. By using liquid stevia, a natural sweetener, as well as organic skim milk instead of cream, you can dramatically lower your calorie intake.

Caffeine also acts as a mild appetite suppressant for many. It helps stimulate *thermogenesis,* which is how your body generates heat. This also helps to raise your metabolic rate. Although there is no evidence that increased caffeine intake either causes or prevents significant weight loss, long-term studies have linked higher coffee intake with a lower risk of developing type 2 diabetes, Parkinson's disease, Alzheimer's disease, cirrhosis, and a number of other diseases.

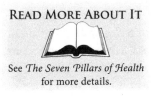

READ MORE ABOUT IT

See *The Seven Pillars of Health* for more details.

Now, before you run out and start drinking three or more cups of coffee a day based on this, realize that there are side effects. Excessive caffeine intake can cause insomnia, a rapid heart rate, and a nervous feeling. People may also experience headaches if they consume too much caffeine or if they suddenly stop consuming it. Therefore, I believe you should play it safe and drink only one to two cups of coffee a day with stevia and perhaps a little organic skim milk.

FRUIT JUICE

We have already exposed the myth that people who switch from regular to diet sodas lose more weight. Ever since the smoothie craze hit a few years ago, I am running into more people now who swear by the same mind-set when it comes to switching to fruit drinks, juices, and smoothies. Even though juices such as orange juice, apple juice, grape juice, and other fruit juices have significantly more vitamins, minerals, antioxidants, and nutrients than sodas, they also contain a lot of calories from sugar (especially fructose). In fact, juice has approximately the same number of calories and sugar content as a soda. For example, 12 ounces of most kinds of juice contain approximately 150 calories, while a regular can of Pepsi, Mountain Dew, or A&W Root Beer yields about the same.

The main problem is that the key ingredient for weight loss and curbing the appetite—fiber—has been extracted from those juices. Often this is compounded by additional sugar being added to the juice during processing. Although the standard serving size of fruit juice is only three-fourths of a cup (6 ounces), many Americans consume 12 ounces or more. Why? Simply because this is how much they have been mentally programmed to consume since soda cans are 12 ounces. Instead of choosing juice, try eating the whole fruit, which is much more satisfying and much higher in fiber. If you insist on drinking juice, I recommend that you drink it in the morning, stick to 4 ounces or less, and add some of the pulp back to it. The fiber in the pulp will lower the glycemic index of the juice and help to decrease your appetite.

A word of warning about smoothies: smoothies are very popular, contain a lot of fruit juice, and are loaded with sugar. If you study the nutritional labels of some of the top smoothies sold in franchises such as Planet Smoothie, Jamba Juice, Smoothie King, and even Dunkin Donuts, you soon realize that the serving sizes are huge, usually ranging from 16 to 24 ounces. A small (16-ounce) order of a Strawberry Banana Smoothie from Dunkin Donuts, for example, packs 360 calories and 69 grams of sugar. In comparison, a small (20-ounce) Immune Builder smoothie from Smoothie King, which also includes strawberries and bananas, contains 384 calories and 80 grams of sugar. These are just two of the hundreds of different smoothie combinations available in the market.

The same warning rings true for many sports drinks, such as Gatorade. While some liquid replenishers may have lower calorie and sugar counts than soda, and come loaded with electrolytes, vitamins, or both, a 12-ounce bottle of Gatorade Performance Energy Drink still has 42 grams of sugar and 310 calories.[14] My advice? Make sure to check the nutritional labels before gulping down a bottle. Without being aware, you can easily sabotage your weight-loss efforts.

LIQUIDATION

Don't depend on your thirst level to determine if you need liquids. During dehydration your thirst mechanism actually shuts off as your hunger increases.[15]

WATER

The best beverage for weight loss is still the world's most natural and abundant: water. Although our bodies are generally made up of almost two-thirds water, it is still the most important nutrient for us to consume—certainly more than soda, coffee, beer, or juice. We lose about 2½ quarts a day just through breathing,

perspiration, urination, and stool.[16] Since we cannot store water in our bodies as a camel can, that water must be replaced throughout the day. Most people need *at least* 2 quarts or 8 cups of water a day. A more accurate figure can be calculated by taking your weight in pounds and dividing it by 2; that is the amount of water in ounces you need on a daily basis for optimal health. Don't forget, however, that if your diet contains adequate amounts of fruits and vegetables (approximately five to seven servings a day), then those foods will contribute approximately one-third of your water needs. Instead of 8 cups of water a day, then, you would need only 5 or 6 cups a day.

Adequate water intake is essential for weight loss because water helps fuel the physiological processes involved in metabolism. But before I go any further on this subject, let me clarify that I am not talking

RULE OF THUMB: H_2O

Drink an 8- to 16-ounce glass either immediately after waking up or half an hour before breakfast.

Drink fifteen to thirty minutes before meals or two hours after (the more you drink, the fuller you'll feel).

With meals, only drink 4 to 8 ounces of water at room temperature.

Avoid drinking large quantities after 7:00 p.m.

about tap water, which typically contains chlorine, fluoride, and many other chemicals. The absolute best water to help you lose weight is clean, pure filtered or spring water. Otherwise, you are contaminating your body with impurities while simultaneously trying to nourish it. Many people grew up drinking tap water. Loaded with chlorine, this usually tastes similar to swimming pool water. I will never forget the time my family was on vacation when I was a child. My parents took us to a restaurant that served sodas from a soda machine that used tap water. The "soda" tasted so heavily chlorinated that my sister and I spit it out of our mouths.

READ MORE ABOUT IT

For extensive information about types of water, water filters, and the like, see *The Seven Pillars of Health* or *Eat This and Live!*

Chlorine is repelling to most individuals' taste buds. When people say they hate the taste of water, it is usually because they've had lousy water most of their lives and have trained their taste buds to be accustomed to sugary sodas, sugary coffees, fruit juices, sweet tea, and so forth. Because of that, they often find it hard to wean themselves from these beverages. I generally switch them over to pure spring or sparkling water such as San Pellegrino and tell them to add a squeeze of lemon or lime and a few drops of the natural sweetener stevia. Others prefer to add 2 ounces of pomegranate juice or 1 or

2 ounces of freshly squeezed ginger (again with a few drops of stevia). The water is then much more flavorful, and most of my patients absolutely love the beverages that they create.

TEAS

Another great way to get adequate water intake is by drinking different teas. When I traveled to England a few years ago, one of the first things I fell in love with was the British tradition of teatime. Every midafternoon we would have a tea break with a few bites of cheese and crackers, along with one or two cups of tea. It left us feeling extremely satisfied for hours afterward. Sadly, in the United States most Americans instead take soda breaks or high-calorie coffee breaks, often with a doughnut, candy bar, or chips.

As I mentioned on page 97, only 3.8 percent of the total U.S. beverage consumption is tea. That is unfortunate since the health benefits of the different types of teas are well documented. Though there are hundreds of teas, the four main groupings are black, green, oolong, and white tea. Each is highly beneficial health-wise, mainly because of its high content of flavonoids. In fact, tea actually provides more flavonoids to the American diet than any other food or beverage. These flavonoids in tea may help to decrease the risk of diabetes, heart disease, and certain cancers, including skin, breast, lung, colon, bladder, ovarian, and esophageal cancers. They assist in blocking oxidation of the bad (LDL) cholesterol, decrease inflammation, and improve blood vessel function. They also help maintain a normal blood sugar, as well as improve immune function. In addition, recent research on tea shows that simply drinking two cups a day decreases the risk of developing ovarian cancer by nearly 50 percent.[17]

The best news for someone struggling with obesity, however, is that tea—especially green tea—helps to burn fat and increase the metabolic rate. Green tea contains a small amount of caffeine but has a specific catechin phytonutrient called epigallocatechin gallate (EGCG) that stimulates the production of norepinephrine, which then boosts the metabolic rate. The EGCG in green tea increases the metabolic rate for as long as twenty-four hours and actually stimulates the body to burn fat. Studies have shown its effectiveness with weight loss, even in those who do not restrict calories.[18]

Green tea also contains an amino acid, L-theanine, that calms and relaxes the body and helps control stress without sedating you. A person typically feels its effect within only a half hour and feels relaxed for approximately two hours. In fact, one study found that drinking five cups of green tea a

day was as effective as taking an antidepressant.[19] Green or regular tea with a few drops of liquid stevia added and water are my favorite beverages for patients desiring to lose weight. It is best to drink the green tea freshly brewed, however, in order to obtain the most catechins. Aim for three to four cups a day to assist with weight loss.

HERBAL INFUSIONS

Herbal infusions look like tea since most are packed like teas; however, the herbs are not tea since they do not come from the Camellia Sinensis bush. They are typically made of barks such as cinnamon bark; flowers, including chamomile and hibiscus; fruits such as orange peal; and grasses such as lemongrass. Herbal infusions with a few drops of stevia are another variety of delicious low-calorie beverages that can help you wean from sodas and other high-calorie beverages.

SEEING RED

Rooibos is actually an herb used as a red tea and is solely grown in the southern tip of South Africa. Red tea has the same antioxidants as green tea but, unlike black tea, doesn't contain tannins, which assist in raising iron levels.

Yerba mate is an herbal infusion that is becoming increasingly popular as more people become aware of its health benefits. While recent headlines have been focused on the weight-loss aspects of yerba mate (it may raise metabolism, regulate appetite, and burn calories), for centuries, Argentinians have consumed yerba mate as an herbal tonic to reduce fatigue, aid digestion, and boost the immune system.

Yerba mate's antioxidant power exceeds green tea, broccoli, and orange juice. The vitamins and minerals in mate include vitamins A, C, E, B_1, B_2, and B complex; calcium; iron; magnesium; selenium; manganese; phosphates; chlorophyll; hydrochloric acid; pantothenic acid; and choline.[20]

HUNGER-SATISFYING BEVERAGES AND LIQUIDS

Vegetable juices, especially tomato juice or V8 vegetable juice, satisfy hunger much better than other beverages. This is because these juices stay in the stomach longer than other liquid beverages, increasing satiety. These are generally on the low-glycemic end of beverages, making them a good alternative.

Dairy products such as organic skim milk and low-fat, low-sugar yogurts and kefir are also more filling since they also remain in the stomach longer and form a semisolid consistency in the stomach. One of my favorite beverages that is extremely satisfying is blending 1 cup of plain organic low-fat kefir with one organic apple. Besides being filling, it is a snack with which you can add other

favorite fruits if desired. As I pointed out in chapter 7, however, yogurts and kefirs that include fruit are usually higher in sugar content, so instead choose low-fat plain yogurts and kefir and add your own fruit. Obviously, if you are allergic or sensitive to dairy, it's best to avoid these foods entirely.

Soups, especially the broth-based (not cream-based) vegetable and bean types, are excellent for weight loss. Soups also stay in the stomach longer and promote satiety. In fact, many times a soup can be so filling that when you finish it, you are less likely to desire additional food. Soup also takes longer to eat, which helps to satisfy the appetite.

As we learned with carbohydrates and fats, the problem most Americans have with beverages is that they consume too much of the wrong type. This double whammy is packing on additional calories and sugar while also stirring up the appetite. In place of sodas and high-calorie coffees, beers, fruit juices, smoothies, and sport drinks, begin drinking more water with lemon and lime, as well as teas—especially green tea since it assists in weight loss. To turn down the appetite, choose vegetable juices, low-fat dairy such as organic skim milk, low-fat plain organic kefir, and yogurt blended with your favorite fruit. And as a final tip, try beginning your evening meal with a broth-based vegetable or bean soup. You will be amazed at how incorporating these little changes will program you for weight loss.

"Can Do" Points to Remember

1. Most Americans are literally drinking themselves obese with sodas.

2. A typical 12-ounce can of soda has about 10 teaspoons of sugar.

3. High-calorie coffees such as lattes and cappuccinos are also typically high in sugar.

4. Fruit juices such as orange juice have approximately the same amount of calories and sugar as similar-sized sodas.

5. The healthiest beverage is clean, pure water.

6. Green tea is one of the best beverages for weight loss; aim for three to four cups a day.

7. Beverages that satisfy hunger include vegetable juice, tomato juice, organic skim milk, and plain, low-fat organic kefir and yogurts.

11

PORTION SIZES

M Y WIFE, MARY, was stuck at a certain weight for years and could not lose additional weight. She would exercise forty-five minutes to an hour about four days a week and ate a well-balanced diet. She cut back on sweets and breads. Despite all the exercise, sweating, and balanced eating, however, her weight did not budge. She grew more frustrated than ever, which then increased her cortisol level and caused even more weight gain.

Then it happened—her "eureka!" moment.

We were eating out at a restaurant one Saturday night and having a great conversation when Mary stopped mid-sentence. She eyed her plate of baked chicken and rice with vegetables, then intensely examined my plate. I could see the change in her face. It suddenly dawned on her that she was eating the same amount of food as I was. I weighed 40 pounds more than she weighed and was more than half a foot taller than she was. In that moment, she became aware that portion sizes could be the reason for her inability to lose weight.

Over the years we had gradually watched our portion sizes increase at restaurants, especially the size of the meats, potatoes, breads, and desserts. The typical vegetable portion, meanwhile, remained about the same but was usually drenched in oil or butter. By dramatically reducing her portion sizes of meats and starches while increasing her portion sizes of vegetables, Mary hoped the weight would finally begin to drop off.

She began by doing a three-day food and beverage diary. She recorded the calories of every food she ate for breakfast, lunch, dinner, and snacks. She also noted the portion sizes using a simple method that you will soon learn. Mary was absolutely shocked by the quantity of food she was consuming. She realized that restaurant servings for meats and starches are typically two to four times the standard serving size. (Some steak restaurants' serving sizes are even five times larger than the standard.) Remember, your unfilled stomach is only about the size of your fist. Mary was putting in multiple fistfuls of healthy meat and healthy starches into her stomach, unaware that the portion sizes of these high-calorie foods were sabotaging her weight-loss efforts.

It was as if she were trying to fill a 10-gallon fuel tank in her car with 20 or 30 gallons of gas. Obviously, if she did this, gasoline would simply spill out onto the ground. A tank can only hold so much. Likewise, Mary realized that she was putting in way more fuel than her body could burn. The fact that it was healthy fuel didn't matter—it was too much. She began to understand that she was exceeding her fuel tank capacity and, as a result, was storing the excess fuel as fat.

THE EXPANDING PORTION

Most people believe that the typical serving in a restaurant or grocery store is standard. Yet if you look at the nutritional facts label on most packaged foods, the given serving sizes are typically small, which means you are likely to eat two or more serving sizes without even realizing it. For example, ice cream usually has a recommended serving size of ½ cup; however, most people eat much more than that. A serving size of Ritz Crackers is only five crackers, while a serving size of chips is typically fifteen to twenty chips. And a serving size of bagel crisps is a mere six pieces.

ALL-YOU-CAN-EAT GAMES

In an effort to earn more money and attract new fans, major league sports franchises are now offering tickets that include unlimited concession snacks. So far, the 50 percent higher tickets have been a hit for almost every sport.[3]

The average American laughs at these meager portion sizes. That's because the amounts we are now eating are drastically different from what they were years ago, and as a result we have what is often called "portion distortion."

A study appearing in the *New England Journal of Medicine* reported that individuals trying to lose weight underestimated the amount they ate by as much as 47 percent.[1] Similar research at Rutgers University reiterated this major disconnect between standard serving sizes and perceived ones. In this study, participants were asked to serve themselves the amount they considered a typical portion size of each meal item on the buffet table. For breakfast, this included eight different items, and for lunch and dinner there were six food options. On average, less than 45 percent of portions selected at breakfast were within 25 percent of the reference portion size. The lunch and dinner meals selected were approximately 30 percent within the 25 percent range. This research again found that portion sizes were extremely distorted and that, more specifically, consumers severely overestimated the standard portion size.[2]

Why are people across America so badly missing the mark when it comes to serving size? One reason stands out: not only have portion sizes changed significantly in the past twenty years, but also so has the *perception* of those portion sizes. In the early 1980s fast-food french fries generally came in one size—2.4 ounces. Today, not only is that considered a small portion, but we also have several variations on the supersized theme: a medium serving runs around 5.3 ounces, while a large portion can get up to 6.9 ounces. (That's a 400-calorie difference, in case you are counting.) A typical take-out order of Chinese chicken stir-fry used to run around 2 cups; today it is closer to 4½ cups.

I have even noticed this portion size increase while eating out at relatively newer midlevel restaurants such as The Cheesecake Factory, Outback, and Carrabba's. If you order pasta or rice in many of these chains, chances are you will be served 2 or more cups of rice, yet a standard serving is

> **MOVIE MESS**
>
> For only seventy-one more cents, upgrading from a small- to medium-sized popcorn at the movies seems like a decent deal—except when you consider you're adding 500 calories. And that additional sixty cents for a large? Not the wisest move, considering your "snack" amounts to 1,160 calories and almost three days' worth of saturated fats.[6]

only ½ cup. A typical serving of chicken, beef, or fish is now 8 to 10 ounces. Potatoes typically weigh ⅔ pound to 1 pound. And steak restaurants are touting even larger portions of steak. (Of course, this is in addition to the salads saturated with dressing and vegetables loaded with butter or oils.)

IN-HOUSE SUPERSIZING

This all highlights the change in eating establishments, but what about at home? Are people necessarily eating bigger portions because of this shift? You bet. A study in the *Journal of the American Medical Association* revealed that the portion sizes of some of the most commonly consumed foods in the home—bread, cereal, pasta, sodas, and cookies—had increased by as much as 16 percent.[4] I believe that may be a low estimate considering other research on this topic. One study from the University of Illinois at Urbana-Champaign found that eating from bigger containers or packages usually causes individuals to consume 40 to 50 percent more. In one case, consumers at a movie theater were given either a small or a large bucket of popcorn. Those given a large bucket ate 46 percent more popcorn.[5]

Grocery shopping has become an expanding adventure as well. Supersized grocery stores and wholesale warehouses offer big discounts on food

packaged in industry-sized containers. Unfortunately, the larger containers simply mean more food intake. We think we are getting a great deal, but we usually consume even more and then later purchase more of the same item. Our waistlines expand while these stores' profits grow.

The bottom line on size comes to this: Americans want bigger homes, bigger cars, bigger furniture, and bigger portion sizes. Most of us have adjusted to our "bigger is better" environment like a frog in a pot of slow-boiling water. We have soaked up our excess to the point of ignoring the fact that it is literally killing us. Restaurants, grocery stores, and discount stores have trapped us in a stewing culture of gluttony. Now we must find a way to break free and take the leap out of our ever-worsening surroundings.

THE HABIT OF CLEANING YOUR PLATE

This can start with a simple way of bucking the system. Since most of us were children, we were taught to clean our plates. Not eating all our food was either impolite or socially unacceptable. "Think of all those starving kids in China," we would often hear as a reason. It was such guilt-laden statements that left us shoving a few more bites down our throats, even though our stomachs had been satisfied long before.

Research has repeatedly shown that obese people are more prone to clean their plates than people of a normal weight. In a survey conducted by the American Institute of Cancer Research, 69 percent of Americans said they finished their entrées either all or most of the time—which, when you think of it, closely correlates with the percentage of overweight and obese people in our country.[7] The truth is we do not have to clean our plate every meal. If your conscience still gets the best of you, ask for a doggy bag or wrap up whatever food you have on your plate for another meal. In fact, these days it is smart to go ahead and plan on splitting any meal you have when eating out because of the supersized portions. And come to grips with the fact that if you do clean your plate, that excess food will usually end up either in the toilet or being stored as fat. It's your choice.

ADDING VOLUME WITHOUT ADDING MANY CALORIES

Most people eat so fast and furiously that they overstuff their stomachs before the appetite center of the brain gets the message that they are full. They are already into their second or third helping before they get that twinge of satisfaction. It becomes obvious, then, that for many people the issue is one of satiety.

Americans like to eat—a lot, and in big quantities, as we've already mentioned. Given the choice between eating more or less, most of us would choose eating more.

Because of this, Barbara Rolls, PhD, introduced the concept of "volumetrics" a few years ago as an answer to dieters who were sick of always feeling hunger. Her premise is simple: rather than eating tiny amounts of calorie-dense foods, eat lots of low-calorie foods that are naturally rich in water and fiber. Instead of bothering with counting calories, or grams of fat, protein, or carbs, Rolls argues that dieters can eat more than they normally do and still lose weight—as long as they eat the right type of foods (ones that aren't energy-dense).

> **SOUP-ER ADVANTAGE**
>
> A study of almost one hundred fifty people found that those who consumed 10.5 fluid ounces of low-fat, low-calorie soup twice a day lost 50 percent more weight than those who ate healthy but carb-heavy snacks such as pretzels or chips.[9]

Though I differ on many of her points, I believe Rolls is onto something by understanding that you can eat large portions of foods with little to no calories. Vegetables are a perfect example of this, which is why in the "I Can Do This" diet program you are essentially able to eat as many vegetables as you want with meals (minus the butter, of course). In fact, there are a few simple volumetric tips you can use at every meal.

I'll share more volumetric tips in later chapters that deal specifically with the eating program.

First, before every meal, drink a tall glass of water with two or three capsules of PGX fiber. (See Appendix H.) The fiber mixed with water forms a thickened consistency that fills the stomach and slows down gastric emptying. This also usually prevents you from overeating and enables you to feel satisfied sooner.

You can also enjoy a bowl of vegetable soup, minestrone soup, black bean soup, lentil soup, or any other broth-based vegetable soup. A study done at Penn State concluded that eating a bowl of soup with an entrée actually reduced the total consumed calories by 20 percent.[8] I also suggest you take one or two Beano tablets before eating any bean soup since it may cause gas.

Precede your entrée with a salad (any size), and make sure you have the dressing on the side or choose a nonfat dressing or use a salad spritzer with only 1 calorie per spray. If you decide to eat your salad with the dressing in a side dish, first dip your fork in the dressing, then pick up the salad with your fork. This way each bite will have a taste of the dressing. Whether eating a salad or your entrée, always remember to chew every bite twenty to thirty

times; this not only helps digest and absorb the food's nutrients, but it also causes you to eat slower and fill up faster.

These are just a few tips, but I hope you can already see that the key is being mindful throughout every meal. It is not difficult at all. When my wife and I dine out, we are able to enjoy a delicious meal bursting with flavor, yet also choose healthy-portion sizes of meats and starches. Our "secret" is simply that we prefill our stomachs with low-calorie bulky foods that take a while to eat and also expand our stomachs so that the appetite center in our brains experience a significant degree of satiety. By the end of the meal, we have actually consumed a large amount of water and fiber and a relatively low volume of fats, starches, and excessive proteins.

So how did things eventually work out for Mary? When she practiced this program by slowing down the eating process, watching and balancing her portion sizes, meal and snack planning, as well as consuming water and fiber, soups, and salads before her main entrée, she not only was full and satisfied for many hours after a meal, but she also had tremendous energy. The weight literally began to melt off of her, and within a few months she was happy and back in her size 6 jeans.

"CAN DO" POINTS TO REMEMBER

1. Restaurant servings for meats and starches are typically two to four times the standard serving size.

2. The amounts we are now eating are drastically different from what they were years ago, and as a result we have what is often called "portion distortion."

3. Eating from bigger containers or packages usually causes individuals to consume 40 to 50 percent more.

4. Obese patients are more prone to clean their plates.

5. "Volumetrics" is the idea that you are more satisfied eating bigger portions of low-calorie foods than consuming smaller portions of energy-dense foods.

6. Filling your stomach can be as simple as drinking water with fiber and eating soup and a salad before you ever begin your entrée. By prefilling your stomach with these low-calorie foods, you are less likely to eat excess amounts of breads, starches, meats, fats, and desserts.

SECTION II

GETTING READY TO BEGIN

12

YOU HAVE A CHOICE

IETING HAS A way of turning life into a roller-coaster ride. You lose weight only to gain it back—or you gain even *more* weight—and after a while it becomes difficult to find yet another reason why you should even bother. In more than twenty-five years of practicing medicine, I have met countless former dieters stuck in this self-defeating mental attitude, and it was sabotaging whatever hope they once had of losing weight.

The truth is, your biggest obstacle for weight loss is your thinking. If you want to lose weight but have been on this yo-yo dieting adventure I am referring to, I'm sure you could come up with 101 different excuses for *not* dieting. After all, who wants to be on a boring, rigid, tasteless diet? It is never fun to deprive yourself. And yet none of us want to be overweight or obese. We want to look good, feel good, and live a healthy life.

TOP TEN EXCUSES FOR NOT DIETING

1. "I just can't resist my favorite foods."

2. "My social life is just too crazy."

3. "I don't have time to lose weight or plan meals."

4. "My family and friends won't support me."

5. "I don't have anyone to hold me accountable."

6. "It's too confusing to find which diet works for me."

7. "I travel too much."

8. "Dieting is too restrictive."

9. "It's too expensive to diet."

10. "I'm just too impatient to diet."[1]

IT'S *YOUR* LIFE

Take a look at the top ten excuses for not dieting listed on this page. Do you see the potential for a downward spiral when you start this type of thinking? It is a self-propelling trap in which so many dieters are caught. They become virtual excuse makers, first blaming circumstances and then themselves for their failures. Most reach a culminating point where they either give in to complete resignation or go see a doctor like me for some last-resort help.

The common problem I see among

repeat dieters is that they do not focus on the simple lifestyle and dietary changes that are needed, but instead they focus on their weight. When their weight does not budge, they then get discouraged and many times stop the program all together. And on the other extreme, when they do hit their target weight, they abandon all reason and quickly slide back into their old eating patterns—the same ones that got them on the diet in the first place!

Why Do You Really Want to Lose Weight?

It's great to set your mind to something and to accept responsibility for your actions, both past and future. Yet such a radical shift in perspective can easily become just another mental pep talk that eventually fizzles out. What must accompany this change of heart is an underlying reason—one that, in fact, comes straight from the heart. To switch to a "can do" kind of lifestyle, you need something that compels you from deep within.

I have found over the years that if your motive for losing weight is for any person other than for yourself, chances are high that you will fail. You should be doing this for *you*, to make *you* healthy, and not to please someone else. Unfortunately, too many women are tempted to lose weight for their spouse or boyfriend. Inevitably, these are the women who find themselves back in the blame-shame-guilt cycle after that person ends up walking out of their life. I hate to sound cynical, but I have seen too many women do this and wind up gradually gaining all their weight back.

Many obese people are the same way. They have heard plenty of reasons from others why they should lose weight, yet they lack a personal driving force for why they should do it. If you are overweight and have never identified this reason, I urge you to do what I suggest to my obese patients: disrobe in front of a full-length mirror at home and analyze yourself from the front and back. While looking at yourself in the mirror, ask yourself what the main things are that concern or bother you about being overweight. Is it the size of your hips, thighs, waist, or buttocks? Is it the way your clothes fit? Is it the way people treat or mistreat you? Is it the embarrassing comments people make about you? Is it the rejection from family members, friends, or co-workers that affects you? Is it being passed over for promotion because of your weight? Is it because your health is being affected by your weight?

For some people these questions are answered more easily by writing in a journal. If that is true for you, take the time to do it. These are important thoughts that, if you are completely honest, may change your life. As you come to grips with why you—and only you—want to lose weight and have

made the decision to do so, you are ready to take responsibility for controlling your weight. Most individuals who have lost weight and kept it off simply took responsibility for their weight loss. It was their choice, and this empowered them to lose weight by developing new healthy habits. You may have unique reasons that only come by looking in the mirror, but the important thing is that you arrive in a new place of hope, determination, and purpose.

VISUALIZING A NEW YOU

As part of securing yourself in this new place, try performing a simple mental exercise involving visualization. Picture yourself at a healthy weight, and then ask yourself a few questions: Will weighing a healthy weight affect your relationships with your family, spouse, friends, and co-workers? You bet it will! Many people never think about this and are shocked when close friends become jealous, or your spouse is intimidated by your weight loss. Family members and in-laws may try to tempt you with your favorite cake, pie, or comfort food. As difficult as it is to imagine, it's possible that some of your close friends or relatives actually don't want you to lose weight. They may be envious and try to sabotage your weight loss. After all, they have gotten accustomed to you being overweight, and when you lose weight, you will be forcing them to come to grips with their own weight problems.

Will your weight loss improve your marriage? You would think that the obvious answer is yes; however, I have treated many overweight couples and often find this not to be the case. When one spouse loses weight and the other one does not lose weight, many times the spouse who has lost weight begins to get much more attention from the opposite sex at work, while shopping, and while running errands. Some men and women have simply never had attention from the opposite sex, and when they lose weight and start looking great in their clothes, the sudden attention is not only flattering but also enticing. Are you and your spouse prepared for these possible feelings of jealousy, intimidation, and flattery? On the other extreme, some people have subconsciously gained weight to protect themselves from the pain of being rejected or from going through another painful relationship or breakup. Have you thought through how these issues affect your current and future health?

Also, will you be ready in a few months to purchase a new wardrobe? While the very thought of shopping makes many women excited, some men get physically ill at the notion that they will have to buy expensive new suits. And are you prepared for the possibility of promotion or demotion at work? Yes, a leaner and trimmer image may be all you need for that promotion, or it

may spark jealousy in your boss who may move you to another department. Understand that by losing weight, people will see you differently and treat you differently.

My point in asking these questions is not to plant fear or worry in your mind but to help you realize that things will change when you lose weight—often drastically. I want you to be prepared to deal with these changes. Some patients with a large amount of weight to lose need psychological counseling to deal with these issues. To me, that is a wonderful sign that they are accepting the drastic change and allowing others to help them walk through it. If you feel you need such guidance, don't hesitate to seek it out before you start losing. The important thing is that you ask yourself these questions now so that you will not sabotage your weight loss later with wrong thoughts.

Timing

This often gets overlooked when people decide to embark on a life-changing journey such as the "I Can Do This" program. It is important that you make sure the timing is right for you and that you have counted the cost before you start this program. In this chapter we have talked a lot about excuses, and the truth is, you only need one real excuse not to do this program. Understand, however, that the very fact that you picked up this book is reason to believe that you are indeed ready for a change. If you are in the midst of a major stressful time in your life such as a divorce, a life-threatening illness, a serious accident, a lawsuit, an IRS audit, a move, a job change, or some other major life event, then this program is *definitely* for you.

Before you question my sanity, hear me out on this. I realize that most diet books would tell you to forgo the diet until the major stress passes. First, you'll soon learn how truly different the "Can Do" mind-set is. Second, this is not only a lifestyle that is easily adaptable, but it is also a lifestyle that can easily bring sanity, peace, assurance, and hope in the midst of a chaotic time of your life. I have found over the years that when these simple dietary and lifestyle principles are practiced regularly, they help you to manage stress and prevent stress eating—not further it. Finally, this is the healthiest program you can be on during such a stressful, up-in-the-air time of your life. I do not want you to follow it during pregnancy, but it can be followed safely for people with heart disease, cancer, type 2 diabetes, type 1 diabetes, and almost any other disease. To top it off, it stabilizes the blood sugar, decreases inflammation in the body, controls hunger, and includes a diversity of tasty foods.

WEIGHT-GAIN MENTALITY

In the early pages of this chapter I stated that your biggest obstacle for weight loss is your thinking. Most of my overweight and obese patients are stuck in what I call weight-gain mentality. They unknowingly have their mental channel set on the weight-gain channel, and as a result, they continue to attract more weight to themselves. I often tell patients dealing with this that their autopilot is stuck on weight gain. You may have the same thing happening, and it is important to remember that the ultimate success of any weight-loss program depends not on how much you eat but what you think and believe.

The Bible repeatedly makes mention of this, often as the law of seedtime and harvest. The Book of Galatians states, "Whatever a man sows, that he will also reap" (Galatians 6:7). In other words, if a farmer plants wheat, he will reap a harvest of wheat; if he plants corn, he will reap a harvest of corn. Elsewhere, Proverbs 23:7 says of a person that "as he thinks in his heart, so is he." This simply means that whatever you think about most, you will eventually become. Similarly, Jesus says in Mark 11:24, "Whatever things you ask when you pray, believe that you receive them, and you will have them."

This means that what you consistently visualize and confess, you will eventually become. This is why it is so important to get a photograph of yourself at or near a healthy or desired weight and place it in different areas of your home, such as on the mirror in your bathroom, on your refrigerator, or as a screensaver on your computers at home and in your office. Some people even tape a copy of the picture to their car's steering wheel or dashboard. Regardless of how many places you want to put your healthy or desired weight photo, it is important to put it in your food journal. As you carry your food journal with you throughout the day and look at the picture frequently, visualize yourself becoming that ideal weight again.

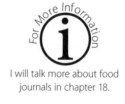

I will talk more about food journals in chapter 18.

It is also important to speak affirmations of your desired weight, pants size, or dress size aloud throughout the day. Even if you weigh 250 pounds, you can state aloud that you see yourself weighing 140 pounds or wearing a size 8, or whatever pant size or dress size you desire. The Bible defines faith in Hebrews 11:1 as "the substance of things hoped for, the evidence of things not seen." Romans 4:17 speaks of calling those things that are not as though they are. So if you hope to weigh 140 pounds or wear a size 8 pair of jeans, start visualizing yourself at that weight and speak it aloud a few times a day.

Do not say, "I have to lose 100 pounds," or you will probably always have

that many pounds to lose. Likewise, don't get in the habit of saying, "I'm planning on losing 50 pounds" or you'll forever be *planning on* doing it. Simply look at the picture of you at your desired weight and speak your desired weight aloud: "I see myself weighing _____ pounds" or "I weigh _____ pounds." (You fill in the blank.) Make that affirmation throughout the day, and as you follow through with your weight-loss program, you will naturally be attracted toward that desired weight, size, or image.

I've had patients who had struggled with their weight for years do this, and they turned around and told me that losing weight became one of the easiest things they've ever done! I believe you will be making the same statement when you reach your ideal weight. This is not difficult. Start by making the decision to lose weight for yourself and no one else. Understand that you are the only one responsible for being overweight. Once you have accepted this and are set in your decision, it is time to take the next step: making a commitment. As we'll discover in the next chapter, decisions come easy, as does lip service. Yet when we make a commitment, we enter into a different arena of long-term planning—one that, by your signed agreement, includes you keeping the pounds off.

"Can Do" Points to Remember

1. Yo-yo dieting takes an emotional toll and eventually makes it difficult to find a reason why you should even bother losing weight in the first place.

2. Your biggest obstacle for weight loss is your thinking.

3. Repeat dieters often do not focus on the simple lifestyle and dietary changes that are needed, but instead they focus on their weight—which is a recipe for failure.

4. You have the choice to lose weight or not—it's completely up to you.

5. If you're losing weight for some reason other than for yourself, you will likely fail.

6. Visualize yourself at a healthy weight and realize that you will be treated differently when you lose weight. Are you prepared to deal with it?

7. The Bible teaches that what you consistently think, visualize, and speak, you will become—and this is especially true regarding your weight.

8. Don't say that you want to lose weight or plan on doing it; speak words affirming that you see yourself weighing _____ pounds (fill in the blank).

13

ALL ABOUT COMMITMENT

WHEN YOU GET married, you make a verbal commitment to your spouse, in front of witnesses, that you will stay together "till death do you part." In addition, you confirm this by signing a marriage certificate that legally binds you together as man and wife. In a similar manner, when you buy a home or a car, you meet with an agent or salesperson and verbally commit to a purchase. To put your money where your mouth is, you sign bank notes, titles, and other legal documents that put the property in your name. In so doing, you commit yourself to paying a monthly mortgage or car payment.

Few dieters ever make such a commitment to lose weight. Sure, we offer plenty of lip service; we moan and groan about how much weight we need to lose, how our clothes continually seem to be shrinking, or how we need to exercise more and eat better—*someday*. Many people even go a step beyond this every New Year's by actually jotting down the well-worn resolution: "I will lose more weight this year." Yet a few weeks later that piece of paper is either misplaced, long forgotten, or sitting crumpled in a trash can.

If you have reached a point of determination in reading this book that is stronger and more resolute than ever before, I am excited for you. I am ecstatic that you have resolved to approach this differently than all your other attempts at losing weight. But I want you to understand an important truth: this is just an emotion, and willpower is simply not enough. Unfortunately, even the strongest of emotions at some point fade away. So how can you use this powerful motivating force to get past those times when there is no more emotion left in the tank? You combine it with commitment.

When you make a commitment to lose weight but slip up and binge or cheat on sweets, junk food, or fast food, your commitment enables you to forgive yourself and get back on the program. A commitment gives you a long-term vision that goes beyond just reaching your targeted ideal weight. A commitment goes beyond a goal. It becomes a framework for your progression in life, not just how many pounds you lost the past week. And when you combine that rock-steady

commitment with positive emotion that propels you to the next level, suddenly succeeding on a daily, weekly, or monthly basis becomes much easier.

Without that commitment, you are more likely to start making excuses and eventually stop the program when your thoughts, feelings, emotions, or attitudes change (which they will, by the way). An uncommitted person does not know what to do when he trips and makes a major dieting mistake. Remember, your biggest obstacle to losing weight and keeping it off is not your choices in food, your exercise schedule, your portion sizes of food, or having regular mealtimes. Your biggest obstacle is your thinking. The majority of chronic dieters and obese individuals have their mental autopilot set on weight gain and do not even realize it. They are doomed to fail from the onset. Unless you make a commitment to lose weight by changing your thinking, changing your feelings, and changing your attitude, you will most likely fail.

WHAT'S WRONG WITH WILLPOWER?

Without commitment, your main driving force to lose weight is sheer willpower. Don't get me wrong; the human will is an amazing thing. Individuals have overcome incredible odds and done amazing feats simply because they set their minds to a task and determined not to fail. But deep down we all know that willpower only takes you so far when it comes to facing a lifelong battle with weight.

Somehow we seem to forget this most when January 1 rolls around—and the health club industry loves us all the more for it. Health clubs currently sign up around 12 percent of their memberships in the month of January—a percentage that has actually gone down in recent years, thanks in part to clubs promoting more long-term vision and working

THE AMAZING HUMAN WILLPOWER

Although he'd survived a house fire that claimed his brother's life, seven-year-old Glenn Cunningham was supposed to die from the extreme burns that covered his lower body. After staying alive longer than doctors thought, he was told they'd have to amputate his legs. When he convinced his mother not to allow this, he was sent home crippled with the assurance that he'd never walk again. Yet after being confined to a wheelchair for weeks, he resolved to walk again, threw himself from the chair, and began daily pulling himself up on the outside fence and dragging his lifeless legs around the yard. Months later he could stand, then within a year he was able to walk, and in his words, "by the grace of God, I learned to run again." Against all odds, the once crippled boy went on to become one of the greatest track stars of all time, setting world records and earning a silver medal in the 1936 Olympics.[1]

on trying to flatten out the traditional bulge in January memberships.[2] Still, if you have ever been to a club in early January, you know what I am talking about. At my local health club, those first two weeks of the year are so busy that I often have to wait in line for a machine. Yet after only two weeks, I usually have easy access to the entire facility and don't have to wait. Meanwhile, the health club is cashing the checks of all those new members who paid their fees but simply gave up.

Willpower temporarily excites, energizes, and pumps you up. But just as a balloon loses air a few days after being pumped up, your excitement and enthusiasm eventually deflate after a few weeks, leaving you unmotivated to continue your diet, go to the gym, or whatever it was you set your mind to. Willpower is like a sprint, while commitment is like a marathon. And contrary to what some diets will tell you, losing weight and keeping it off is a marathon. It requires commitment for long-term success.

The good news is that making this adjustment from depending on willpower to relying on a commitment is not as hard as it may sound. Just as you were programmed for weight gain, you can also be programmed for weight loss, but this involves changing your thinking, feelings, and attitudes and aligning them with a solid commitment.

We will address what exactly this commitment entails in just a bit, but first we need to explain what to do with those old mind-sets that continue to pull us down.

STINKIN' THINKIN'

Stinkin' thinkin' is simply thinking thoughts that sabotage your weight-loss commitment and program you for weight gain. However, faith calls those things that are not as though they are (Romans 4:17). Some call it the *law of attraction*. This law states that everything coming into your life is the result of what you have been attracting to your life: "Do not be deceived, God is not mocked; for whatever a man sows, that he will also reap" (Galatians 6:7).

The law of attraction involves saying and believing. Everything coming into your life is a result of what you have been attracting to your life by thinking, feeling, saying, and believing. Another way to look at it is how you live your life is like a magnet that draws the events that occur into your life, both good and bad. Words and thoughts are like magnets, but emotions and feelings are like super magnets. Everything around you, including the things you are complaining about, you have attracted.

Every time you think a thought, including negative thoughts, you are

attracting similar thoughts to you. The law of attraction works both ways: positive attracts positive, and negative attracts negative.

Unfortunately, most yo-yo dieters and obese individuals share a few common negative thoughts, and often they are not even aware that they have these. By thinking these negative thoughts, they are subconsciously attracting other similar thoughts and locking themselves into a weight-gain mentality. Like a virus that infiltrates a computer and takes hold of its operating software, these thoughts are sabotaging their weight-loss efforts, reprogramming their outlook, and enabling them to make excuses for why they fail.

Look at the first column of the chart below to see some of these sabotaging "stinkin' thinkin'" thoughts.

"Can Do" Thinking

The stinkin' thinkin' lines in the left column of the chart below are the most common ones that I hear. Without a doubt, they can sabotage your weight loss. Although combating them often goes beyond the surface to some deep-seated beliefs, you can start by identifying them and contradicting them. It's important to understand that for every negative thought, there is a positive one. As you identify these virus-like thoughts that want to ruin your weight-loss efforts, I challenge you to write down a positive statement for each of the negative ones that pertain to you. As you do this, you will eventually remove the virus, figuratively speaking, from your mind or your computer's operating software. (See Appendix C or www.thecandodiet.com for more affirmations.)

Stinkin' Thinkin'	"Can Do" Weight-Loss Thoughts
I hate myself.	I love myself, accept myself, and forgive myself.
I look terrible.	I look great and feel great.
I am so fat; I do not fit into any of my clothes.	My favorite jeans fit perfectly.
I will never lose weight.	I am at my ideal or healthy weight and size, and I will remain at my ideal or healthy size for life.
I can just look at food and gain weight.	I can resist the temptation for junk food or foods high in sugar and calories.
My whole family is fat, so I have the genes to be fat and I will be fat.	I have inherited genes that will help me lose weight.

Stinkin' Thinkin'	"Can Do" Weight-Loss Thoughts
I have no willpower.	I have the ability to say no to unhealthy food.
I cannot give up junk food.	I no longer crave junk food—it's out of sight, out of mind.
Eating healthy is too expensive.	Eating healthy is very affordable.
If I lose weight, I always gain it back.	I have lost weight, and I am able to keep it off.
I love junk food and hate healthy food.	I love whole grains, fruits, vegetables, and other healthy foods.
I hate to exercise.	I love to exercise.
It is not safe for me to lose weight; I may attract the opposite sex and cheat on my spouse.	I can safely lose weight and choose to remain faithful to my spouse.
It is not safe to lose weight; I may be hurt again by another relationship.	I can safely lose weight and surround myself with supportive, healthy relationships.
I am too busy to eat healthy.	I have time to eat healthy.
I am too bored to exercise.	I am excited about exercise.
I am too tired to exercise.	I have energy to exercise.
I have a slow metabolism.	I have a healthy metabolism.
I am too old to lose weight.	I am never too old to lose weight and feel great.
It is too late for me to lose weight.	Now is the perfect time to lose weight.
My friends and family will not change their poor eating habits and will make it impossible for me to change mine.	My friends and family see how easy it is for me to lose weight and want to join me.
I am not motivated to exercise or eat healthy.	I am motivated to eat healthy and exercise.
I am a failure and have failed at every diet.	I am a winner, and I am successful at losing weight.

Write these positive affirmations, these "Can Do" thoughts, in your weight-loss journal next to a picture of yourself at a healthy weight or a lower weight. And always write them in present tense, alongside your ideal weight's affirmative statement ("I see myself weighing _____ pounds"). Do not write, "I am going to look great" or "I will be at a healthy weight or pants size." It is critically important that you affirm the positive and

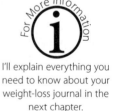

I'll explain everything you need to know about your weight-loss journal in the next chapter.

express this through your present-tense visualization. Start every day looking in your mirror and saying, "[Your name], I forgive you, I accept you, and I love you." Then read your "Can Do" thoughts aloud, and read them again before bedtime. I also recommend that you carry the list of "Can Do" thoughts with you and read them a few times a day, especially when you feel discouraged. I also recommend that you read the weight-loss affirmations in Appendix C.

Thoughts are also visually driven. They rely on images or imaginations. For instance, when I say the words "pink elephant," your mind doesn't go to the words *pink elephant*; it immediately paints a picture of a pink elephant. Likewise, when your thoughts are filled with "I look terrible," "I hate myself," or "I am fat and ugly," it's not the words that are making an imprint on your mind; it is the images. You are training your thoughts to visualize a fat, reproachable you. Those images or imaginations eventually become mental strongholds and mind-sets. And that, of course, leads to the exact opposite outcome of what you desire. It actually attracts that image to you.

Think of it in terms of programming your radio to preset stations. When your radio is programmed, all you do is press a button, and it jumps to your favorite station. Unfortunately, after years of being stuck in a cycle of failed diets, most overweight individuals have their minds preprogrammed to negative thoughts and feelings. Every time a negative thought enters their mind, they automatically punch a button and tune in a station that is singing a similar song—

READ MORE ABOUT IT

For more information, please read my book *The New Bible Cure for Depression and Anxiety*.

namely that they are fat, ugly, hopeless, a failure, and so on. And as we all know, the blues love company! Sing a single line of negativity, and you will hear a chorus of negative thoughts and feelings echoing…all to the tune of more weight gain.

Loving Your Body: Is It Possible?

Before you dive into this section, let me forewarn you: you may not like, believe, or agree with what I am about to share with you. Nevertheless, I ask that if you are challenged by my words, you should at least extend the courtesy of mulling them over. If it takes reading this section a few times so you can process it better, please do so. Having said that…

Every person needs to be grateful for the body he has. Every overweight or obese person needs to be grateful for the body he has. Yes, even if you are overweight or obese, it is crucial that you express gratitude for the body you

currently have, not your ideal or healthy body weight that you are now diligently holding captive in your thoughts. I am referring to your current body, regardless of how many extra pounds are on it.

Let me take this one step further: I strongly recommend that you accept your body, forgive your body, and love your body—and that you do this every single day. Why all the self-love, even if you do not think it is possible? I have been treating overweight patients for more than twenty-five years, and I have come to realize that their negative programming completely sabotages their weight loss. Many chronic dieters find it hard to love themselves, accept themselves, or forgive themselves. That is normal. Yet what I find is that even though these people say they want to lose weight, commit to losing that weight, and try to follow through with the program, subconsciously they are programmed to not lose weight. Beneath the surface, they actually don't want to do whatever it takes to lose weight. In fact, their subconscious has already assured them that they *do not* want to lose weight.

It took me years to realize that this unseen negative programming is sabotaging most chronic dieters. Understand that there is no machine or organism ever made in this world that is as wonderful as the human body. The Bible describes us as being "fearfully and wonderfully made" (Psalm 139:14). We have already been defined in these terms. Yet the combination of culture and human nature does everything it can to change that perception. For many overweight or obese people, it starts in childhood. A traumatic event such as parents divorcing or a loved one's death. A best friend's betrayal or rejection. A classmate's piercing, public words about their looks. These are the types of instances that, big or small, shape them at a young, impressionable age. And as they continue on in life, they simply accumulate emotional baggage and mental arguments for why they *aren't* "fearfully and wonderfully made." After years of fighting this internal battle, most obese people give up and become upset, angry, frustrated, resentful, depressed, and embarrassed over their bodies. They eventually despise the way they look.

This, obviously, is a guaranteed recipe for weight gain. If you hate your body and continually feel bad about it, you attract more bad feelings about your body. Let me reemphasize that: being critical or fault-finding toward your body actually causes more weight to be attracted to you. As strange as it sounds, you must start by forgiving, accepting, and loving your body. Then and only then will you be able to effectively program your mind for weight loss and allow the law of attraction to bring it to pass.

This can begin with the relatively simple step of identifying how you are feeling. Our emotions and feelings are indicators of our thoughts. For example,

if the engine light on your car comes on, it is a signal that something is wrong with the vehicle. If you continue to ignore that signal, it is likely that something worse will happen. Our emotions operate in the same manner. When we feel bad, it is an indicator that we are thinking bad thoughts. Generally speaking, if you are feeling positive, you are thinking positive thoughts; if you are feeling negative, you are thinking negative or toxic thoughts.

Obviously, things can get somewhat cluttered in our minds. Considering that we have tens of thousands of thoughts each day, it can sometimes be difficult to discern which thoughts are making us feel bad. Instead of focusing on your thoughts, then, a much simpler method to get to the bottom of things is to focus on the way you are feeling. Check your warning signals. By stopping and asking yourself throughout the day how you are feeling, you make yourself aware of whether you are feeling good or bad—which, in turn, indicates whether your thoughts are good or bad. It is impossible to feel bad and still be thinking about happy thoughts.

READ MORE ABOUT IT

If you think I am oversimplifying this aspect of the battle with weight loss, I challenge you to read my books *Deadly Emotions, Stress Less,* and especially *The New Bible Cure for Depression and Anxiety.* In all three of these books I discuss the power of being grateful in more detail.

For years I have taught my patients how to turn the channel of their minds off the constant messages of worry, fear, hate, and weight gain and on to those of gratitude, love, joy, and peace. Refocus your attitude to thoughts of gratitude. The more you can be appreciative, the better you will feel and the more positive feelings you will attract to you—including attracting weight loss.

Believe me when I say I have seen this affect hundreds, if not thousands, of lives. It is not a complex notion. When you ask yourself how you feel throughout the day and you discover you are feeling bad, you can literally turn your mental mind-set over to the gratitude channel. When you practice gratitude, you automatically start smiling more, singing more, laughing more, moving more, playing more...and weight starts dropping.

SEALING THE DEAL

Let's now go back to the core issue of this chapter: commitment. Again, without commitment, all of this is just activity that will eventually wear thin. If you are running on sheer willpower to shed your pounds, you are running on empty fumes and will eventually end up in the same place you have been before—stalled on the side of the road. The difference, then, is going beyond

a verbal commitment and, as a salesman would say, "sealing the deal." Just as a marriage license or mortgage is not official until there are signatures, so it is with a commitment to the "I Can Do This" diet.

I have included in Appendix A such a document for you. This is a weight-loss contract that you can sign and date in the presence of a witness. You can also print a copy at www.thecandodiet.com. Obviously, there is nothing legally binding with this piece of paper. This is purely for your benefit. Yet it has long been proven that a commitment becomes more official and takes on additional weight (pardon the pun) when it is in the form of a written document and signed in the presence of one or more witnesses.

I promise you, even though this is technically only a piece of paper, it means something more—and signing it makes a difference. If you take to heart what you are committing yourself to, you will understand the actual freedom it offers. Your weight loss is no longer a failed-diet issue. You have now begun a lifestyle that is headed directly to a healthier you!

"CAN DO" POINTS TO REMEMBER

1. A commitment enables you to forgive yourself and get back on the program when you falter.

2. Willpower only takes you so far when it comes to facing a lifelong battle with weight.

3. Long-term weight loss only occurs through a commitment to lose weight.

4. Stinkin' thinkin' sabotages your weight-loss commitment and programs you for weight gain.

5. You can reverse negative thoughts by writing out positive ones in present tense and reading them aloud upon awakening and before going to bed.

6. A traumatic childhood event and years of repeated dieting failure can often lead to despising your body.

7. Generally speaking, if you are feeling positive, you are thinking positive thoughts; if you are feeling negative, you are thinking negative or toxic thoughts.

8. Signing an official weight-loss contract can make a difference in your commitment level to losing weight.

14

SETTING REACHABLE GOALS

T IM REMEMBERED FITTING into his favorite suit. It was the dark blue one his wife had bought for him on their anniversary trip to Paris, the one she even asked him to wear sometimes when they would attend a special banquet or dinner function. A naturally muscular guy from playing sports throughout his younger years, Tim had always had a hard time finding a suit that fit him just right. But this one had, and he had to admit, it boosted his confidence every time he wore it.

Not anymore. Now forty-six, Tim had not worn the suit for at least eight years. His gut was now significantly larger, his body shape completely different. He had also lost most of that confidence, as I could easily tell when he walked into my office weighing 275 pounds—despite standing only five feet eight inches. Tim had experienced a heart attack only a year prior and had two stents in his coronary arteries. He also had hypertension and hypercholesterolemia and was on numerous medications. It didn't take a doctor to see he was not in good health.

I told Tim that if he wanted to decrease his chances of dying early from another heart attack, he needed to lose weight—especially in the abdominal area. His obese, apple-shaped frame held a protruding belly full of toxic fat. Because of this, he was putting himself at risk for ongoing heart disease, hypertension, type 2 diabetes, hypercholesterolemia, metabolic syndrome, and a host of other diseases. Fortunately,

GASTRIC BANDING SURGERY

As you set your weight-loss goals, you might be thinking of restrictive surgery—gastric bypass, gastric banding, lap bands—as a weight-loss solution. When a person elects for this type of surgery, a silicone band is placed around the upper part of the stomach so that it can only hold about an ounce of food. The person feels full faster and eats less. The band can be tightened or loosened, depending on the person's needs. Most people lose about 40 percent of their excess weight with gastric banding; therefore, I believe it is a viable solution for some people. However, it is not the entire solution. Making healthy choices on a daily basis is the only way to maintain weight loss. If you opt for gastric banding, remember that you must change your eating habits or you may gain the weight back.

my warnings motivated him and his wife, and they were committed to losing weight. But Tim admitted to me that he needed a goal, something he could challenge himself with and strive to meet.

GET REAL

The same is true for any person hoping for weight-loss success. When you are about to embark on a significant lifestyle change to lose a significant amount of weight, it's crucial to establish attainable goals. After all, you want your results to be attainable, don't you? I have seen countless people dive headfirst into a new diet with no set goals in mind. I have seen just as many people launch into a diet with unrealistic goals. Both end up as failures. Success requires vision, and when it comes to controlling your weight, that vision must also incorporate reality.

An unrealistic goal for weight or clothing size sets you up for discouragement. People who become discouraged will usually stop the program altogether and eventually gain back all their weight. If you are a five-foot-two-inch female weighing 300 pounds, for instance, understand that you will not be a size 2 or 4 in a year—maybe never. Realistically, look to be a size 10 or 12 with a waist

CALCULATING YOUR IDEAL WEIGHT

In 1871 a French surgeon, Dr. P. P. Broca, created the first ideal body weight formula, often called Broca's index. It looked like this:

Weight (in kg) = Height (in cm) - 100, plus or minus 15 percent for women or 10 percent for men.

If we translate it into pounds and inches, and simplify it slightly, it looks like this:

Ideal weight for women = 100 pounds + 5 pounds per inch over 5 feet

Ideal weight for men = 110 pounds + 5 pounds per inch over 5 feet

If you are a five-foot-seven-inch woman, for instance, then your ideal weight would be about 135 pounds (7 inches over 5 feet = 35 pounds, which when added to 100 = 135 pounds).

Broca's index is likely to have influenced the Metropolitan Life tables of height and weight, which were developed in 1943. The Met Life tables were commonly used by doctors as an indicator of "ideal" weight until 1974, when Dr. B. J. Devine published the following formula for medical use:

Ideal weight for women (in kg) = 45.5 + 2.3 kg per inch over 5 feet

Ideal weight for men (in kg) = 50 + 2.3 kg per inch over 5 feet[1]

However, this formula has been abandoned for the BMI. For many obese patients, this ideal weight calculation is an unattainable goal. Therefore, I do not use it.

measurement of 34 inches instead of 45 inches. That is an attainable goal. And when you reach that goal, then you can set another.

Likewise, if you hate going to the gym but have set a goal to work out five days a week for an hour each time, you have just created an unrealistic goal and have paved the way for discouragement and failure. Instead, set a goal of ten thousand steps a day on a pedometer, which simply means more movement or more walking. Also, avoid making promises that can be easily broken. For instance, do not tell yourself that you will never have another piece of cake, pie, cookie, or whatever food

I'll explain more about the importance of waist measurements in just a few pages.

weakness you have. Whenever you say that, you have just set your autopilot on desiring that food and will most likely want that food even more. Instead, as you learn how to develop good eating and discipline habits, avoid using the word *never*.

None of this means that you have to settle for a lowered expectation. You can and will look better than you ever have. But the important thing is to first set a goal and then keep it in perspective—both of which can come through taking a few initial measurements.

MEASURING UP

To help Tim establish his goal, I weighed him on the scale, then measured his waist, hips, body mass index, and body fat percentage. His BMI was more than 40, his body fat was 32 percent, and his hip measurement came in at only 34 inches. But these were all secondary to what mattered most at that point for Tim: his waist measurement of 46 inches. I have discovered that weighing a person weekly is probably one of the worst motivators for weight loss.

The first few weeks can seem almost miraculous for some individuals as they

BABY STEPS

One of the most important keys to losing weight is establishing attainable goals rather than ones that will leave you frustrated, angry, and most likely *gaining* weight. That's why virtually every physician says that when starting a diet, aim for a goal of losing no more than 10 to 15 percent of your total body weight. Once you've reached that, set a new goal—but don't jump the gun. While you can dream big (or in this case small), remember that traveling on the road to weight loss happens one step at a time.

watch the pounds fall off and assume this is all "fat-related" weight. The problem, however, is that many people are in fact losing muscle or water weight, which is guaranteed to lower your metabolic rate and eventually sabotage your

weight loss. When these people hit a plateau a few weeks or months later, they wind up discouraged and often quit the program entirely—all because they are rating their efforts and results based on a daily or weekly scale reading.

For Tim, I simply had him measure his waist and his weight each month and try on different pants in order to gauge his shrinking waistline. I also checked his body fat percentage each month. It didn't take long before he was lining up all his old pairs of pants that he had saved, hoping to one day fit in them again. Most important, of course, was getting back into those favorite suit pants he'd worn when he weighed almost 100 pounds less and had a 35-inch waist. Because of that, he originally said he wanted to get down to a weight of 185 pounds and a BMI of 28. Although those numbers would have technically kept him in the "overweight" category, I explained to him that because of his naturally muscular frame, even those numbers might cause him to lose muscle and subsequently lower his metabolic rate. Instead, the better way was to establish a goal based on his waist measurement. Keeping this in mind, he set his waist measurement goal at 39 inches, which meant he would be losing 7 inches of fat from his abdomen.

> ## A FEW EXCESS POUNDS = LONGER LIFE?
>
> According to the journal *Obesity*, a study that followed 11,326 Canadian adults for twelve years surprisingly found that people who were overweight but not obese—meaning they had a BMI of 25 to 29.9—were 17 percent less likely to die than people whose BMI put them in what has been considered "normal" weight category (a BMI of 18.5 to 24.9). This is why I want you to focus on your waistline and not your BMI or your weight.[2]

IT'S ALL IN THE WAIST

If you are overweight or obese, I advise you to take the same approach in establishing your own weight-loss goals. Measure your waistline at your navel or belly button. If you are a man and your waist measurement is greater than or equal to 40 inches, you are at a much greater risk of heart disease, hypertension, type 2 diabetes, metabolic syndrome, and many other diseases. If you are a woman and your waist measurement is greater than or equal to 35 inches, you're

> ### EXPANDING WAISTS
>
> Over the past four decades, the average waist size for men has gone from 35 inches to 39 inches; among women, it's increased even more, from 30 inches to 37 inches. According to the NIH, nearly 39 percent of men and 60 percent of women are carrying too much belly fat.[3]

prone to the same risks. In fact, after years of linking only weight and BMI to higher mortality rates and serious illnesses, scientists are beginning to understand—once again—that abdominal fat is a major contributor to the onset of these diseases. Belly fat is highly toxic, and, after bubble-wrapping itself around internal organs, it secretes powerful inflammatory chemicals that set the stage for type 2 diabetes, heart disease, cancer, and a host of deadly diseases, as well as even more weight gain.

That is just one of the reasons why your first goal should be to decrease this area of your body that is holding all this toxic fat and keeping you susceptible to disease. Your first goal, if you are a man, should be to get your waist measurement to less than 40 inches and eventually to 37.5 or less. If you are a woman, your first goal should be to get your waist measurement to less than 35 inches and eventually to 32.5 inches or less. I also recommend that women initially get their body fat percentage to less than 33 percent and eventually less than 30 percent. For men, I recommend that they initially get their body fat percentage to less than 25 percent and eventually to less than 22 percent. However, waist measurement is the most important measurement.

BODY FAT PERCENTAGE

By now it should be clear that I believe the waist size is the most important measurement by which to establish your goals for weight loss. This does not mean, however, that you can't or shouldn't take other types of measurements beyond those you can do with a tape measure. Part of my time with patients during their goal-setting stage is spent getting a body fat percentage. I do an initial measurement and then one each month until they reach their goal.

MEASURING TOOLS

Although skin calipers are the easiest devices for measuring body fat percentage, they can also be the most inaccurate. For a more precise (albeit it sometimes expensive) measurement, try:

Underwater weighing: Fat floats, while lean tissue sinks—making it easy for specialized hydrostatic weighing equipment to get a highly accurate read on how much fat you're actually carrying.

Dual X-ray Absorptiometry (DEXA) scan: Using low-level X-rays, this machine takes into consideration your bone mass and muscle mass to calculate your body fat percentage.

The Bod Pod: A highly accurate (but again expensive) machine that measures how much air you displace.

Bioelectrical impedance: Less expensive than the other high-tech tools but pricier (and more precise) than a skin caliper, this method measures the speed of an electrical current as it passes through your body. Unfortunately, numerous variables (e.g., full stomach, recent exercise) can sway your results.[4]

There are many ways to measure body fat percentage, including a bioimpedance analysis, underwater weighing, and using skinfold calipers. Whatever method you decide to use, you need to measure your body fat percentage the same way throughout the program. Consistency is the key here since body fat percentage can fluctuate dramatically with inaccurate measurements.

I hold more stock in body fat percentage than I do BMI, and the reason is simple: accuracy. BMI uses only height and weight to judge how overweight or obese a person is. For example, a twenty-three-year-old football linebacker and a fifty-six-year-old executive may both be five feet ten inches tall and weigh 220 pounds. This gives both men a BMI of approximately 35, which is considered obese. In reality, however, the linebacker has a 32-inch waist and a remarkable 6 percent body fat, while the executive has a 44-inch waist and carries around 33 percent body fat. That's an astounding 27 percent differential in body fat percentage alone that is never considered using only BMI.

Hopefully, you are beginning to see some of the confusion that patients, doctors, and other health-care workers deal with when it comes to varying measurements. Although many physicians simply use BMI to determine if a person is overweight or obese, I strongly believe the more accurate assessments come from using body fat percentage and waist measurements.

Rating your body fat percentage

Finding your ideal body fat percentage involves two main factors: sex and age. Initially, obese men should aim for a reading of less than 25 percent, while obese women should shoot for less than 33 percent. If you are not obese but just overweight, then aim for a body fat of less than 21 percent if you are a male and less than 31 percent if you are a female.

Remember, however, that this is secondary to your main initial focus, which is reducing your waist measurement. And don't worry; you will find that your body fat percentage will naturally decrease as your waist measurement does. Also consider that women should have a higher body fat percentage than men because of their hormones. Female hormones cause fat to be distributed in the breasts, hips, thighs, and buttocks. A typical woman should have between 7 percent to 10 percent higher body fat than an average man.

Many health clubs, nutritionists, and physicians have the equipment to measure your percent body fat. Once you have this initial number, log it in your food journal and have it checked each month.

You can go online and find many Web sites that have helpful tools to calculate your BMI, your body fat percentage, and other information. Visit www.thecandodiet.com or refer to Appendix G to calculate your BMI. But for

now, do not worry about your weight, your BMI, or your body fat percentage. Simply focus on one thing and one thing only: your waist measurement.

Yes, it's that simple. You really do not need a scale or any other fancy tools—just a simple tape measure. By focusing on your waist measurement

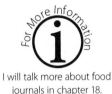

and achieving your goal measurement, you will eliminate one of the main risk factors for disease, the toxic fat located in your abdominal area. Along the way, you can track other measurements such as body weight and body fat percentage once a month. Log these in your food journal so you will have a clearly established

I will talk more about food journals in chapter 18.

goal. I will advise you, however, to measure yourself *each month* and not every week. When locked into measuring every seven days, many people can become obsessed with each fraction of an inch that's not lost soon enough. Remember, the goal here is to lose in your waist area. This will eventually work wonders on the rest of your body—trust me!

Let me also remind you of something: your waist starts at your navel (your belly button), not your lower abdomen or hips. I have worked with many people who confused the two and shot themselves in the foot because they never took helpful, accurate measurements. A man can have a 46-inch waist around the navel but still wear 34-inch-waist pants simply because he keeps his pants fastened below his bulging belly. (Come on, now…you know what I'm talking about.) The popularity of low-cut jeans and saggy pants in recent years really has some people confused about the true location of their waistline!

WAIST SIZE AND TYPE 2 DIABETES

The larger your waist, the greater your chances of having type 2 diabetes. For men, however, it's been proven that waist size is an even better predictor of diabetes than BMI. A thirteen-year study of more than twenty-seven thousand men discovered:

- A waist size of 34 to 36 doubled diabetes risk.

- A waist size of 36 to 38 nearly tripled the risk.

- A waist size of 38 to 40 was associated with five times the risk.

- A waist size of 40 to 62 was associated with twelve times the risk.[5]

A MATTER OF WEIGHT

For some dieters, the idea of not looking at a scale every day is foreign. Others feel strange without checking at least once a week. Yet after helping thousands of individuals lose weight for good, I have discovered most people do better

when they either pack up their scale or get rid of it entirely. The reason is almost purely psychological. As I mentioned earlier, dieters can often lose the wrong type of weight, such as water weight or muscle weight. As a result, their skin may sag or wrinkle, their cheeks and eyes may appear hollow, and their muscle mass may melt away. In the meantime, their metabolic rate decreases, their weight plateaus, and they wind up discouraged because each time they get on the scale the numbers are still the same. Most often, these are the same people who quit the program and gain their weight back.

Weight is important—don't get me wrong. That is why I always get an initial weight on every patient. But because of our weight-obsessed culture, the numbers on a scale can easily become the only measure of success. It becomes too tempting to monitor your progress by regularly hopping on a scale. This is not a reliable indicator of fat loss, which should be your primary concern as you start to lose weight. Avoid the potential depression, guilt, shame, or hopelessness by putting your scale away temporarily; rely more on an old-fashioned tape measure, a pair of old jeans, a food journal, a monthly body fat percentage measurement, and committing to only weighing yourself once a month.

> ### FIVE "NON-DIGIT" WAYS TO MEASURE YOUR WEIGHT LOSS
>
> 1. Overall attitude
> 2. Energy level
> 3. Fit of clothes
> 4. Friendly comments
> 5. Feeling of taking up less space

Also, weigh yourself at the same time of day on the same day of each month, and make sure you are fully disrobed. If you are a woman, keep in mind that your weight will fluctuate each month based on hormonal fluctuations and on your menstrual cycle. So do not get discouraged when this occurs.

Once you reach your goal weight, then I recommend that you weigh yourself daily. That is the only time that I recommend weighing daily, which is the best way to maintain your weight loss.

DAY BY DAY

Now that you have your waist measurement goal and have recorded your body measurements, weight, BMI, and body fat percentage (if desired) in your food journal, you don't have to think about these numbers. Your focus should simply be on taking one day at a time. Too many people pay so much

attention to the final result that they forget to focus on what they are doing day by day. As a result, they battle discouragement.

If you get nothing else from this chapter, understand this: Losing weight takes time. Not only that, but everyone is different and loses weight at different rates. Men usually lose weight much faster than women since they typically have more muscle and a higher metabolic rate. Most individuals will lose between 1 and 2 pounds a week on this program; however, some may only lose ½ pound or ¼ pound a week. Others may gain muscle in the process of trying to lose fat, which often causes their weight loss to go even slower. Also, some individuals are severely metabolically challenged due to chronic dieting, insulin resistance, low thyroid, hormone imbalance, and other factors. These and other factors all come into play, making each weight-loss experience unique.

You may not be able to control how fast you will reach your goal, but you can control how you follow the "I Can Do This" diet program day to day. When you focus on implementing these dietary and lifestyle choices

I will discuss these potential roadblocks in the last section of this book.

each day, they will eventually become habits. Many experts say that it takes twenty-one days to form a habit. Others agree upon forty, while still others say it takes ninety days to make that habit a natural part of your lifestyle. However long it takes, the point is that when you simply focus on applying the principles of this program for today—without worrying about how you'll face tomorrow or next week—then after a while, after doing this over time, it becomes part of your daily life. And when that begins to happen, you will find your mind's autopilot set on losing weight rather than gaining it.

Obviously, having established, reasonable goals is essential to losing weight. That is what this chapter is about. But many people get so focused on the goal that they forget the process and, as a result, constantly fight discouragement. By focusing on one day at a time, you consistently make the right choices every day. Obviously, there will be some exceptional days such as birthdays, holidays, and anniversaries. You may cheat and eat too large a portion size or too many high-glycemic foods. But do not get discouraged; simply realize that you are just one meal away from getting back on the program and again choosing to make the right choices for weight loss.

Tim reached his initial goal waist measurement of 39 inches—a loss of 7 inches—in just six months. Because he had reached that goal, it gave him the momentum and perseverance to establish another goal. This is often the case with obese people, which is why I strongly emphasize setting realistic, attain-

able goals. Tim's second goal was getting to a waist measurement of 35 inches. He attained that in just four months.

Although his weight only decreased from 275 pounds to 210 pounds, he lost a total of 11 inches of waist girth in less than a year. As a result, his blood pressure and cholesterol normalized without any medications. He was more active and had more energy than he'd had since he was young.

"Can Do" Points to Remember

1. Success requires vision, and when it comes to controlling your weight, that vision must also incorporate reality.

2. Measure your waist at the navel and make decreasing this your primary goal. If you are a male, aim for a waist measurement of less than 40 inches; if you are a female, shoot for less than 35 inches.

3. Establish a weight-loss goal by choosing a clothes size you wore when you were at a healthy weight.

4. Focus on one day at a time and not on your final weight.

5. Because of our weight-obsessed culture, the numbers on a scale can easily become the only measure of success—which can lead to frustration or depression at the slightest hint of a plateau.

6. When you focus on daily implementing the dietary and lifestyle choices found in this book, they will eventually become habits.

SECTION III

THE PROGRAM

15

THE EATING PLAN

O NE OF THE first things people think of when they hear the word *diet* is something they *can't* eat. For many, the word immediately brings to mind celery-stick meals and hunger pangs. If you haven't already discerned by now, the "I Can Do This" program is designed to keep you satisfied all day. You won't be starving yourself or eliminating a major food group from your diet—yes, carbohydrates are welcome. This program is not boring and does not use the same foods repeatedly, but instead it offers a variety of foods from which you can choose. It even allows you to eat out whenever you want, as long as you stick to some basic guidelines. In fact, even if you're forced to eat most of your meals at restaurants for a while, you can still learn which foods and the right portion sizes to choose to stimulate your body for weight loss. Likewise, if your busy schedule does not allow time to cook, you will learn how to quickly select foods that will fill you up and burn fat.

The key to this program is that it is amazingly simple, easy to follow, and, most importantly, doable. You now have a basic understanding of calories, fat grams, carbohydrate grams, glycemic index values, and even glycemic load. However, you won't be tracking any of these things while you're losing weight. Instead, you will learn to select the right amount of low-glycemic carbohydrates and combine them with the right amounts of healthy proteins and fats. This combination will literally program your body to burn fat, particularly the toxic fat in your belly.

Up to this point we have touched on many of the other fundamental principles of this program. I have even gone into detail on some elements to help you gain a better understanding of what is actually going on in your body as you shift to a healthier dietary lifestyle. As we begin this third section of the book, we are now ready to dive into the "nuts and bolts." Over the next few chapters you'll find an extension of much of what we have briefly alluded to—such topics as portion size, snacking, and choosing low-glycemic foods. You'll notice we've printed a tab on the edge of the pages in this section. That's because as you embark on this journey, I expect you to continue to use these chapters as mile-marker references whenever you are a bit unsure of what

to do. Think of them as the "how to" pages. But first let's spend this chapter nailing down the four basic components of the "I Can Do This" eating plan.

WHAT TO EAT

When it comes to food, your body ultimately needs three components of food every day to stay healthy:

1. Carbohydrates (low-glycemic carbohydrates such as vegetables, fruits, and whole grains)
2. Proteins
3. Fats

All of the calories you consume can be attributed to one of these three groups. Healthy, low-glycemic carbohydrates should comprise about 40 percent of your total calorie intake per day. Proteins need to make up about 30 percent of this daily intake, while healthy fats should also cover about 25 to 30 percent of all the calories you consume each day. You should also consume 5 to 10 grams of fiber per meal and 3 to 5 grams of fiber per snack. (I'll explain more about fiber in chapter 21.) For now, all you need to remember is that every meal should have a carb-protein-fat ratio of about 40:30:30. That's easy enough, now isn't it?

> ### SKIP NOW, PAY LATER
> A University of Massachusetts study of almost five hundred people found that those who regularly skip breakfast are four and a half times more likely to be obese.[1]

Yes and no. Although the ratio is easy to comprehend, I've found that many dieters are confused over which foods belong in which group. After all, many foods include *all three* components. Therefore, knowing what to eat requires going beyond the three components. And for that reason, I've developed the sample menus you will find later in this book and online at www.thecandodiet .com. In the meantime, here are a few key rules of thumb to keep you eating the right types of carbs, proteins, and fats:

- Sprouted bread, such as Ezekiel 4:9 bread (no sugar or raisins), is a good carb to have before 6:00 p.m. However, it tastes better when it is toasted. You can also have a sweet potato or a small serving of

brown rice. If you make instant brown rice, be sure to check the sodium content. You can use Uncle Ben's Whole-Grain Brown Rice; this is sold in microwavable packets that contain two servings. A serving is ½ cup for women and ½ to 1 cup for men. Also, double-fiber bread and ½ to 1 cup of thick whole-grain pasta (cooked al dente) are good choices. Women will usually have ½ cup of a starch, whereas men may have ½ to 1 cup for breakfast and lunch.

- Good protein includes extra-lean meats such as bison, beef, venison, skinless chicken, turkey breast or turkey breast burgers, wild Alaskan salmon, tongol tuna (packed in water), wild tilapia, and eggs. Lean pork and shellfish may be eaten in moderation.* Men should be eating 3 to 8 ounces of protein per meal, and women should have 2 to 6 ounces per meal. If unable to choose organic or range-fed meat, simply choose extra-lean cuts.
- Cut down on white salt as well (less than 2,300 milligrams a day, which is about 1 teaspooon). It is best to use Himalayan sea salt (purchased from the health food store) in moderation, less than 1 teaspoon a day. Herbs or seasonings, such as lemon pepper or garlic powder, that do not contain salt are excellent choices.
- Avoid all white flour, as well as white sugar.
- Campbell's Select Harvest soups are an excellent choice before lunch or dinner at only 80 calories. Be sure to always choose broth-based soups rather than cream-based soups.
- You can add a large salad with a salad spritzer before lunch and dinner. A salad spritzer contains 1 calorie per spray and 10 calories per serving.
- As I mentioned in chapter 10, your beverage choices can be just as important as your food choices when it comes to weight loss. For beverages, choose spring water, filtered water, sparkling water, green tea, white tea, or black tea. You can add lemon or lime to your tea or water and sweeten it with stevia to taste.
- *When* you drink is also important: drinking 1 cup of hot tea three to four times a day can aid in weight loss. Also, you should drink 8 to 16 ounces of water upon waking.
- Last but not least, avoid beverages and food products with artificial sweeteners such as NutraSweet and Splenda.

---

* If eating pork or shellfish bothers you for religious reasons, I recommend that you avoid it. However, there is no scientific research to prove that these foods are harmful if organic, free-range selections are eaten in moderation.

We'll go over the specific foods to eat later in this chapter and in the next. In fact, I give you plenty of examples of how to apply the proper ratio of foods to every meal. You'll learn how to break down every single meal according to our 40:30:30 ratio. And you'll quickly see that the world is your oyster when it comes to what you can eat. (OK, not *literally*.)

WHEN TO EAT

One of the most important principles of this program is one you have probably heard all your life: eat three meals a day. It's a basic concept, yet you would be amazed at how many people—even health-conscious folks—do not adhere to it. For losing weight, this is absolutely fundamental—a nonnegotiable, if you will. The reason is that these three meals provide the fuel at just the times your body needs it most. And it all starts with the most important fueling time, breakfast.

In chapter 2, we took a look at the habits of those who have been successful at weight loss and are able to keep off the weight. One of those habits was that they ate breakfast every day. Other studies have gone a step further, proving that people who skip breakfast are prone to eating more food and snacks during the day.[2] Unfortunately, most Americans have their meals backward. We skimp on breakfast, eat a medium-size lunch, and then pig out come dinnertime.

We have always heard how important it is to eat a healthy, well-rounded breakfast, and yet we rarely make the effort to make one. In our frantic rush to get out the door, we scarf down a high-glycemic breakfast such as a processed cereal, bagel, doughnut, toaster pastry, muffin, or piece of toast (with jelly, of course) alongside a cup of coffee with sugar and cream or a large glass of juice. As we have already learned, these high-glycemic breakfast foods and beverages increase blood sugar

> ### SLOW COOKERS: NOT JUST FOR DINNER ANYMORE!
>
> Try preparing traditional breakfast foods such as oatmeal or scrambled eggs with turkey sausage the night before in your slow cooker. This will save time in the morning and eliminate one more excuse for not eating a hearty breakfast.

short-term. When your blood sugar level starts to fall, your energy level drops, your thinking becomes foggy, and your appetite is triggered. These foods and beverages also program us for fat storage. And most of us wonder why we cannot lose weight while we're riding on a sugar, carbohydrate, and caffeine merry-go-round.

Before seeing me, many of my overweight patients would skip breakfast,

lunch, or both, and then wound up consuming most of their calories for dinner. They would get frustrated when exercise and diets did not help them lose weight. Yet when I had them spread out their meals during the day so they ate about every three to three and a half hours—with a healthy mid-afternoon snack in between—their appetites were almost always controlled, they lost weight, and their work performance improved. Some of my patients have actually received promotions at work while following this program because of improved work performance.

The correct fuel mixture should control your hunger for three to four hours. Yet even if your lunch consisted of a good fuel mixture and you ate it at noon, by 4:00 p.m. your blood sugar will naturally drop. This causes a noticeable decrease in energy and mental clarity, and you are also likely to become irritable and hungry. That is why a midafternoon snack (usually around 3:00 p.m. to 4:00 p.m.) of the correct fuel mixture will enable you to remain hunger-free and productive for several hours. The importance of snacking cannot be overlooked. In fact, eating healthy, energy-boosting snacks is so crucial for maintaining blood sugar levels—and ultimately a successful weight-loss lifestyle—that I have an entire chapter dedicated to this subject.

See chapter 17 for more information on snacking to support your weight-loss lifestyle.

Often my patients will argue that they don't have time to eat breakfast, lunch, or a midafternoon snack. Because their work requires nonstop attention once they arrive, they say there is no way to stop for these "fuelings." My reply is almost always the same: "If you can carve out just five to fifteen minutes from your busy schedule each day to refuel the right way, you'll not only continue to lose weight, but you'll also discover an immediate payoff in energy and effectiveness during your workday."

MISSING OUT

About 25 percent of Americans skip breakfast, with the average person forgoing the morning meal at least once per week.[3]

Eating at the right times is crucial, and it has immediate benefits. You'll find yourself energized, mentally sharper, and more emotionally stable. Even your job performance will go up as a result.

You should eat breakfast like a *king* (within thirty minutes of waking up), lunch like a *prince*, and dinner like a *pauper*; eat every three to three and a half hours to avoid hunger. Your snack should be like a mini-meal consisting of protein, good carbs, and good fats.

Your breakfast should have a good balance of carbs, protein, and fat. You should go "carb-free" after 6:00 p.m. If weight loss is stalling, you need to

meal plan and rotate your carbohydrates according to page 242. Vary your carb intake by cycling a maximum of 200 grams of carbs for men, 150 grams for women, a day to a minimum of 50 grams of carbs a day. This will help keep your body "guessing" and keeps your metabolic rate high, increasing your weight loss. After 6:00 p.m., you can have all the "green carbs" you want, including broccoli, green beans, and lettuce, and any nonstarchy vegetables, but no starchy carbohydrates like bread, pasta, rice, potatoes, corn, and so forth. (Starchy vegetables are primarily root vegetables and include beets, carrots, parsnips, potatoes, rutabagas, and sweet potatoes/yams.)

It is important to control your appetite by eating the correct meal and snack composition every three to three and a half hours; if not, you could possibly go on a sugar or carb binge. This will cause your insulin level to increase, programming you to gain weight. Choosing low-glycemic, high-fiber foods is important to help stabilize the blood sugar and the insulin levels to stop any sugar or insulin fluctuations.

How Much to Eat

Chapter 11 showed us how distorted our views of portion sizes have become in this country. While recommended serving sizes on food labels say one thing, we've trained our stomachs (and brains) to say another. It's time to train them correctly.

Figuring out the correct portion size for a food isn't rocket science. All it takes is a little visual imagery. Most people like to keep things simple, so rather than track every ounce, I suggest you pick your portion sizes using visual measurements. Imagine a deck of cards or a man's wallet. That's the equivalent to how much protein should be consumed per serving for a woman. If you want to get specific with numbers, this usually amounts to 3 to 3½ ounces of food. A man needs more protein and will need

> ### SWITCH YOUR PLATES!
>
> One patient on the "Can Do" diet came up with a great idea. She began serving her salad on her dinner plate and her dinner on her salad plate!

protein equivalent of one and a half to two decks of cards or two wallets, or eat meat approximately the size of the palm of your hand. For instance, a serving of chicken, beef, or pork should be about 3½ ounces—again, roughly the size of a deck of cards. A 3½-ounce piece of fish is roughly the size of a thick checkbook. Most men will actually need one and a half to two serv-

ings of this per meal, or two decks of cards or two thick checkbooks. Almost all women will stick with one serving. (We'll touch on both cases in a bit.)

Your serving size of starches and fruits is about the same as it is for proteins. You can go slightly bigger—about the size of a tennis ball for women and one to two tennis balls for men—but don't overdo it. (Remember from the 40:30:30 ratio that you'll be eating more carbs than proteins, so upping each portion size beyond that of a tennis ball could potentially turn into a case of "portion distortion.") For low-glycemic starches, a tennis ball measurement amounts to about half a cup (4 ounces) per serving. Women need to stick to the ½ cup of low-glycemic starch for breakfast and lunch; men can usually have 1 cup of low-glycemic starch for breakfast and lunch. Since men's protein portion is larger, his starch will also be larger. Remember, it's a 40:30:30 ratio. For fruits it's the same, like a medium-size apple.

For vegetables…ah, vegetables. (You'll like this part.) Most vegetables are made of mostly water and fiber, which means you can go to town on most of them. I've rarely met anyone who overdid it on vegetables like lettuce, spinach, broccoli, asparagus, green beans, and such. I do have two warnings, however:

- First, make sure what you are eating is actually a vegetable. I've had plenty of patients go crazy with corn on the cob, only to wonder why they weren't losing any weight! (In case you need a reminder, corn is *not* a vegetable even though you find it with the fresh produce and frozen vegetables at the grocery store. It's a grain!) Remember, farmers feed cows and pigs corn to fatten them up.
- Second, be careful with the butter or oil those vegetables are cooked in, especially when you are eating out. (I prefer to steam or lightly stir-fry my vegetables, or eat them raw.)

As for fats, serving size can be a little tricky for some people. The main reason for this is because fats are found in most of the foods we already consume (particularly condiment-type foods like butter or salad dressing), and when your goal is losing weight, you have to especially guard against eating too many bad fats, especially in the evening. Fats are also highly dense. For instance, if you sat down to each meal and

I'll list the fats you need in your diet, with specific amounts for each item, in the next chapter.

ate the equivalent of a tennis ball in butter, I would be worried. (I hope you would be too!) The rule of thumb for fats actually involves using your thumb.

You only need about 100 to 120 calories of fat per meal, which is the equivalent of ten to fifteen nuts, 2½ tablespoons of light ranch dressing, or approximately 1 tablespoon of oil or butter. That's about the size of your thumb. A serving of nuts, meanwhile, is simply a small handful. Can you see how quickly these fat calories can add up?

Now, let's see how healthy complex carbs, proteins, and fats combine together to make up the correct fuel mixture.

WHAT FUEL *MIXTURE* TO EAT

Just as important as what, when, and how much you eat is how to *mix* what you're consuming. Every meal and snack needs to have the right fuel mixture of foods so that you can stay energized and continue to burn fat. For instance, if you only had a couple of toaster pastries and a glass of orange juice for breakfast (which hopefully you know by now is definitely not a good meal), you'd be eating nothing but sugary carbohydrates. As a result, you would be setting yourself up for the munchies and a serious drop-off in energy. Or even if you were more knowledgeable about what foods to eat, yet still had the wrong ratios of foods, you'd still be shooting yourself in the foot with your weight-loss goals.

> ### FATS CAN BE FISHY
>
> Just because a dish has fish doesn't mean it's automatically healthy. On the Border's Dos XX Fish Tacos with Rice and Beans carries a hefty 2,100 calories, 130 fat grams, 169 grams of carbs, and a whopping 4,750 milligrams of sodium.[4]

Putting it together on your plate

Now let's place your food on your plate—your protein, your low-glycemic starch, and your veggies. This percentage breakdown on your plate is different from the 40:30:30 ratio of carbohydrates, protein, and fats because you will get enough fat in your diet without filling 30 percent of your plate with it! This is simply how to combine foods on your plate at each meal. A man will have an 11-inch plate, and a woman will use a 9-inch plate. That's because men typically require more calories and will need larger portion sizes for proteins and low-glycemic starches.

For men, I recommend two low-glycemic starch servings for breakfast and lunch and none for dinner. For women, I recommend one low-glycemic starch serving for breakfast and lunch and none for dinner. The low-glycemic starch will be "A" on the plate and will take up approximately one-fourth of the plate.

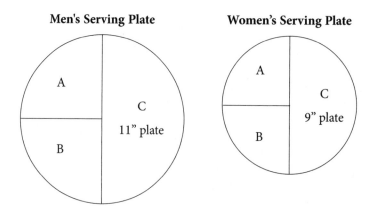

Men's Serving Plate   **Women's Serving Plate**

A = Low-glycemic starch   B = Protein   C = Nonstarchy vegetables

A woman will have one protein serving per meal for breakfast, lunch, and dinner, whereas a man may have one and a half to two protein servings per meal. The protein serving is "B" on the plate and will take up approximately one-fourth of the plate.

The vegetable portion should take up approximately one-half of your plate for lunch and dinner. The vegetable portion can actually be as many nonstarchy vegetables or "green carbs" as you desire, such as green beans, broccoli, asparagus, salad, and so forth. For each meal, the composition should be approximately 40 percent carbs, 30 percent protein, and 30 percent fat, except for dinner, in which your carbs will be lower since you can only have nonstarchy vegetables or green carbs. Your fats should also be lower for dinner.

"Can Do" Points to Remember

1. Your carb-protein-fat ratio should be around 40:30:30.

2. Each meal should contain healthy complex carbohydrates (low-glycemic starches), proteins, and fats, except dinner, which will only have nonstarchy veggies.

3. One of the most important principles of this program is to eat three meals a day and two to three snacks, eating every three to three and a half hours. (And remember, people who skip breakfast are prone to eating more food and snacks during the day.)

4. Every meal and snack needs to have the right fuel mixture of foods so that you can stay energized, control your appetite, and continue to burn fat.

5. The most important component in the fuel mixture is choosing low-glycemic starches.

6. The simplest way to put it all together is to visualize your plate divided like a pie chart into three sections—50 percent veggies, 25 percent protein, and 25 percent low-glycemic starch.

16

MIX-A-MEAL

I N THE LAST chapter I broke down the components of the program. I hope you are beginning to understand how you literally program your body for fat loss by eating three regular meals a day and snacks between meals with the correct fuel mixture. Keeping your body fueled with the right mix of healthy foods also maintains your energy level, gives you mental clarity, and prevents hunger.

Let's now tackle each meal of the day separately and see what foods you can combine to make for a delicious, healthy eating experience. I have divided up each meal according to the five groups we emphasized in the last chapter: low-glycemic starches, fruits, vegetables, proteins, and fats. Although these lists are by no means comprehensive, you can use them to give you ideas for tailoring your own program to fit your own preferences. These food choices have been used by many of my patients over the years and are extremely easy to implement into your meals.

A.M. MEAT

It's doubtful morning cereal pioneers such as John Harvey Kellogg, Will Keith Kellogg, Dr. James Caleb Jackson, and Charles William Post ever imagined their creations would one day fill an entire aisle at grocery stores. That's because their original purpose in the late 1800s was simply to provide a fiber-rich remedy for the gastrointestinal disorders that were often a result from all the pork and beef people ate for breakfast.[1]

BREAKFAST

Breakfast is by far the most important meal of your day and should be treated as such. For more than twenty years, I've told my patients to eat breakfast like a king, lunch like a prince, and dinner like a pauper. Breakfast not only sets the tone for the rest of your day, but it also gets your body revved up to burn calories and continue on your path to losing weight. Ever since I began implementing the "I Can Do This" program, one constant has stood out: the people who are most successful with losing their weight and maintaining it are the ones who understand the importance of breakfast.

Before we dive into the list of breakfast foods, let me address an issue that helps explain why breakfast is so unique and essential. So far, I've periodically mentioned fiber and its role in controlling your appetite. However, getting enough fiber at breakfast is instrumental to keeping your blood sugar stabilized for many hours, turning down your hunger, boosting your energy, and keeping your mind sharp. It also is fundamental for keeping your digestive system working optimally. I often call fiber nature's street sweeper for your GI tract. It removes waste products, food toxins, pathogenic microbes, and bile and the toxins it contains; it also prevents toxins from being reabsorbed into the bloodstream. Generally speaking, the less fiber you eat, the hungrier you will be.

To control your hunger and keep your GI tract functioning optimally, you should aim for eating 5 to 10 grams of fiber in each meal, along with at least 3 to 6 grams in a snack. This should be a mixture of soluble and insoluble fiber. This will also help to provide you with plenty of energy and mental clarity, especially if you make sure you eat an adequate amount at breakfast. To help you with this, I've included the fiber amounts for some of the low-glycemic starches listed below.

> ## CAN I EAT WHAT I WANT AND JUST EXERCISE MORE OR TAKE SUPPLEMENTS?
>
> Many people think it's OK to simply eat whatever you want as long as you exercise or take supplements that aid you with weight loss. But I believe exercise and taking supplements do not have nearly the same impact on your weight as your food choices do. I believe that to successfully take weight off and keep it off:
>
> - Seventy percent depends on meal planning and eating the right foods every three to three and a half hours.
>
> - Twenty percent depends on doing both resistance exercises and aerobic exercise.
>
> - Ten percent depends on taking the correct nutritional supplements.

Since most people consume so little fiber, let me also offer a word of caution. Starting with 10 grams of fiber a meal may cause some excessive gas and abdominal discomfort. Don't worry—your body will adjust to the high-fiber diet. However, you may need to gradually increase your intake by starting with 5 grams of fiber per meal and working up to 10 grams per meal. You can also take one or two Beano capsules if needed until your body adjusts.

Low-glycemic carbs (remember, these are your healthy carbs)

Breads
- Bagel (Sara Lee Heart Healthy)—one bagel or 3.3 ounces (6 g fiber)

- Double Fiber Bread (Orowheat)—one slice (6 g fiber)
- Double Fiber Wheat Bread (Nature's Own)—one slice (7 g fiber)
- Ezekiel 4:9 Whole-Grain Bread—one slice (3 g fiber)
- Multigrain Manna Bread—one slice (5 g fiber)
- Ezekiel 4:9 Organic Sprouted 100% Whole-Grain Flourless Tortillas (for wraps)—1 tortilla (5 g fiber)
- Multigrain (Earth Grains)—one slice (5 g fiber)
- Multigrain (Sara Lee Heart Healthy Plus with honey)—one slice (5 g fiber)
- Pita, whole-wheat (Sahara)—one slice (5 g fiber)
- Whole-wheat (Earth Grains and Earth Grains honey)—one slice (5 g fiber)

Cereals
- All-Bran cereal—½ cup (10 g fiber)
- All-Bran Complete Wheat Flakes—¾ cup (5 g fiber)
- All-Bran Extra Fiber—½ cup (13 g fiber)
- Ezekiel 4:9 cereal—½ cup (6 g fiber)
- Fiber One Caramel Delight cereal—1 cup (9 g fiber)
- Kashi Vive cereal—1¼ cup (12 g fiber)
- New England Muesli, natural—½ cup (8 g fiber)
- Old-fashioned oatmeal—½ cup (4 g fiber)
- Quaker Oat Bran cereal—½ cup (6 g fiber)
- Quaker Oat High-Fiber Instant Oatmeal (plain or cinnamon)—1 packet (10 g fiber)
- Steel-cut oatmeal (preferred oatmeal)—½ cup (8 g fiber)

Fruits (fresh)
- Apple—one medium (5 g fiber)
- Banana (not overripe)—one medium (4 g fiber)
- Blackberries—½ cup (3.6 g fiber)
- Blueberries—½ cup (2 g fiber)
- Cantaloupe—one-fourth medium (1 g fiber)
- Cherries—½ cup (1.5 g fiber)
- Grapefruit—one-half medium (6 g fiber)
- Grapes—1½ cups (1 g fiber)
- Kiwi—two medium (4 g fiber)
- Mango—one-half medium (1 g fiber)
- Orange—one medium (3.4 g fiber)
- Peach—two medium (4 g fiber)

- Pear—one medium (4 g fiber)
- Pineapple—1 cup, diced (1.8 g fiber)
- Raspberries—½ cup (4 g fiber)
- Strawberries—sixteen medium (8 g fiber)
- Watermelon—2 cups, diced (2 g fiber)

Most fruits are acceptable; however, limit or avoid fruit juice as well as dried fruit (no more than 2 ounces per meal). The best fruits for weight loss are the high-fiber fruits such as apples, pears, all berries, grapefruit, and kiwis. Since berries are high in fiber, low in calories, and low-glycemic, you may consume up to 1½ cups per meal. You can also mix berries to equal up to 1½ cups. Remember, the higher the fiber content of your fruit, the better the fuel mixture to control your appetite. These "power fruits" are also excellent energy-boosters to have for breakfast so you can start your day off right. You can also freeze them and add them to smoothies.

Vegetables
- Asparagus—½ cup (2 g fiber)
- Bell peppers—½ cup (0.85 g fiber)*
- Broccoli—½ cup, chopped (1.3 g fiber)
- Celery—½ cup, diced (1 g fiber)
- Cucumbers—½ cup, sliced (0.4 g fiber)*
- Eggplant—½ cup (1 g fiber)*
- Green beans—½ cup (2–3 g fiber)
- Lettuce—½ cup, shredded (0.5 g fiber)
- Onions—½ cup, chopped (1.4 g fiber)
- Spinach—½ cup (2 g fiber)
- Summer squash—½ cup, sliced (1.1 g fiber)*
- Tomatoes—one medium (1 g fiber)*
- Zucchini—½ cup, sliced (0.7 g fiber)*

Most people do not eat vegetables for breakfast, which is why I usually don't require them as part of the meal. However, as with other meals, they are an excellent source of volumetric eating, especially if you deal with severe hunger in the morning (which you shouldn't once you have been on the program for a while, since each breakfast is already high in fiber). The vegetables above can all be added to an omelet, steamed, or eaten raw. And remember, because of their low caloric content, you can eat as many vegetables as you desire.

---

* While technically considered a fruit, the low-glycemic value is more like a vegetable.

Proteins

Cheeses

(Note: 1 ounce of cheese is equal to about four dice, four small cheese squares, or the size of your thumb. Also, use caution when eating cheese since most cheese is high in fat. It is best to choose nonfat cheese.)

- Cheddar cheese (Cabot Light 75% Reduced Fat)—1⅓ ounce (18 g protein, 5 g fat)
- Cottage cheese, nonfat plain—½ cup (13 g protein, 0 g fat)
- Cream cheese (Philadelphia, fat-free)—4 tablespoons (10 g protein, 0 g fat)
- Farmer cheese (Friendship)—two slices (10 g protein, 5 g fat)
- Feta cheese (Alpine Lace Reduced Fat)—two slices (12 g protein, 6 g fat)
- Laughing Cow Light—two wedges (5 g protein, 4 g fat)
- Mozzarella cheese (Alpine Lace Reduced Fat)—two slices (16 g protein, 6 g fat)
- Provolone cheese (Sargento Reduced Fat)—two slices (10 g protein, 7 g fat)
- Ricotta cheese (Polly-O Nonfat)—½ cup (16 g protein, 0 g fat)
- Swiss (Kraft Singles 2% Milk)—two slices (8 g protein, 5 g fat)

Dairy and eggs
- Eggs (omega-3 or organic preferred)—two large eggs (12.6 g protein), or one egg yolk with two egg whites (10 g protein), or three egg whites (12 g protein)
- Low-fat plain kefir (organic preferred)—8 ounces (14 g protein)
- Low-fat plain yogurt (organic preferred)—8 ounces (12 g protein)
- Organic skim milk—8 ounces (8 g protein)
- Undenatured whey protein powder—two scoops (19 g protein)
- Life's Basics Protein Powder—one scoop (22 g protein)
- PureLean Protein—one scoop (15 g protein)

Meats
- Canadian bacon—3 ounces (18 g protein)
- Extra-lean ham—3 ounces (15 g protein)
- Salmon, smoked—3 ounces (18 g protein)
- Turkey bacon—three slices (9 g protein)
- Turkey sausage—3 ounces (18 g protein)

Fats

- Almond butter—2 tablespoons (16 g fat)
- Almonds—½ ounce or twelve whole almonds (9 g fat)
- Avocado—¼ cup, puréed (16 g fat)
- Butter (organic)—1 tablespoon (12 g saturated fat—avoid all trans fats such as margarine)
- Cashew butter—2 tablespoons (15 g fat)
- Cashews—twenty medium cashews (14 g fat)
- Extra-virgin olive oil or any other type oil—1 tablespoon (14 g fat)
- Flaxseeds—4 tablespoons (13 g fat)
- Hummus—8 tablespoons or ½ cup (10 g fat)
- Peanut butter—2 tablespoons (16 g fat)
- Peanuts—1 ounce (14 g fat)
- Pecans—½ ounce (10 g fat)
- Pumpkin seeds—¼ cup or 2 ounces (16 g fat)
- Sunflower seeds—3 tablespoons or 1 ounce (15 g fat)
- Walnuts—½ ounce (10 g fat)

LUNCH OR DINNER

I've grouped lunch and dinner together for two reasons. First, because most of us eat the same types of foods at lunch and dinner, from meats to vegetables to pastas and breads, it makes little sense to repeat these listings. Second, I want to promote a different mind-set in you (if you haven't already adapted it) that understands these meals are indeed somewhat secondary to breakfast. Although there may be more items listed in this section than the previous one, that is simply because most of our "taste buds" are a little more expansive later in the day than they are in the morning. We don't naturally wake up craving mahimahi, asparagus, or sweet potatoes.

Low-glycemic carbs

Beans
- Beans (kidney, lima, navy, pinto, red, black)—½ cup (5–8 g fiber)
- Black-eyed peas—½ cup (4 g fiber)
- Butter beans—½ cup (5 g fiber)
- Lentils—½ cup (4 g fiber)
- Chickpeas—½ cup (5 g fiber)

Breads
- Bagel (Sara Lee Heart Healthy)—one bagel or 3.3 ounces (6 g fiber)

- Double Fiber Bread (Orowheat)—one slice (6 g fiber)
- Double Fiber Wheat Bread (Nature's Own)—one slice (7 g fiber)
- Ezekiel 4:9 bread—one slice (3 g fiber)
- Ezekiel 4:9 Organic Sprouted 100% Whole-Grain Flourless Tortillas (for wraps)—one tortilla (5 g fiber)
- Multigrain Manna Bread—one slice (5 g fiber)
- Multigrain (Earth Grains)—one slice (5 g fiber)
- Multigrain (Sara Lee Heart Healthy Plus with honey)—one slice (5 g fiber)
- Pita, whole-wheat (Sahara)—one slice (5 g fiber)
- Whole-wheat (Earth Grains and Earth Grains honey)—one slice (5 g fiber)

Pastas and rice
- Pasta (choose a thicker pasta variety, cooked al dente and preferably whole-grain)—½ cup
  - Plain (2.8 g fiber)
  - Whole-grain, 100 percent (Eden Organic) (12 g fiber)
  - Whole-wheat (Westbrae Natural Organic) (18 g fiber)
- Rice (long-grain brown and wild rice)—½ cup (1–3 g fiber)
- Uncle Ben's Instant Brown Rice—½ cup, dry (2 g fiber)

Vegetables
- Asparagus—½ cup (2 g fiber)
- Beans (green or string)—½ cup (2–3 g fiber)*
- Broccoli—½ cup (1.3 g fiber)
- Brussels sprouts—½ cup (1.8–3.4 g fiber)
- Butternut squash—½ cup (1.1 g fiber)
- Cabbage—½ cup (2.1 g fiber)
- Carrots—½ cup (2.6 g fiber)
- Cauliflower—½ cup (1.7 g fiber)
- Celery—½ cup (1 g fiber)
- Collard greens—½ cup (2–3 g fiber)
- Cucumbers—½ cup (0.4 g fiber)*
- Eggplant—½ cup (1 g fiber)*
- Lettuce—½ cup (0.5 g fiber)
- Okra—½ cup (2 g fiber)
- Onions—½ cup (1.4 g fiber)
- Sauerkraut—½ cup (3 g fiber)

* While technically considered a fruit, the low-glycemic value is more like a vegetable.

- Spinach—½ cup (2 g fiber)
- Summer squash—½ cup (1.1 g fiber)*
- Sweet potatoes—½ cup (3–4.5 g fiber)
- Taro—½ cup (3.4 g fiber)
- Tomatoes—one medium or ½ cup, diced (1 g fiber)*
- Turnips—½ cup (2 g fiber)
- Watercress—½ cup (0.4 g fiber)
- Yams—½ cup (2.7–3.1 g fiber)
- Zucchini—½ cup (1 g fiber)*

Fruits (fresh)
- Apple—one medium (5 g fiber)
- Banana (not overripe)—one medium (4 g fiber)
- Blackberries—½ cup (3.6 g fiber)
- Blueberries—½ cup (2 g fiber)
- Canteloupe—one-fourth medium (1 g fiber)
- Cherries—½ cup (1.5 g fiber)
- Grapefruit—one-half medium (6 g fiber)
- Grapes—1½ cups (1 g fiber)
- Kiwi—two medium (4 g fiber)
- Mango—one-half medium (1 g fiber)
- Orange—one medium (3.4 g fiber)
- Peach—two medium (4 g fiber)
- Pear—one medium (4 g fiber)
- Pineapple—1 cup, diced (1.8 g fiber)
- Raspberries—½ cup (4 g fiber)
- Strawberries—sixteen medium (8 g fiber)
- Watermelon—2 cups, diced (2 g fiber)

Remember: no carbs such as pasta, rice, bread, or starchy vegetables for your evening meal. However, you can have as much nonstarchy vegetables as desired at each meal. You may also sprinkle Butter Buds or Molly McButter or use Smart Balance Butter Burst spray to improve the taste and flavor of your vegetables, or you may season them with spices.

---

* While technically considered a fruit, the low-glycemic value is more like a vegetable.

Proteins

Cheeses

(Note: Regular cheese is simply too high in fat, with about 10 grams of fat per ¾ ounce. However, you may lightly sprinkle regular cheese over a salad or main dish. It is also best to choose nonfat cheese.)

- Cheddar cheese (Cabot Light 75% Reduced Fat)—1½ ounce (18 g protein, 5 g fat)
- Cottage cheese, nonfat plain—½ cup (13 g protein, 0 g fat)
- Cream cheese (Philadelphia, fat-free)—4 tablespoons (10 g protein, 0 g fat)
- Farmer cheese (Friendship)—two slices (10 g protein, 5 g fat)
- Feta cheese (Alpine Lace Reduced Fat)—two slices (12 g protein, 6 g fat)
- Laughing Cow Light—two wedges (5 g protein, 4 g fat)
- Mozzarella cheese (Alpine Lace Reduced Fat)—two slices (16 g protein, 6 g fat)
- Parmesan cheese (Kraft Reduced Fat)—2 teaspoons (1 g protein, 1 g fat)
- Provolone cheese (Sargento Reduced Fat)—two slices (10 g protein, 7 g fat)
- Ricotta cheese (Polly-O Nonfat)—½ cup (16 g protein, 0 g fat)
- Swiss (Kraft Singles 2% Milk)—two slices (8 g protein, 5 g fat)

Dairy and eggs
- Eggs (omega-3 or organic preferred)—two to three large eggs (12.6 g protein) or one egg yolk with three egg whites (10 g protein)
- Low-fat or nonfat plain kefir (organic preferred)—8 ounces (14 g protein)
- Low-fat or nonfat plain yogurt (organic preferred)—8 ounces (12 g protein)
- Organic skim milk—8 ounces (8 g protein)
- Undenatured whey protein powder—two scoops (19 g protein)
- Life's Basics Protein Powder—one scoop (22 g protein)
- PureLean Protein—one scoop (15 g protein)

Meats

(Note: Generally, most meats and fish contain approximately 7 grams of protein per ounce. I recommend 2 to 8 ounces of protein per serving. Women

only need about 2 to 6 ounces, whereas men require 3 to 8 ounces, depending on their lean body mass and their activity level.)

- Beef, extra lean (preferably organic or free-range; remove all visible fats)—2 to 6 ounces for women, 3 to 8 ounces for men (limit your total red meat consumption to less than 18 ounces a week)
- Buffalo, bison, elk, caribou, venison, goat, ostrich—2 to 6 ounces for women, 3 to 8 ounces for men (limit your total red meat consumption to less than 18 ounces a week)
- Chicken and turkey (remove skins)—2 to 6 ounces for women, 3 to 8 ounces for men
- Fish—3 to 6 ounces; examples: cod, flounder, haddock, herring, halibut, mahimahi, sea bass, tilapia, perch, snapper, tongol tuna, orange roughy, salmon, trout, sardines, mackerel
- Pork* (lean ham, lean pork chops, pork tenderloin, Canadian bacon)—3 to 6 ounces (limit to one to two servings week)
- Shellfish* (i.e., shrimp, crab, lobster, scallops, oysters, mussels)—3 to 6 ounces (limit to one serving a week)

Some species of fish contain more mercury, PCBs (polychlorinated biphenyls), and other contaminants than others. Fish that are higher in mercury

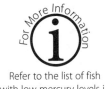

Refer to the list of fish with low mercury levels in chapter 8.

include shark, swordfish, king mackerel, and tilefish. Albacore tuna and canned tuna contain moderate amounts of mercury. Fish low in mercury include haddock, herring, Atlantic mackerel, perch ocean, Pollock, salmon (both fresh and canned), sardine, tilapia, trout, and tongol tuna.

Young children, pregnant women, women who may become pregnant, or women who are nursing should be careful to avoid eating fish high in mercury. Remember, the American College of Obstetricians and Gynecologists recommends only two 6-ounce servings of fish each week for pregnant women. For children and nursing women, the American Academy of Pediatrics recommends that both children and nursing mothers consume no more than 7 ounces of high-mercury level fish per week. Realize that all fish increasingly contain more mercury, which is toxic to fetuses and to chil-

---

* If eating pork or shellfish bothers you for religious reasons, I recommend that you avoid it. However, there is no scientific research to prove that these foods are harmful if organic, free-range selections are eaten in moderation.

dren's brains. In addition, farm-raised fish are generally prone to having more PCBs than wild fish.

Fats

- Almond butter—2 tablespoons (16 g fat)
- Almonds—about eighteen almonds (14 g fat)
- Avocado, fresh—½ cup, puréed (16 g fat)
- Butter—1 tablespoon (12 g fat)
- Cashew butter—2 tablespoons (15 g fat)
- Flaxseeds—3 tablespoons (10 g fat)
- Hummus—8 tablespoons or ½ cup (10 g fat)
- Mayonnaise (Smart Balance Light)—2 tablespoons (10 g fat)
- Mayonnaise (Smart Beat fat-free)—2 tablespoons (0 g fat)
- Mayonnaise, regular—1 tablespoon (11 g fat)
- Oil (extra-virgin olive oil, extra-virgin coconut oil, or any other healthy oil)—1 tablespoon (about 14 g fat)
- Peanut butter—2 tablespoons (16 g fat)
- Peanuts—1 ounce (14 g fat)
- Pecans—½ ounce (10 g fat)
- Pumpkin seeds—¼ cup (16 g fat)
- Smart Balance Butter Burst Spray—5 sprays (0 g fat)
- Smart Balance Omega spread—1 tablespoon (14 g fat)
- Sunflower seeds—3 tablespoons (15 g fat)
- Walnuts—½ ounce (10 g fat)

Salad dressings

(Note: It is best to choose light dressings or one part extra-virgin olive oil with four parts vinegar in a salad spray or spritzer. I also recommend the new salad spritzers sold in supermarkets, including Wishbone and Ken's Lite Accents brands. They have only 1 calorie per spray and are superior to other salad dressing options, in my opinion. Nonfat dressings are also an option, but most people do not enjoy the taste of these—and enjoying what you eat is crucial to the success of the "I Can Do This" diet program. If you do not enjoy the taste of light dressings, either put the regular dressing in a salad spritzer and spray it on (to reduce the amount you use), or put the dressing in a side dish and limit it to 1 to 2 tablespoons.)

- Balsamic vinaigrette (Wishbone Salad Spritzers Balsamic Breeze)—10 sprays (1 g fat)
- Blue cheese dressing (Litehouse Lite)—4 tablespoons (12 g fat)

- Blue cheese dressing, regular—2 tablespoons (12–16 g fat)
- Caesar dressing (Cains Light)—4 tablespoons (10 g fat)
- Caesar dressing (Wishbone Salad Spritzers Caesar Delight)—10 sprays (1 g fat)
- Caesar dressing (Wish-Bone Just 2 Good, Light)—4 tablespoons (4 g fat)
- Caesar dressing, regular—2 tablespoons (12 g fat)
- Olive oil (extra virgin) and vinegar—1 tablespoon of olive oil with 4 tablespoons of vinegar (balsamic or apple cider vinegar) (12 g fat)
- Ranch dressing (Wishbone Salad Spritzers Ranch Vinaigrette)—10 sprays (1 g fat)
- Ranch dressing (Cains Light)—4 tablespoons (12 g fat)
- Ranch dressing (Wish-Bone Just 2 Good, Light)—4 tablespoons (4 g fat)
- Ranch dressing, regular—2 tablespoons (16–18 g fat)
- Thousand Island dressing (Wish-Bone Just 2 Good, Light)—4 tablespoons (4 g fat)
- Thousand Island dressing, regular—2 tablespoons (14 g fat)

Putting It All Together

As an example, let's construct either a lunch or dinner using some of the items just listed. (See Appendix F for a week's worth of sample menus that include suggestions on each part of the meal.) For a beverage, you can drink a glass of spring, filtered, or sparkling water with a squeeze of lemon or lime. You may also drink tea sweetened with stevia or Just Like Sugar, if preferred, and a squeeze of lemon or lime.

Salads

When eating out, skip the bread and begin your meal with a salad made of large, dark-green leaves and plenty of cucumbers, tomatoes, and onions. You may add brussels sprouts or broccoli spears to your salad and top with a little low-fat cheese and some sunflower seeds (no croutons). Then add 2 to 4 tablespoons of light

Caesar Savvy

Though a few low-fat choices exist, be extra careful when buying any type of Caesar dressing. The notorious fat-laden dressing is often the worst choice on the condiment aisle, yet brands like Ken's Steak House (which contains 9 grams of fat and 80 calories per tablespoon) still often tack a "0 g carbs" label on their products. A better choice: Wish-Bone's Caesar Delight Vinaigrette Salad Spritzer, which packs only 2 calories and minimal fat per spray.

salad dressing, 2 to 4 tablespoons of fat-free salad dressing, or ten or more sprays of a salad spritzer. Or if you prefer an oil-and-vinegar dressing, mix 1 tablespoon of extra-virgin olive oil with 4 tablespoons of balsamic vinegar. I believe the easiest way to cut fat is to use a salad spritzer with only minimal fat per spray. Another good suggestion is to have your server put 1 to 2 tablespoons of regular salad dressing in a small dish and simply dip your empty fork in the salad dressing before eating each bite of salad. But be careful not to eat more than this amount since it is not low-fat or fat-free.

Most people forget that 10 cups of romaine lettuce only has about 100 calories, while a mere 1½ tablespoons of most salad dressings contains the same amount of calories. I see a lot of dieters getting into trouble by eating salads smothered with high-calorie salad dressings. A large Caesar salad may have only 20 calories worth of salad leaves yet more than 1,000 calories worth of dressing. Do you get the picture? Go easy on regular dressing; instead, opt for a light or—if you don't mind the taste—fat-free dressing. Better yet, use a salad spritzer.

Soups

Next up for your meal is a soup. Select a soup that is broth-based, such as vegetable or bean soup. These are very filling and will usually prevent you from overeating. Avoid cream-based soups, such as broccoli cheddar, which are high in calories. Make sure your soup is low in sodium (preferably less than 500 milligrams) and low in fat (preferably less than 10 grams). One of the key ingredients for a healthy soup is fiber, so look for those that have at least 3 grams of fiber. When it comes to fiber, the higher the better. Finally, don't overdo it on the carbohydrate content. Many soups are loaded with high-glycemic carbs such as white rice and pasta. Choose vegetable soups such as minestrone or bean soups such as black bean soup. Make sure for dinner you choose only vegetable soups.

SOUP STRIKES AGAIN

A recent study from Penn State University found that consuming a bowl of low-calorie soup before a meal reduced total calorie intake by a whopping 20 percent.[2]

If, by chance, you are still extremely hungry after eating your salad and soup, then you can take some fiber capsules. Take two to three PGX fiber capsules—again with 16 ounces of water. (See Appendix H.) When you do this before you eat your entrée, you fill your stomach faster and are less likely to overeat the wrong types of foods.

Entrées

For your entrée, choose a 2- to 6-ounce serving of protein if you are female and a 3- to 8-ounce serving if you are male. For example, a common choice is a grilled chicken breast flavored with a few low-sodium seasonings. (Watch out for those high-carb, high-calorie marinades.) Along with your main source of protein, add a serving of vegetables such as broccoli, which should take up about half of your plate. These can also be flavored with a sprinkle of Mrs. Dash, Butter Buds, Molly McButter, Smart Balance Butter Burst spray, garlic, lemon pepper, or other spices.

Next, select a low-glycemic starch such as a piece of whole-grain bread (with 3 to 6 grams of fiber per slice) or half a cup (the size of a tennis ball) of whole-grain rice, pasta cooked al dente, corn, sweet potato, or beans. Women can have one serving and men one and a half to two servings of starch for breakfast and lunch, but no starch or fruit for dinner. In addition to this, you can also end your meal, except dinner, with a piece of fruit such as a medium-size pear.

If you are eating out, remember that most entrée serving sizes are double or triple what is recommended. Most of the time you can simply eat half of the protein and starch provided and save the rest for another meal or snack. And if you enjoy sandwiches and want to incorporate them in this weight-loss program, you can. Again, men may usually be able to eat two starch servings per meal; however, women should limit their serving to just one. Remember, a serving of a starch is only the size of a tennis ball or one slice of regular bread. However, women may eat two slices of Ezekiel 4:9 bread since it has a lower carbohydrate content than regular bread.

Desserts

After being on this diet for one to three months, on occasion you may eat a treat such as some dark chocolate or another small dessert. Prior to enjoying this, however, I recommend that you take two to three PGX fiber capsules with 16 ounces of water. This not only lowers the glycemic index value of the dessert, but it also helps satiety. With desserts, it is especially important to practice mindfulness and savor each bite (which I'll explain more in chapter 19) so that you do not overeat and sabotage your weight-loss efforts. If you do eat dessert, it's best to eat it for lunch or early dinner (4:00 p.m. or earlier) and decrease your starch intake for that meal. Also, take PGX fiber afterward. Remember, fiber covers a multitude of dietary sins!

Now you have the idea of what each meal looks like. Using the principles laid out in the previous chapter and the examples in this one, you are ready

to design meals and practice meal planning specific to your preferences and taste buds. (Remember, enjoy what you eat—don't make this a boring chore!) Again, if you need more examples or help for planning meals, Appendix F in the back of this book will provide a full week of sample menus. You can also find additional weeks of menus at www.thecandodiet.com.

Let's continue our eating plan by looking at the incredible benefits of snacking. The right snacks will keep you from being hungry, prevent you from binge eating, and help you continue to burn fat.

"Can Do" Points to Remember

1. Eat breakfast like a king, lunch like a prince, and dinner like a pauper.

2. The people who are most successful with losing their weight and maintaining it are the ones who understand the importance of breakfast.

3. Aim for 5 to 10 grams of fiber in each meal and 3 grams in each snack.

4. Excellent "power fruits" that boost energy in the morning include apples, blackberries, blueberries, pears, raspberries, and strawberries.

5. Limit your intake of certain types of fish, especially those high in mercury.

6. Remember to start lunch and dinner with a large salad (with light or low-fat dressing) and a bowl of a broth-based vegetable soup.

17

THE POWER OF SNACKING

W HEN I WAS in the Boy Scouts, we would go camping at least one weekend out of every month. Before nightfall we would build a large campfire that could be seen for miles as it lit up the pitch-black sky. Everyone loved huddling around the fire, staring at its glow while talking and enjoying the warmth against the cool night air. We knew that if we wanted to continue enjoying that warmth, someone had to keep the fire burning through the night. I can remember many times waking up shivering from the cold weather and walking over to the fire to put more wood on it. Every Boy Scout understood that the more wood you put on the fire, the hotter and longer it burned. If this was done throughout the night, you could wake up warm and with a fire still burning just as strong.

Your body works in a similar way with snacking. By consuming "mini-meals" in between your three main meals or eating every three to three and a half hours, you keep your body's metabolic fires burning, allowing you to burn more calories throughout the day. If it were just a matter of keeping your dietary fires burning, however, many would not have an issue with weight. The problem starts with craving.

WAGING WAR WITH A SNACK

If you are like many people, at some point during the day you probably experience an overwhelming desire for a particular food—usually a food you know you should avoid. On those days when you do not feel like fighting the battle, the craving quickly goes from a thought to a simple bite to an all-out binge session. You then feel guilty, ashamed, and maybe even hopeless over the thought that you'll forever be locked into this grueling appetite struggle.

Sound familiar? I encounter this with patients every single day. They may be doing everything right—eating three healthy meals a day, exercising regularly, practicing portion control, and avoiding sodas and sweets. Yet without fail, usually between 3:00 p.m. and 6:00 p.m. or 8:00 p.m. and 11:00 p.m., it's

172

as if someone flips an appetite switch and all they can think about is food—and typically the wrong type of food.

The truth is that no matter how many carrot or celery sticks you eat, your cravings probably will not go away. But before you put down this book and think that there's no point in fighting, understand this: even though you may not be able to *eliminate* cravings, you *can* control them and eventually overcome them. The key is *controlling* them. And one of the most important and effective ways to do this is by snacking.

SNACKING RIGHT

Many people do not understand that a good snack not only can turn off the appetite, but it can also prevent it from being triggered in the first place. And though it seems counterintuitive to some, snacking can actually help you burn more calories in the process. Researchers have determined that snacking on the right amount of healthy foods in addition to eating three meals a day boosts the metabolic rate more than if you only eat three meals each day.[1] Snacking stimulates the body to burn more energy. Like adding more logs on a campfire to make it burn hotter and longer, a proper quantity of healthy snacks keeps the body's metabolic fires stoked throughout the day.

I hope you caught my emphasis on both the quantity *and* quality of snacks. It does you no good to eat healthy snacks if you are consuming too many of them. According to a survey conducted by the Calorie Control Council, one-third of all adults put "snacking too much" as a main reason their weight-loss efforts had failed.[2] I have had to correct many patients who used the power of snacking as an excuse to eat a fourth or fifth meal. Even when they chose healthy foods as snacks, they wound up eating massive portions of each item, plus it was the wrong fuel mixture. This obviously defeats the purpose and should be a no-brainer. Snacking is important for losing weight. However, snacking on too much will definitely sabotage your efforts.

Likewise, just because you happen to throw the right amount of something on the fire to prevent it from going out does not mean the fire will necessarily burn longer. You have to throw the right *kind* of fuel on the fire, or in this case eat the right kind of snack. Twinkies don't count as a good snack. Nor do Krispy Kreme doughnuts, kettle corn popcorn, or even some high-sugar granola bars. Each of these is similar to putting hay on a fire; it burns up quickly. In fact, as we will discuss later in the chapter, eating these kinds of wrong snacks will usually cause you to crave more of these high-sugar, processed snacks. In other words, when you habitually down an entire pack

of Oreo cookies for a "snack," you not only fill yourself with the wrong fuel, but you also make it so that you're bound to crave the same thing again. That's why overweight and obese people can often eat their favorite foods and yet never really feel satisfied.

HEALTHY SNACKS

So what makes for a healthy snack to ward off these cravings? Many people immediately picture carrots, celery sticks, and broccoli. Even though these are healthy foods, they will definitely not satisfy your appetite or hunger. You may eventually binge on sugary foods and carbohydrates after eating these. The best type of snack food is a mini-meal consisting of some healthy protein, some high-fiber, low-glycemic starch, and some good fat. When mixed together, this food fuel or fuel mixture is digested slowly, causing glucose to trickle into your bloodstream, which controls your hunger for hours.

> ### FIVE SNACK DUDS
>
> 1. Cookies (even if they're fat-free, watch out for those calories and sugar)
>
> 2. Granola bars (some pass the test, but most are loaded with sugar)
>
> 3. Chips and nachos (fat, fat, fat…and the bad kind too)
>
> 4. Cakes and pastries (tons of calories, lots of sugar and fat, and zero nutrition)
>
> 5. Crackers (although many are doable, keep your eye on the serving size)

To know which protein, fat, and low-glycemic carbohydrates to choose for a mini-meal snack, you can refer to chapter 16 for the food lists. Select half a serving size of either a low-glycemic starch or one serving size of a fruit. Then add 1 to 2 ounces of a protein and half a serving size of fat. Typically this mini-meal should only amount to a total of 100 to 150 calories for women and 150 to 250 calories for men. A few examples of these well-rounded snacks include:

Morning or afternoon snack

- A piece of fruit, 6 ounces of plain low-fat yogurt or kefir, five to ten nuts (fruit can be eaten whole or blended into kefir), and one scoop of vanilla or banana protein powder
- 2 tablespoons of hummus with one small piece of whole-grain, high-fiber pita bread (4 inches in diameter) and 1 to 2 ounces of sliced chicken or turkey

- Six Wheat Thin Fiber Selects crackers with 1 to 2 wedges of Laughing Cow Light cheese and 1 to 2 ounces (for men) of smoked salmon or tongol tuna, 1 ounce for women
- Half a slice for women, one slice for men of Ezekiel 4:9 bread or high-fiber whole-wheat bread with 1 teaspoon of almond butter, cashew butter, or natural peanut butter, and 1 to 2 ounces of organic beef jerky
- Half a cup of nonfat cottage cheese, one piece of fruit, and five to ten nuts
- One low-glycemic, high-protein food bar such as a FitSmart bar or Jay Robb JayBar (full bar for men; half a bar for women)
- A small salad with a 1 to 2 ounces of sliced turkey and 2 tablespoons of avocado; use a salad spritzer
- A bowl of broth-based vegetable or bean soup with 1 to 2 ounces of boiled chicken
- Dr. Colbert's "Can Do" Smoothie (page 276)
- Protein smoothie made from protein powder (1–2 scoops) mixed with 8 ounces of skim milk, coconut milk, or low-fat plain or coconut kefir (option: dilute the skim milk, coconut milk, or kefir by reducing it

BAR NONE

Countless dieters go wrong by assuming a snack bar is healthy just because the words *health, protein,* or *low-carb* appear somewhere on the wrapper. In fact, it's hard to find a tasty, healthy, balanced snack bar on the market right now. Most are either loaded with sugars and carbohydrates or with fats—and should be classified as cookies rather than snack bars. Others are loaded with low-quality proteins but have no healthy ratio of complex carbohydrates, good fats, and fiber. In addition, many use soy as their protein, which is certainly not the best for weight loss. Very few have adequate fiber, and most leave you craving more, so you end up eating two or three—or the whole box—to satisfy your craving.

Unfortunately, there is no perfect snack bar that currently exists. The four I recommend are Jay Robb JayBar, any FitSmart bar, the NuGo Free Dark Chocolate Crunch bar (www.nugonutrition.com), and the Nutiva Hemp Chocolate Bar (www.drcolbert.com). The best option is still to eat a "mini-meal" using real food rather than a man-made substitute, but always have a snack bar in your purse or briefcase for emergencies. Most of these snack bars can be found in health food stores and not in supermarkets. Avoid the snack bars sold in most supermarkents since they are high in sugar and refined carbs. Remember, as with every meal, a good fuel ratio for a snack bar is 40 percent carbs, 30 percent fats, and 30 percent proteins, along with 5 grams of fiber per bar.

I also allow one "cheat" bar: a Fiber One bar.

to 4 ounces and combining with 4 ounces of filtered water or spring water)

Be sure to add two to three PGX fiber capsules with 16 ounces of water along with your snack. Also remember that you can also add as many non-starchy vegetables as you want to this snack. To top it off, I recommend a cup of green or black tea with your snack, using natural stevia as a sweetener.

Evening snacks

- Protein drink
- Lettuce wraps
- Salad with meat
- Vegetable soup with meat

Healthy "Cheats" for Your Evening Snack

For most people, the evening is the hardest time to stay on the straight and narrow. I've come up with a few healthy versions of popular evening snacks that I'll allow if you are really craving chocolate or a scoop of ice cream before bed.

- Homemade frozen yogurt: blend plain Greek yogurt (such as Oikos or Choboni brands) with ice, pure vanilla extract, and stevia or Just Like Sugar (to taste). This will taste like ice cream and satisfy your craving without throwing you off the "Can Do" wagon.
- Hot chocolate made from Green & Black's Cocoa Powder with skim milk, and stevia or Just Like Sugar.

A Fiber One bar can also help curb your late-night craving if you don't have these other approved "cheat" snacks on hand.

A Healthy Snack Stash

I have already urged you to clean out all the junk food, chips, crackers, candies, cookies, ice cream, sodas, and high-sugar beverages from your refrigerator, freezer, pantry, and cabinets. The second part of that equation, however, is keeping these places stocked with healthy snacks, including plenty of fruits, seeds, nuts, Ezekiel 4:9 bread, hummus, low-fat cheese, avocados, Wheat Thin Fiber Selects crackers, and the like. Get a large bowl

and fill it with your favorite fruits, especially high-fiber fruits such as apples, pears, kiwi, grapefruit, and all types of berries. Keep different deli meats, such as nitrite-free, free-range turkey, chicken, lean roast beef, lean ham, and organic nitrite-free beef jerky, in the refrigerator. I also recommend always having a supply of organic skim milk; nonfat, low-fat, or part-skim cheese such as Laughing Cow Light cheese; nonfat cottage cheese or cream cheese; nonfat or low-fat plain yogurt; and kefir. All of these are simple items that you can take on the go.

> ### GOOD FRUITS
>
> A Brazilian study found that women who ate three small apples or pears a day lost more weight on a low-calorie diet than those who didn't add fruit to their diet. Because of the high fiber in these fruits, those fruit-eating females also ate fewer overall calories.[3]

In addition, buy different nut butters, including almond butter, cashew nut butter, and natural peanut butter. Have a supply of hummus, avocado, guacamole, seeds and nuts, tomatoes, and cucumbers readily available so you can mix these with different salads and nonfat or light salad dressings or salad spritzers. (Most salads can now be bought in ready-to-serve bags.) For those who often find themselves restricted for time, you can also have a stash of healthy snack bars, such as the JayBar, the FitSmart bars, Nutive Hemp Chocolate Bar, or NuGo Free Dark Chocolate Crunch Bar. Keep black and green tea with stevia around as well as lemons and limes.

Along with making sure your home is stocked with these easy snack items, be prepared at work and other places as well. I tell all of my female patients to always carry a healthy snack in their purses, such as a Hemp Chocolate Bar, a small bag of nuts, an apple or a pear, and PGX fiber capsules. Keep items that are not perishable in your desk drawer at work. Always be prepared by having plenty of healthy snacks at home, in the office, and on the road. And don't forget that it is important to get snacks that you truly enjoy.

CONTROLLING SEVERE SUGAR
AND STARCH CRAVINGS

We have already discussed how sugary foods and processed carbohydrates are digested within only a couple of hours. This rapid digestion causes the appetite to be triggered again and again, raising the blood sugar and insulin levels and ultimately causing you to store fat and gain weight. Even obese people have a natural sense for this process because they know firsthand how

quickly a sugar high fades away, only to be met by another irresistible craving for more sugar.

Yet what do you do if your cravings are naturally for these high-sugar, starchy items? What happens when the different snacks listed above do not turn off your tremendous cravings for these foods? This is usually the case for those who have low serotonin levels in the brain. As we learned early in this book, serotonin is an important neurotransmitter that calms us down, helps us control our appetite, and gives us an overall feeling of well-being. Having a low serotonin level is what causes us to crave sugary foods, chocolates, carbohydrates, and starches.

To find out if you have low serotonin levels, take the test in chapter 22. You can also go online to take the test.

For many individuals, this is a serious matter, not just an occasional hankering for a chocolate bar. These people typically have been under long-term chronic stress and have probably had high cortisol levels for years. They may be chronic low-carb dieters, or they may battle insomnia, depression, or PMS. Some may also be compulsive eaters and bingers. They typically think about food all the time and are emotional eaters who use food as a comforter whenever they are lonely, bored, sad, anxious, or angry. Women are more prone to be in this category than men because the female brain produces 50 percent less serotonin than the male brain.[4] This is also why women often go through "carbohydrate withdrawals" more often than men.

A duo of scientists researched this physiological need for serotonin in some people and identified the problem. Judy Wurtman, PhD, and her husband, Richard Wurtman, MD, both neuroscientists at the Massachusetts Institute of Technology, discovered among other things that there were carbohydrate snacks that could boost serotonin levels in the brain.[5] These could ultimately decrease cravings and help control the appetite. Similar to water helping to relieve thirst, eating the right amount of carbohydrates can help to relieve cravings for sugar and carbohydrates by ultimately enabling the body to produce serotonin.

While the Wurtmans' findings are good news, I need to add a caveat that especially pertains to those who struggle with these "hyper-cravings" for sugars and starches. Make sure the carbohydrate you choose to prevent such cravings is not one that you actually crave. This is a case where the correct amount of carbohydrate has to be taken at the right time each day. If you love the carbohydrate you choose to snack on, you will probably binge on it—or at least be tempted to—and probably will not lose weight. Too much serotonin

will also cause you to become lethargic and sleepy. The more mundane and boring the snack, the less tempting it usually is for you. Also, it is important to realize that no serotonin is produced in the brain when you either eat protein alone or have too much protein with a carbohydrate.

BRAIN-BOOSTING SNACKS

Any of these snacks will jump-start your brain's serotonin levels.

- Fiber One Oats and Chocolate Chewy Bar
- Fiber One Oats and Peanuts Chewy Bar
- Fat-free premium saltine crackers (twelve small crackers)
- Fat-free pretzels (1½ ounces)
- Air-popped popcorn, no oil (1½ cups)
- Rice cakes, regular size (four pieces)

SEROTONIN-BOOSTING SNACKS

If you normally binge on sugars and carbohydrates, it's possible for you to learn to choose certain carbohydrates in the proper amount and at the correct time of the day to stop your cravings, improve your mood, and help you lose weight. To boost serotonin levels I recommend one or two snacks each day. About three to three and a half hours after lunch, eat a mix of approximately 30 to 40 grams of a starchy whole-grain carbohydrate with less than 3 grams of fat and less than 3 grams of protein. Although this seems like a scarce amount of protein, this is because too much protein can interfere with serotonin production. As you lose weight, you can decrease the carbohydrate grams in your snack from 40 to 30 grams, to 30 to 25 grams, and eventually from 25 to 20 grams. These snacks should be eaten on an empty stomach in less than ten minutes; they can be eaten again an hour before dinner if needed. Keep in mind that it usually takes about thirty minutes for the serotonin effect to lower your appetite and improve your mood.

Once you figure out the snack that works best for you, I recommend that you put the amount equal to 30 to 40 grams of the snack in a resealable plastic bag. Then carry the bag with you in your car, purse, or briefcase. By eating this snack at the specified times, you will not only boost your serotonin levels, but you'll also notice your weight beginning to drop.

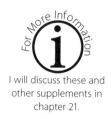

I will discuss these and other supplements in chapter 21.

To further help with this, I also recommend taking 50 to 100 milligrams of a 5-HTP supplement or one Serotonin Max along with these snacks and again at

bedtime. (See Appendix H.) I also recommend consuming 16 ounces of water and two to three PGX fiber capsules before eating your serotonin-boosting snack. The PGX fiber helps to fill you up.

Whether you deal with low serotonin levels or not, the snack is a powerful thing for any successful weight-loss program. It helps to control the appetite, which is one of the strongest forces that can come against your efforts to lose pounds and keep them off. In special cases, such as having low brain serotonin levels, this force can seem overwhelming. Let me assure you, it is not. In fact, with simple preparation you will soon learn it can be easily managed—even to the point of becoming routine.

"Can Do" Points to Remember

1. By consuming "mini-meals" of the correct fuel mixture between our three main meals, we keep our bodies' metabolic fires burning, allowing us to burn more calories throughout the day.

2. Even if you eat three healthy meals a day, snacking on the wrong types of foods or too much of the right types can sabotage your weight loss.

3. Healthy snacks include the correct fuel mixture of quality proteins, healthy fats, and low-glycemic, high-fiber carbohydrates.

4. A typical snack should only amount to a total of 100 to 250 calories.

5. It's important to keep healthy snacks readily available at all times.

6. Having a low serotonin level is what causes many to crave sugary foods, chocolates, carbohydrates, and starches.

7. You can choose some serotonin-boosting snacks to control your cravings and boost your serotonin level.

GUT CHECK: KEEPING TABS ON WHAT YOU'RE REALLY EATING

R ETIRED ARMY CAPTAIN John Harrison was already four months into being an identity theft victim before he got his first warning sign. In October 2001, he received a phone call from a credit union about an account in his name. Since he had never opened an account with them, he quickly assumed it was their error and dismissed the incident.

A call the following month, however, wouldn't be forgotten so easily. A detective in Beaumont, Texas, informed Harrison that a Harley Davidson motorcycle had been purchased with a Bank of America check signed "Jhon Harrison." After researching Harrison's credit report, the detective had no doubt Harrison was the victim of an identity thief and guided the retiree on the first steps he should take.

Harrison immediately began working to do whatever was required of him to clear his name. Yet sadly, the thief's short-lived spending spree still haunts Harrison—years later—on a daily basis. In barely six months, a twenty-one-year-old soldier named Jerry Wayne Phillips ran up more than $260,000 worth of debt, opened sixty-one credit or bank accounts, and wrote at least 112 checks for such things as motorcycles, trucks, time shares, and beach rental properties.

Although Harrison obviously can't be blamed for being victimized, his lack of keeping tabs on his financial records cost him dearly. Not until after the second call had Harrison ever looked at his credit report. He had failed to take notice of his standing with banks, yet in the time it took various institutions to detect and notify him of the fraudulent activity, Phillips had already done the damage.[1]

For many dieters, similar havoc has already been wreaked on their bodies as the pounds continue to pile on. Understandably, these people are left frustrated and wondering what they're doing wrong. They try diet after diet, exercise faithfully, and avoid fatty foods, yet they still can't shed the extra

weight. And often, as it was with the unfortunate retired captain, it's simply a case of not keeping track—on paper—of what's *really* going on.

The Value of Journaling

I've alluded to a food journal at various points in the last few chapters, yet in this one I want to show you how simple and worthwhile it is to keep one. We keep a diary to record our thoughts. Likewise, we keep a file (often both hard copy and soft) of our various financial dealings so that we have official records. In the same way, keeping a food journal can help those hoping to lose weight, especially as they begin the "I Can Do This" diet program. I have found that 70 percent of your success on this program depends on your food choices.

One of the first things I do with my weight-loss patients after I've taken their medical history is to ask them to keep track of their eating for a four-day period. This involves three weekdays and one weekend day (to indicate if there is a major difference between the two). As you'll see, it isn't a complicated process—I don't expect them to log every calorie or fat gram consumed. My main concern is to see *what* they're eating and *how much* of it. Those basic things almost always reveal a deeper issue.

Diaries Double Your Weight Loss

A study of 1,700 participants conducted by Kaiser Permanente found that keeping a food diary can double a person's weight loss. The participants followed a diet rich in fruits, vegetables, and low-fat dairy. After six months, those who kept a diary lost an average of 13 pounds; those who didn't lost only 6 pounds.[2]

Rather than explain the dry details of how to use a food journal to begin keeping tabs on what you eat, let me show you how it works by sharing Pam's story.

Losing Track of Size

After having her first child five years earlier, Pam had gained 60 pounds and could not get it off, no matter what diet she tried. The thirty-year-old home-maker was up to 200 pounds and carried most of it in her abdomen, which unfortunately made her appear seven to eight months pregnant. As you can imagine, that led to several embarrassing situations at malls or restaurants, where people would undoubtedly stop to ask her when her baby was due. Pam had no health problems and was not on medication, which made her even more perplexed as to why her weight did not budge.

When she came to see me a few years ago, we took our time going over her detailed dietary and exercise history. She was exercising four times a week for thirty minutes. She generally ate healthy foods and included plenty of fruits and vegetables, as well as lean meats—either grilled or broiled, but never fried. Added to the mix were whole-wheat bread or whole-wheat pasta, brown rice, high-fiber cereal, low-fat milk, and no desserts. Pam could not understand why, after doing everything she knew to do, she still could not lose weight.

I then asked her what portion sizes of food she ate. She said that she ate normal portion sizes, and then added that she never went back for seconds or thirds as her husband did. Her husband was also a patient of mine and, as a former college football player, was a very large, muscular man who still played sports regularly at his church. This gave me a hunch of what was really going on with Pam's inability to lose weight.

MORE PORTION DISTORTION

Twenty years ago, a restaurant's typical serving of spaghetti and meatballs contained a single cup of spaghetti noodles with sauce and three small meatballs, totaling 500 calories. Today, the same "regular" serving includes twice as much pasta with sauce and totals an average of 1,025 calories.[3]

I instructed her to purchase a small, inexpensive notebook that she could easily carry in her purse. She was to record everything she ate and drank in a food journal for three days during the week and one weekend day. "Don't just write down what you eat and drink," I told her, "but also *how much* you eat and drink." I then added that I wanted her to note the day of the week, the time of each meal and snack, and, most importantly, the calorie content of each food she consumed.

When Pam came back the next week, we were both stunned at her four-day food diary. Sure, she was eating a healthy, high-fiber cereal with a banana in the morning. But her serving size of cereal was a little more than a cup, and instead of drinking skim milk she was drinking 2 percent milk. Rather than a 4-ounce glass of orange juice, she was drinking a 12-ounce glass of orange juice. And along with two pieces of turkey bacon, she ate a piece of whole-wheat toast with 1 teaspoon of butter and 1 teaspoon of jelly, in addition to an 8-ounce cup of coffee with 1 tablespoon of coffee creamer and an artificial sweetener. Pam believed she was eating a low-calorie breakfast; her food diary showed otherwise.

Day 1—Monday

Breakfast

Food/beverage	Time	Portion size	Calories
Whole-wheat toast	8:00 a.m.	1 slice	69
Raisin Bran cereal		1 cup	380
Banana		½ banana	52
2 percent milk		1 cup	122
Orange juice		12 ounces	165
Turkey bacon		2 slices	70
Butter		1 teaspoon	33
Jelly		1 teaspoon	13
Coffee		1 cup	5
Coffee creamer		1 tablespoon	40
Artificial sweetener		1 packet	0
Total calories			**949**

For lunch, Pam typically would go to Subway and would eat a Subway Club sandwich with a Diet Coke and a small bag of baked potato chips.

Lunch

Food/beverage	Time	Portion size	Calories
Subway Club sandwich	12:00 p.m.	6 inches	320
Baked potato chips		1 ounce	120
Diet Coke		12 ounces	0
Total calories			**440**

Around 3:00 p.m. each afternoon, Pam would eat an energy bar and a Diet Coke for a snack.

Snack

Food/beverage	Time	Portion size	Calories
Kashi energy bar	3:00 p.m.	35 grams	140
Diet Coke		12 ounces	0
Total calories			**140**

Dinner was by far Pam's largest meal. She prided herself on fixing a big dinner for her husband and children every night. Typically, she had meat, such as a lean 8-ounce porterhouse steak on the grill, grilled or baked chicken breast, or grilled salmon. She usually accompanied that with a baked potato, mashed potatoes, or corn, as well as some other type of vegetables such as green beans, broccoli, or asparagus. About twice a week she would fix brown rice or whole-grain pasta and usually served whole-grain rolls or whole-grain pita bread along with the meal.

Even though Pam rarely had seconds or thirds like her husband, her plate was an 11-inch plate and filled to capacity. It contained an 8-ounce piece of meat; a cup of potatoes, rice, or corn; half a cup of vegetables; and two whole-grain rolls or slices of pita bread. She started dinner with a large salad, usually smothered with blue cheese dressing or Caesar dressing. She also added a lot of butter to all her vegetables, including her corn, her baked potatoes, her broccoli, and even her asparagus.

Staying true to the task I had assigned her, Pam measured out the typical amount of salad dressing she used and discovered that she used 10 tablespoons of blue cheese dressing on her salad—which amounted to 850 calories alone! It didn't take long for her to see that her portion sizes were too large and that she used too much butter and salad dressing.

Dinner

Food/beverage	Time	Portion size	Calories
Porterhouse steak	8:00 p.m.	8 ounces	641
Mashed potatoes		1 cup	200
Lettuce		1 cup	8
Blue cheese salad dressing		10 tablespoons	850
Whole-wheat pita bread		Two 6½-inch slices	340
Broccoli		½ cup	27
Butter		2 tablespoons	200
Total calories			**2,266**

Pam was consuming 2,266 calories just for dinner and then went to bed at 10:00 p.m. Although she was eating healthier foods, the sheer volume of food and calories, especially for dinner, was locking her body into obesity without

her realizing it. Her total calorie intake for just one day was a whopping 3,795 calories. She consumed 949 calories for breakfast, 440 calories for lunch, 140 calories as a midafternoon snack, and 2,266 calories for dinner. She was not eating dinner like a pauper but like a queen.

How Much Do You Need to Burn?

After discovering how many calories Pam was consuming on a daily basis, our next step was to calculate the number of calories she needed to maintain her weight at 200 pounds. In chapter 5 we discussed how to calculate your basal metabolic rate (BMR) both as a rough estimate and using a more precise method. We applied this to Pam and discovered that to lose a pound a week, she would need to either decrease her calorie intake by 500 calories a day or increase her physical activity to burn off 500 calories a day. A third option was to combine the two for the same reduction in calories.

Since she already worked out four times a week and did not have room in her schedule to do much more than that, Pam decided to decrease her portion sizes. It started with the simple move of changing dinner plates. Instead of eating off her usual extra-large dinner plate, she began to eat off a 9-inch plate. She switched to blue cheese

Swim Hard

To burn off the 952 calories and 80 grams of fat found in a single Bob Evans Bacon and Cheese Omelet, you'd have to swim in rough waters for 112 minutes.[4]

salad dressing in a spritzer (with 1 calorie per spray) and decreased her butter and bread intake. Instead of consuming more than 2,000 calories for dinner, she only consumed 500 to 600 calories. And instead of consuming more than 900 calories for breakfast, she chose low-glycemic foods and decreased her portion sizes. By doing this, Pam was able to decrease her calorie intake for breakfast to around 400 to 500 calories.

Pam also practiced mindful eating and actually maintained control of her eating when she was stressed. By adjusting her portion sizes, eating off a smaller plate, choosing low-glycemic foods, eating a healthy midafternoon snack, and prefilling her stomach with broth-based vegetable and bean soups and more salad before meals (but with low-calorie dressings), she had an easy plan to lose weight and keep it off. She also began eating dinner at 6:00 or 6:30 p.m. instead of 8:00 p.m. In just nine months, Pam was able to lose 55 pounds of weight, and her waist measurement went from 39 inches to 31 inches. She was no longer mistaken for a pregnant woman—which suited Pam just fine.

THE FOOD JOURNAL

The most helpful thing Pam did to lose weight was record what she ate in her four-day food journal. This allowed her to realize that she was consuming more calories than she could possibly burn. Much as a diary reveals personal thoughts and insights, food journals can reveal a lot about what you are actually eating rather than what you *think* you are eating.

I have discovered this is a common problem for dieters. We try our best to eat healthy foods and exercise, but we never bother with the details of exactly how much we are putting in our bodies. Pam was guilty of this, and as a result, her surplus of intake was being stored directly in her belly as toxic belly fat. Once she saw exactly what and how much she was putting in her body, she realized that her portion sizes, her choices in food, as well as her late-night eating were sabotaging her weight-loss efforts. Keeping a food journal was also a great motivator for Pam, and instead of stopping after four days, she actually continued using her food diary for the duration of her weight loss.

SIX WAYS TO STAY ACCOUNTABLE

1. Meet regularly with a friend or family member.
2. Talk on the phone daily with someone else trying to lose weight.
3. Write a blog.
4. Join an online weight-loss community.
5. Take daily or weekly photographs and post them around the house.
6. Meet as a group each week at work, church, or at someone's house.

THE ACCOUNTABILITY FACTOR

Keeping a food journal while losing weight is a tremendous motivator for most individuals because it creates accountability. This is why weight-loss programs such as Weight Watchers are largely successful. Accountability is built into their programs, and as a result, you have a team of people surrounding you with support. I have found the same level of accountability is created when you maintain a food diary. It not only helps you to control portion sizes, but it also challenges you to continually practice mindfulness.

I am not recommending that you track your calories every day during the program. That, like many dieting techniques, can become such a burden that it is more harmful than helpful. To get an idea of how many calories you are ingesting daily, however, you need to start this program by journaling at least

for three weekdays and one weekend day to calculate your calorie intake. Like Pam, you may discover your meal portions are too big. Or you may find out your calorie count for a particular meal is much higher than you thought. It will be easy to distinguish such characteristics if you simply take the time to record them in a food journal.

Don't worry; this does not have to be a complicated thing. At this stage, you do not have to concern yourself with tracking every gram of fat, sugar, or carbohydrate. For these four days, simply keep tabs on what you are eating, how much you are eating, and how many calories that amounts to—all of which can be easily calculated by looking at food labels. If you do not have the time to fill out your food diary, simply take a picture of each meal with your cell phone for three weekdays and one weekend day. Then figure out your calories by going to www.thecandodiet.com. Write on a napkin next to each meal "Day 1, Breakfast," and so on. This will help you identify each meal and help you to calculate the calories for each day.

I have included a blank sample journal page on the next page that you are free to photocopy for your own journal. You can also download the journal pages from www.thecandodiet.com. This should help you get started on being honest with what you are actually eating.

"Can Do" Points to Remember

1. You can eat all the right foods and exercise enough, but without keeping tabs on how much of what you're eating, it's possible you'll never lose weight.

2. Much as a diary reveals personal thoughts and insights, food journals can reveal a lot about what you are actually eating rather than what you *think* you are eating.

3. Prepare a four-day food journal, tracking what you eat for three days during the week and one day on the weekend.

4. Keeping a food diary not only helps you to control portion sizes, but it also challenges you to continually practice mindfulness and provides accountability.

FOOD DIARY

Day of the week:_____

Breakfast

Food/beverage	Time	Portion size	Calories

Lunch

Food/beverage	Time	Portion size	Calories

Snack

Food/beverage	Time	Portion size	Calories

Dinner

Food/beverage	Time	Portion size	Calories

THE PROGRAM

189

19

MINDFUL EATING

A FEW YEARS AGO my wife and I went to a buffet-style restaurant. I will never forget the couple sitting at the table next to us who looked like they each weighed more than 350 pounds. Their bellies were so large that they prevented them from getting close to their table. When they went to the buffet line, they grabbed large plates and stacked them with food about 4 to 5 inches high. By the time they returned to sit down, their waitress had brought them each a huge glass of sweet iced tea. They took a couple sips, then for the next ten minutes, neither one said a word. The couple simply sat and ate. Nonstop.

When they finished, it was on to round two. Once again they filled their entire plates with food stacked equally as high as the first time. Again, they ate nonstop without saying a word or even once putting their forks down. They chewed each bite one or two times and, on occasion, reached over to wash it down with a swig of iced tea.

After cleaning their second plates, they then moved on to the dessert bar, where they piled their 12-inch plates full of a vast assortment of desserts. And of course, they again ate nonstop. No conversation,

HOW TO EAT MINDLESSLY

Walk into a Chili's restaurant and order an Awesome Blossom, or what *Men's Health* editor in chief David Zinczenko calls "easily one of the worst things you can put in your body." Why so harsh? Maybe it's the appetizer's 2,710 calories. Or the incredible 203 grams of fat (36 of which are saturated). Or the 194 grams of carbohydrates. Or the jaw-dropping 6,360 milligrams of sodium.[1]

barely any eye contact. Simply bite after bite of food. In a matter of twenty to twenty-five minutes, this couple probably consumed more than 10,000 calories—*each*!

MINDLESS EATING

If you live in the United States, it goes without saying that you have watched a similar scene unfold in front of you. Maybe you have even been the one guilty

of the all-you-can-consume-and-then-some gluttony. We eat with no regard for what or how much we are putting in our mouths. All we care about is pleasing an appetite that, over time, never really goes away.

The tragic fact is that most of this nation's obesity problems could disappear if people just ate mindfully. One of the biggest pitfalls that most overweight and obese individuals unknowingly fall into is the habit of mindless eating. This is simply when you stop paying attention to or being aware of the amount and taste of the food you are eating. Mindless eating is an automatic or unconscious type of consumption that most people fall prey to while they are watching their favorite TV show, a ball game, a movie, working on the computer, or talking on the phone. Even if they are not hungry, these individuals slide into the habit of eating on autopilot, oblivious to the amount of calories they are consuming.

FOOD, FOOD . . . IT'S EVERYWHERE!

Part of the problem, as we touched on in chapter 1, is the complete barrage of tempting junk foods. Unless you live in the country, you are most likely within a five-minute drive of some type of fast-food "haven." Once you pass that, you're bound to run across a Starbucks, Dunkin' Donuts, or Krispy Kreme—and if you don't, you can always run to the nearest convenience store (open 24-7, of course) to find their offerings. Past the gas station is likely to be a wholesale club that would be honored to pack your car with industry-sized portions of these same tempting items. If you are itching for a movie instead, you can always head to the mall, where first you'll encounter the ever-lingering smell of fresh-baked cookies and cinnamon buns. If you manage to avoid that temptation, next up is facing the movie ads touting barrel-sized tubs of popcorn, Milk Duds, and gallons of soda—with free refills.

Whether it is while we're shopping at the grocery store, walking in the mall, or just taking a breather in the office break room, we are constantly surrounded by lousy food options. Sadly, our culture has made it so that finding what is actually good for us takes a little bit of effort and some purposeful thinking. Because of this, the easier option is to eat without regard to the amount, quality, calorie density, or even taste of the food we are consuming.

To combat this takes mindful eating—being aware of the taste of the food and how much of it you are eating. When practicing mindful eating, you can enjoy a food while being fully aware of its calorie content. You can savor each bite without being distracted by a mind-numbing form of entertainment. Awareness of eating is a common trait of people who lose weight and keep it

off. Too many people multitask while they are eating, which brings about a disconnect with whether or not they are enjoying and savoring each bite.

French Lessons

For years I told patients to look to the French for an example of mindful eating. Even within Europe, they were always the model culture of how to eat mindfully. Despite a diet that included many high-fat, starchy foods, as well as plenty of wine and sweets, the French were a lean culture. Studies proved that this was largely due to their approach to eating. Instead of multitasking like Americans, they sat, relaxed, enjoyed pleasant conversation, and savored each bite of food as they ate. They knew the pleasure of most foods is in the first few bites and were then able to stop eating when they were satisfied. By slowing down while eating, they were less likely to be hungry at the end of the meal and were content with only a bite or two of dessert.

> ### Everyday Mindfulness
>
> Being mindful can start with something as simple as breathing. When you awake, rather than rushing into your thoughts for the day, concentrate on the process of breathing, and allow your mind to center in on your deep, replenishing breaths. Hear, smell, and slowly observe the things around you as you let all your senses take in the moment. Practice this throughout the day whenever you find yourself sitting at a stoplight, walking to an appointment, or facing a stressful situation.

Then a strange thing happened. The French got fat.

In the past ten years, the number of overweight or obese people in France has almost doubled. More than 42 percent of the French are now considered overweight.[2] Between 1997 and 2003 alone, obesity levels among both men and women rose from 8 percent to around 11.4 percent,[3] which is still much lower than the overweight/obesity levels in the United States, which is 34 percent.[4] The national average, meanwhile, has increased even more as a new generation of obese French children has emerged. Researchers now estimate that 16 percent of all French children between the ages of five and eleven are obese. To make matters worse, it is believed this could rise as much as 20 percent by the year 2010.[5]

What could cause such a relatively sudden change in a culture's dietary habits? French doctors and health experts chalk it up to both a change in eating habits and a people suddenly enamored with "convenience foods." The French now eat more fast-food meals—previously unheard of for most of the country—as well as snack more on processed foods. McDonald's, Kentucky

Fried Chicken, and other American fast-food chains are experiencing booming growth throughout the country.

Dr. Jean-Michel Cohen, a French nutritionist and author of *Understanding Eating*, explained this widespread cultural shift: "The rise in obesity is probably a result of the fact that the French don't understand how to eat properly with commercial food, since they have never had to do it before. We need to teach them how to use supermarket food to put a balanced diet together."[6]

As a result of all this, the French now enjoy fewer sit-down meals in the traditional manner with fresh-cooked vegetables and meats. In 1978, the notoriously slow-eating French took an average of one hour and twenty-two minutes to eat a meal; today, that number has decreased to thirty-eight minutes.[7]

Slow Down!

Sadly, the French are becoming more like us by losing the very thing they first perfected: the art of slowing down. In America, we live life at a hundred miles an hour, and this is reflected in most everything we do. We use a microwave oven to rapidly heat our microwavable frozen dinners and toaster pastries. We eat at fast-food restaurants that, on the rare occasion, make amends if their food isn't prepared in a few minutes. We have "fast lanes" for traffic, self-serve gas stations with rapid credit card payment, fast checkout lines at the grocery store, and countless other fast and convenient services. Rampant in our society, this hurry-up mentality has already shown its effects via our obesity epidemic. What does eating too fast have to do with obesity? Let's explore the science that explains why eating in a hurry is a sure way to get stuck in the trap of mindless eating and gradual weight gain.

Chew, Then Spit?

Health-food faddist Horace Fletcher, also known as "The Great Masticator," is famous for claiming, "Nature will castigate those who don't masticate." Fletcher's weight-loss programs in the early 1900s advocated that food be chewed at least thirty-two times—once for each tooth—and then spit out. Fletcher believed by doing this you could absorb the essential nutrients without having to gain the weight.[8]

The Autonomic Nervous System

The autonomic nervous system regulates automatic body functions, including heart rate, digestion, and sweating. This system has two different branches:

the sympathetic (or fight-or-flight response) and the parasympathetic (or relaxation response). Our autonomic nervous system is supposed to be balanced with just the right stimulation of the sympathetic nervous system, as well as the parasympathetic nervous system. If the sympathetic system is overstimulated, our system may get stuck in a fight-or-flight pattern. If our parasympathetic system is stimulated, our bodies become very relaxed. In other words, the sympathetic nervous system is similar to the accelerator of your car, while the parasympathetic nervous system is akin to a car's brake. When we are stressed, upset, uptight, or in a hurry, our sympathetic nervous system is stimulated and blood is shunted away from our digestive tract to our muscles so that we can fight or flee.

In everyday life, this means that when we eat while standing up, eat in our car, rush through our meal, or feel stressed and in a hurry, we do not digest our food properly. This also causes our cortisol levels to rise, setting us up for weight gain. We are also more likely then to have heartburn and indigestion, since blood is shunted away from the digestive tract and digestion is impaired.

On the other hand, when we sit down, take a few deep breaths, bless our food, and enter into an attitude of gratitude, our autonomic nervous system shifts from sympathetic dominant to parasympathetic dominant. As we keep our conversation pleasant and slowly eat our meal, chewing each bite twenty to thirty times, our body is able to then digest our food properly and secrete sufficient amounts of digestive enzymes.

Part of learning the art of slowing down involves approaching the very act of eating differently. I recommend that my patients put their forks down between bites in order to slow down their eating. I also encourage them to savor each bite of food. By savoring each bite of food and enjoying the flavor, texture, and taste of the food, they are practicing mindful eating and will be less likely to overeat. Remember that when we slow down our eating, our appetite center in the hypothalamus is able to get the message that we are no longer hungry but are instead satisfied and full.

Saboteurs of Mindful Eating

Unfortunately, most of us have certain habits that sabotage mindful eating. One of the worst yet most common habits found in almost every household across America is eating while watching TV. In fact, one online survey found that a whopping 91 percent of respondents said they typically watch the tube whenever they eat meals at home.[9] We have a rule in our house at dinnertime that the TV must stay off while eating so that we can enjoy valuable family time.

THE PROGRAM

By practicing this, we are able to gain control of our mindless eating. Other families or individuals find themselves distracted by movies, the computer, or the telephone—all of which can cause us to lose touch with what and how much we are consuming. (This can easily be curtailed by designating a single specific place in the home to eat such as the kitchen or dining room.)

Other saboteurs of mindful eating are skipping meals or eating a meal when you are starving. First, do not skip meals, or else you will most likely become extremely hungry, and eat every three to three and a half hours. I recommend having a bowl of broth-based vegetable soup and a large salad (using a salad spritzer) before a meal, especially if you feel like you are starving. Buffet restaurants are another culprit of mindless eating, as they lead to way too large portion sizes and having multiple servings. Finally, social events, stress, or other emotional eating habits where food is used for comfort can all lead to mindless eating.

ZONED OUT

Eating while watching television adds an average of seventy extra minutes to your tube time.[10]

THE FINAL FOUR

To practice mindful eating, always ask yourself four questions before putting any food or beverage in your mouth:

1. *Is this beverage or food healthy, or is it high in calories?* I trust you are smart enough to never buy a suit, car, or house without first asking the price. The same check should be put in place for the food that goes in your mouth. Consider the cost of the food, whether it is high in calories or not. You should also know if the food you are eating is healthy or unhealthy. If the food is unhealthy or high in calories, then the next step is developing the fortitude to say no, regardless of how tempting it is.

2. *Am I hungry?* Many people, particularly obese individuals, eat constantly throughout the day without ever realizing that they were never hungry in the first place. They become eaters—or grazers, to be more precise—by habit. I once had a patient who was frustrated with his obesity, yet I found out that whenever people offered him food at work, he never refused it. This happened throughout the day. When I asked him if he was hungry each time he was offered food, he admitted he was not. The problem was that he did not want to refuse for fear that he might offend the individual. I told him to start by

offering a "no, thank you" whenever people offered him food and he wasn't hungry. If people were ever offended when he said no, he could explain that he was not rejecting them but was simply not hungry. And if they persisted, he could explain that his weight-related health issues now required him to say no to most high-calorie foods.

This may happen to you at times. It's Murphy's Law that whenever you set your mind to losing weight, someone will wind up baking your favorite cake, pie, or casserole. If you are able to say no to their offer (which I hope you can), sometimes these people can take it as a personal rejection. I always have my patients blame me for saying no: "I'm sorry, Dr. Colbert said that I couldn't have that food now. However, it sure looks delicious." By saying no in this manner, the person does not feel rejected but is actually complimented.

3. *Do I truly enjoy the taste of this food?* I love a nice juicy steak on occasion, but I've noticed that the first few bites are always my favorite. I savor and enjoy those initial bites. My wife's favorite is anything chocolate, and like me, she has learned that the first bite of chocolate is absolutely awesome, the second bite is good, and the third bite is just average. She has learned how to savor those first few bites and quickly become satisfied. After all, even the most incredible taste of your favorite food can become boring once you get used to having it. Why not savor the flavor and enjoy it every time by only eating a few bites?

4. *How will this make me feel in a few hours?* Many years ago, I used to allow pharmaceutical representatives to bring lunch for my staff and me once or twice a week. Many times the lunches consisted of Italian food with a great deal of creamy pastas and breads. An hour or so after eating a large amount of this lunch, I would usually get so tired that I could barely stay awake, even though I had to see my patients who were scheduled for the afternoon. I did not realize that the starchy foods were making me feel this way since the pharmaceutical representatives brought different types of food each week.

After about six months of going through this, especially after eating pasta and bread, I finally put one and one together and discovered that a large consumption of starch made me sleepy. I then began associating what I ate with how I felt an hour or so later. I discovered that if I ate starches or sugars for lunch, my work performance, energy level, and mental clarity decreased dramatically. I also found out that if I ate the correct fuel mixture and practiced mindful eating, then

my energy level, mental clarity, and work performance were excellent. Little did I realize back then that this fuel mixture was also the best fuel mixture for weight loss.

If you find that you are groggy, irritable, fatigued, or grumpy an hour or two after a meal, I can guarantee you that you chose the wrong fuel mixture and are probably not practicing mindfulness. Begin to judge how you feel a few hours after a meal so you can improve your work performance and lose weight.

GROWING IN THE PRACTICE

None of us are born with the skill of eating mindfully. This is a habit that must be developed. And like all habits, you must start practicing on a regular basis. Commit to being intentional with every bite of food you put in your mouth. Slow down as you eat. If you have a sudden craving for a food, stop yourself and ask the four questions. Remember, habits can be broken.

THE MORE, THE MERRIER

Children who eat with their families only two nights a week or less are 50 percent more likely to try alcohol than those who share family meals at least five nights a week.[11]

When Mary and I were first married, she used to eat her food in such a hurry that she would almost always be finished with her entire meal by the time I was barely beginning. One night we were dining in a nice, fancy restaurant that served a five-course meal. As soon as the first course was served, Mary tore into it like someone who hadn't eaten in days. The servers then brought out the second course, and she again tore into her food, eating as fast as she could. She ate so fast that I jokingly reassured her I was not going to eat her food. In a loving manner, I asked her to try slowing down, chewing every bite twenty to thirty times, and even putting her fork down between bites.

It had never even dawned on Mary that she ate this way. She began to explain to me that it was something she had done as long as she could remember. When she was growing up, she had three older brothers with ravenous appetites who would eat their food in a hurry and then try to eat her food. She had learned at an early age to eat her food as fast as possible so that her older brothers would not eat it. Little did she realize that when she was wolfing down her food, it was actually causing a stress response in her body that impaired her digestion and increased her cortisol level. When she made a conscious effort to slow down, chew her food slowly, and put her fork down

between bites, she discovered that she did not desire nearly as much food. She also began to enjoy her food more, while I enjoyed the fact that because it now took her longer to eat, we could enjoy our meal together.

When my son, Kyle, was young, we got in a bad habit of discussing stressful topics at the dinner table. Sometimes I would discuss the bad grade he received at school. Other times I would reprimand him for something he had or hadn't done, or we would wind up arguing over some other stressful topic. Undoubtedly, this left Kyle, Mary, and me upset. A wonderful dinner would turn into a verbal argument. I later learned that one of the most important things that we can do when we eat is to keep our conversation pleasant. In simple terms, do not argue, fuss, or fight. The problem isn't just that it leaves you emotionally wrecked; it is also a surefire way to raise your cortisol level and forget about what you are eating. As we would argue, my wife, son, and I would mindlessly shovel food into our mouths without enjoying each bite. Worse still, I can remember many times when one of us would develop an upset stomach after the meal.

Mindfulness keeps you paying attention to what is happening to you from moment to moment. Renowned cardiologist Herbert Benson once said, "To be mindful, you must slow down, do one activity at a time, and bring your full awareness to both the activity at hand and to your inner experience of it."[12] You do this through the simple practice of slowing down your eating, enjoying and savoring each bite, and keeping the conversation pleasant. The more you do it, the better you will become at it and the more pounds you will lose, so make a commitment to practice mindful eating—and practice it until it becomes a habit.

"Can Do" Points to Remember

1. Mindless eating is simply when you stop paying attention to or being aware of the amount and taste of the food you are eating.

2. Awareness of eating is a common trait of people who lose weight and keep it off.

3. When you rush through a meal, you usually don't digest your food properly, which may cause your cortisol levels to rise and may set you up for weight gain.

4. Mindful eating starts by asking yourself four questions: Is this food or beverage high in calories? Am I hungry? Do I truly enjoy this food? How will this make me feel in a few hours?

20

ACTIVITY TIME

I F YOU HATE working out, know that you are not alone. Even these big-name celebrities, all known for their ultra-fit bodies and sex appeal, disdain it.

> I hate working out—and *hate* is a strong word, but I cannot stand working out.[1]
>
> —JANET JACKSON

> I'm lazy, I hate working out, I only do it for films and I think of it as work.[2]
>
> —BRUCE WILLIS

> I hate working out more than anything, but I have to—when I'm running, I think about how much I want to win. That's the only thing that keeps me going....I guess everyone has to find that one thing that encourages them and just think about it the entire time you're working out. But I have to be honest, I hate going to the gym. I don't like running. I hate doing anything that has to do with working out.[3]
>
> —SERENA WILLIAMS

> I hate working out. I just get very bored. It kills me. But when its part of the work it's another avenue to get into the character.[4]
>
> —COLIN FARRELL

> If I wasn't in this industry, I wouldn't work out. But I have hips and a butt and everything that goes along with that, including cellulite.[5]
>
> —KATHERINE HEIGL

There's definitely a love-hate relationship between most Americans and exercise. We know it's necessary, but we would rather avoid it at all costs.

We like the fruit of it and, at times, even enjoy the burn that comes from a great workout; yet we dread taking time from our already cramped schedules. Why else do you think there are so many late-night television infomercials for time-saving exercise gadgets that promise the pounds will "instantly" fall off if we use their product? When it comes to exercise, it seems we're always looking for the easy way out.

The result is that two-thirds of all Americans are not physically active on a regular basis, while less than half get less than the recommended amount of exercise. Sadly, a full 25 percent—a quarter of the population!—get absolutely no exercise at all.[6] The top reason why? Time. Almost every survey conducted finds this atop its list of excuses.[7] People feel they are just too busy to exercise.

WHAT'S IN A WORD?

We know the truth: exercise is essential. That applies universally to not only every human being but also especially to anyone hoping to lose pounds. You can restrict your diet and eat less than your daily requirement, yet without burning off calories through physical activity, you only have half the equation. After working with thousands of overweight and obese individuals, I have discovered that almost without exception, they struggle with their perception of exercise. Essentially, it comes down to the single word *exercise*.

MARATHON BURN

To burn off the 1,510 calories in a Quiznos large Chicken Carbonara, you'd have to expend the same calories it takes to bike across the state of Delaware (thirty miles).[8]

When many people hear the word, it immediately conjures up negative feelings, much as the word *diet* does. Those who are overweight or obese think of dread, pain, sweating, humiliation, embarrassment, anxiety, and so forth. They may visualize themselves in a health club surrounded by people with perfect bodies, or a physical education instructor testing their lack of physical capabilities, or a threatening coach. In another words, many overweight and obese individuals literally dread the very thought of exercise. So instead of using the term exercise, I use a different word: *activity*. For some, this seems a bit silly. It's just a word, after all—what difference could substituting a word possibly make? Isn't it still referring to the same thing?

I cannot explain all the various reasons this has worked, but it has. *Activity* seems to be less intrusive. It usually does not trigger any emotional symptoms or anxiety; it is a safe and nonthreatening term for most overweight or

obese individuals. It also does not overwhelm a person with thoughts of time commitment, discipline, or early-morning alarm clocks.

I won't say that whether you use the word *activity* or *exercise* makes no difference, because in my experience, it has. It is up to you whether you want to adapt a change of vocabulary. But the bigger issue that cannot be overlooked is that both are absolutely crucial for weight loss. Plain and simple, the reason why people successfully lose weight and keep it off is because they are physically active on a regular basis.

The Perks of Regular Activity

In case you needed a reminder, here are just a few of the tremendous benefits that come with regular activity:

- It decreases the risk of heart disease and stroke, as well as the development of hypertension.
- It helps prevent type 2 diabetes.
- It helps protect you from developing certain types of cancer.
- It helps prevent osteoporosis and aids in maintaining healthy bones.
- It helps prevent arthritis and aids in maintaining healthy joints.
- It slows down the overall aging process.
- It improves your mood and reduces the symptoms of anxiety and depression.
- It increases energy and mental alertness.
- It improves your digestion.
- It gives you restful sleep.
- It helps prevent colds and flu.
- It alleviates pain.

READ MORE ABOUT IT

For more details on each of these reasons, see *The Seven Pillars of Health.*

And the favorite reason among overweight and obese people...

- It promotes weight loss and decreases appetite.

The Weight-Loss Supplement

There is no better way to complement a weight-loss dietary program than by being physically active on a regular basis. How does activity specifically help with losing weight? The ways are just as plentiful as the overall benefits of activity. First, regular physical activity helps raise the metabolic rate both during exercise and for hours afterward. It also enables you to develop more

muscle, which raises the metabolic rate all day long and even while you're sleeping. Daily activity decreases body fat and improves your ability to cope with stress by lowering the stress hormone cortisol (which, if you recall, is a major cause of weight gain).

Such activity also raises serotonin levels, which helps to reduce cravings for sweets and carbohydrates. It assists in burning off dangerous belly fat and improves your body's ability to handle sugar. Finally, regular physical activity can even help control your appetite by boosting serotonin levels, lowering cortisol, and decreasing insulin levels (which can also decrease your chances for insulin resistance).

Muscles, Metabolism, and Aging

Everyone wants to look young and fit forever. That's particularly true in this country, where we plaster our magazine covers, TV ads, and movie screens with buff, sculpted, trimmed, toned, and *youthful* bodies. But did you know the reality is that

> ### Strength in Years
>
> In 2004, Connecticut resident George Brunstad became the oldest man to swim the English Channel when he crossed the twenty-five-mile stretch at age seventy. Though he swam an extra seven miles due to strong currents, Brunstad completed the grueling journey just a minute shy of sixteen hours. Just as admirable was the former pilot's underlying purpose for swimming, which was to let people know about a ministry his church sponsors in Haiti.[9]

adults typically lose approximately ½ to 1 pound of muscle tissue every year past the age of twenty-five? Stated another way, our bodies naturally progress toward more fat and less muscle. That isn't the greatest news for those who are already struggling with bodies overloaded with fat. But it can be a driving force for turning your body from flab to fit. Understand that the more muscle mass you have, generally the higher your metabolic rate and the more calories you will burn at rest. For each pound of muscle mass that you either gain or do not lose, you will burn approximately 30 to 50 calories a day.

I will never forget a patient I saw years ago while in residency on orthopedic rotation. He was a star running back on a high school football team who had fractured his left thigh. Part of the reason he played running back was because of how powerful his legs were. His thighs were extremely muscular. Before he fractured his leg, he said he had been able to leg press more than 1,000 pounds for ten repetitions. But because of his injury, this football star had a full leg cast placed on his left leg for approximately two months.

When the cast was removed, we were shocked at how much his left leg had

atrophied. After measuring his thighs, we found that his right thigh was 32 inches in circumference at mid-thigh, but his left thigh was only 24 inches. It was such a huge discrepancy that his left leg didn't even look like it belonged with his big, muscular body. In only two months' time, this young man had lost 8 inches of muscle just because of inactivity.

A similar process happens to most adults, albeit not as fast. If you are inactive most of the time, your muscles are slowly melting away. Your metabolic rate is decreasing, while your muscle tissue is (typically) being replaced with fat. Many people do not notice this because the size of their arm or leg remains the same, when in fact it is simply a case of fat replacing muscle tissue, similar to the marbling of meat.

This is particularly true for women. A woman's metabolism typically begins to decrease at the age of twenty at a rate of about 5 percent per decade of life. To understand this more, let's use the example of an average fifty-year-old female—we'll call her Sarah. Since her late twenties, Sarah's weight has gone from around 120 to her current weight of 150 pounds. During those years, she gained 30 pounds of fat, but she also lost around 15 to 30 pounds of muscle. That may sound like it averages out except when you consider the corresponding drop in metabolic rate. When she was twenty, Sarah could eat 2,000 calories a day and maintain her 120-pound frame. At the age of fifty, however, if she eats 2,000 calories a day, she will most likely gain weight because of the muscle tissue she has lost. Remember, for each pound of muscle tissue lost, your metabolic rate decreases by 30 to 50 calories per day. So in addition to losing 15 pounds of muscle, Sarah also lost the ability for her metabolic rate to burn about 450 to 750 more calories a day.

Now you can see why maintaining or gaining muscle mass is so crucial. Muscle does not just look better than fat; it is essential for maintaining a healthy body. And the only way to keep muscle intact is to use it and keep it strengthened on a regular basis, which means increasing your activity level. When you decide to do the opposite and remain inactive, you put yourself in a body cast, so to speak, as your metabolic rate nose-dives and you become a fat magnet.

RECOMMENDED AMOUNT OF ACTIVITY

Are you convinced yet of how crucial it is to stay active? Great. Now let's tackle the natural follow-up question: How much activity do you need? Unfortunately, this cannot be answered with a single universal number. There are many factors

involved when you engage in activity to lose weight, yet all of them start with the heart.

Every activity either requires or can be performed at a different level of intensity. Given that, it makes sense, then, that every person hoping to lose weight has an ideal intensity at which they should work out. This is called your target heart rate zone.

To calculate the low end of this zone, start by subtracting your age from 220. This is your maximum heart rate. For example, if you are forty years old:

220 − 40 = 180 beats per minute

Now multiply this number by 65 percent to find the low end of your target heart rate zone.

180 x 0.65 = 117 beats per minute

To figure out the high end of your zone, multiply your maximum heart rate by 85 percent.

180 x 0.85 = 153 beats per minute

This means if you are forty, you should keep your heart rate between 117 and 153 beats per minute when exercising. That is quite a range, however, which prompts the next question: Which end of the zone do you aim for to lose more weight? Experts have debated this ever since the "target zone" idea came about more than fifteen years ago. To find out the real answer, let's look at the types of activity that push the heart to these two extremes of the zone.

BURNING FAT WITH AEROBIC ACTIVITY

The word *aerobic* means "in the presence of air or oxygen." Aerobic activity is simply movement that strengthens the lungs and the heart. It involves steady, continuous movements that work large muscle groups in repetitive motion for at least twenty minutes. The key point for weight loss with aerobic activity is to maintain a moderate pace, which triggers your body to burn fat as its preferred fuel.

One of the biggest and most common workout mistakes I see among overweight people is the tendency to get on a treadmill and run as hard as they can for as long as possible. Their intent is to burn off more fat by doing this,

but in the long run (pardon my pun), they won't. Sprinting, running, or jogging at a high intensity for long periods of time so that you are short of breath actually makes you burn less fat as fuel. For those used to being inactive who are just beginning a workout routine, it's also the quickest way to sure-fire burnout.

NOT JUST NERVOUS

Fidgeting or getting up from your seat frequently can cause you to burn an additional 350 calories a day—which amounts to 36 pounds lost in a year![10]

Remember, aerobic means with oxygen; therefore, the activity that you choose must be of moderate intensity for your body to use oxygen in order to burn the fat as fuel. That usually translates to about 65 to 85 percent of your maximum heart rate. When you exercise to the point that you are severely short of breath, you are no longer performing aerobically but have shifted to an anaerobic activity, which is activity without oxygen. Anaerobic activity burns glycogen, which is stored sugar, as the primary fuel rather than fat. When you run out of glycogen and have not eaten for a while, you then may begin breaking down your muscle tissue and burning muscle protein as fuel. (Notice that burning fat still has not been mentioned.) Many marathoners and triathletes burn a significant amount of their muscle as fuel, which is often why they remain so lean.

If you are overweight and aim to burn primarily fat, you need to work out at a moderate intensity, which again is around 65 to 85 percent of your maximum heart rate. This is the fat-burning range of your target heart rate zone. As you approach the high end of your zone, you near anaerobic activity, which does you less good in burning fat. This might be a completely revolutionary idea to you, and if so, it may be a struggle to change your ways. Most people believe that to the hardest worker—meaning the guy who runs the fastest and sweats the most—goes the spoils. Not true. In fact, if you are overweight or obese, working out at a higher intensity for long stretches may not only sabotage your ability to burn fat, but it may also increase cortisol levels, which can cause more belly fat to accumulate.

When beginning an activity program, start by working out around 65 percent of your maximum heart rate. As you become more aerobically conditioned, increase your intensity gradually to 70 percent of your maximum heart rate. Then after a few more weeks, increase to 75 percent, and so on. You may never be able to work out at 85 percent of your maximum heart rate, especially if you are huffing and puffing. Be sure that as you increase the intensity of your workouts, you remain able to converse with another person. That is a fairly good sign that you are training aerobically and are burning fat.

HOW MUCH?

This brings us back to the original question of how much activity is needed. A recent Duke University study sheds some light on this.

Over a period of eight months, researchers at Duke studied a group of overweight men and women from ages forty to sixty-five. Participants were split into four main groups: those who walked twelve miles a week, those who jogged twelve miles a week, those who jogged twenty miles a week, and those who did nothing. None of the groups changed anything about their diets, and all exercised at different maximum heart rates. As you might expect, the sedentary group gained weight, added to their waistline, and upped their body fat percentage. Those who walked twelve miles a week (or thirty minutes a day) did so at 40 to 55 percent of their maximum heart rate. Their results were minimal. The group that jogged this same distance each day kept their heart rates between 65 to 80 percent the maximum rate, meaning they exercised within their target heart rate zone. Though some of their results were similar to the walking group, they did lose more body fat and gained more lean muscle. Finally, those who jogged for twenty miles each week kept within their target heart rate zone and saw by far the best results. On average, group members dropped 3.5 percent of their weight, 3.4 percent of their waist measurement, 4.9 percent off their body fat measurement, and added 1.4 percent of lean muscle.[11]

> ### DOG LOVERS?
> Approximately 60 percent of dog owners do not walk their dogs but simply let them out in the backyard.[12]

Clearly, it pays to be active. In this case, the longer you engage in activity at a moderate intensity, the more fat you burn as fuel. I am not going to ask you to jog twenty miles a week, but you can get started by choosing enjoyable, fun activities that you and your family can do daily to obtain similar results. Unless you have already been working out consistently, I suggest that you initially set a goal of twenty minutes of aerobic activity a day, which may be split into ten minutes, twice a day. (You can do this by simply walking your dog!) Once you have adapted to that time, then you can gradually increase to thirty minutes and eventually forty minutes or longer. To minimize soreness, begin by doing this aerobic activity three days a week every other day to start with, and then work up to five or even six days a week. And remember, a brisk walk can accomplish almost the same thing as jogging, provided your maximum heart rate is maintained at 65 to 85 percent. The key is staying

within your target heart rate zone and being able to carry on a conversation, which, again, usually ensures you are training aerobically.

TYPES OF AEROBIC ACTIVITY

There are countless aerobic activities that will help you lose weight. The easiest activity, as I just mentioned, is taking a brisk walk. I am not referring to a leisurely stroll but rather a lively, relatively fast-paced walk. Other good aerobic activities include bike riding (either on a stationary bike or a real one), jogging slowly, aerobic dancing, hiking, cardio-yoga, and using an elliptical machine or stair stepper. Sports such as basketball, volleyball, soccer, football, racquetball, tennis, and squash are all considered aerobic. Pilates, ballroom dancing, washing the car by hand, working in your yard, and mowing the grass are other activities within this category. Swimming and water aerobics are also good, but unless done as sport (rather than leisure) they often do not burn as much fat as other activities.

The key is finding something that you enjoy and that you will do on a regular basis four to six days a week. For some of you, that may be playing hoops with your children when you get home from work. For others, it may be as simple as walking your dog thirty minutes a day.

Remember, you do not have to work out vigorously to burn fat. Too many of us think that we have to suffer and sweat to burn fat, but that is simply not the case. A simple rule of thumb is to walk slow enough so that you can talk but fast enough so that you cannot sing. If you are walking and singing, then speed it up; if you are unable to carry on a conversation while walking, then slow it down. You may want to purchase a heart rate monitor so you can adjust your intensity to enter and stay in the fat-burning range. These can be purchased at most sporting goods stores, while most cardio equipment at health clubs are already equipped with them.

Working out with a buddy greatly improves compliance and usually adds enjoyment to the activity. I encourage all my patients to get an activity buddy, such as a spouse, friend, neighbor, or child.

STRENGTHENING ACTIVITIES

Just as aerobic activity is important for weight loss, so are strengthening activities. We have already talked about the importance of increasing and maintaining muscle mass, which helps to decrease body fat. Strengthening

activities do just this. They also boost the metabolic rate, enabling you to burn more calories throughout the day and night.

Strengthening activities include weight training with free weights or machines, calisthenics, Pilates, resistance band activities, core-specific activities, and balance ball activities. To eliminate the risk of injury, you must maintain good posture and form while performing these exercises. In addition, it is important to learn the correct lifting techniques, the correct range of motion, correct breathing, and the correct speed of the movement in which muscles are being trained. I recommend getting a certified personal trainer to teach you this valuable information in order to maximize your results. I have worked out in health clubs for many years and I am still appalled at the large percentage of individuals who lift weights incorrectly.

You should typically perform ten to twelve repetitions per set. When starting out with strength training, I recommend only performing one set per activity. This reduces soreness, which is common in beginning any type of strengthening program. As you become better conditioned over time, you can then increase to two or three sets per activity for each body part to strengthen and tone your muscles. But remember, go slow! Strength training causes microscopic tears in muscle fibers, which eventually causes them to become stronger and larger. This in turn increases your metabolic rate. You never want to overdo it and train the same muscles every day because the muscles will not have time to repair and rebuild.

Eventually, after a couple of weeks of strength training, you will be able to

THIGH CIRCUMFERENCE

Thin thighs (less than 24 inches in circumference) are associated with significantly increased risk of death and cardiovascular disease. The risk increases as thigh circumference decreases. This makes it important to maintain a thigh circumference greater than 24 inches.[13]

The thigh muscles are the largest in the body and need to be exercised both aerobically and with repetitive exercises. I have found that as my patients with diabetes increase the muscle mass in their thighs, their blood sugar typically decreases.

increase your workouts to three or four days a week. By following the correct lifting techniques, you will prevent injury, build muscle, and burn fat.

PRACTICE MINDFUL LIFTING

Mindful lifting is similar to mindful eating. It involves concentrating on maintaining the correct lifting techniques, proper posture, correct form, good

breathing technique, and keeping the muscles engaged in the full movement, all in order to train the specific muscles. Too often I see individuals in the gym going through their strengthening program on autopilot. This entirely defeats the purpose, and I'm sure if you asked them, they would probably admit to hitting a plateau.

The important thing is focusing as you work out. When I do curls, for instance, I maintain correct form and posture by holding my shoulders back, lifting the weight slowly, and concentrating on flexing my biceps muscles with each repetition. I also let the weight down very slowly with each repetition. Unfortunately, many people lift with their shoulders slumped forward, swing the weight, and end up working their lower back more than their biceps. Instead of slowly lowering the weight, which keeps the muscles engaged in the movement, they let it drop rapidly. These individuals are not practicing mindful lifting, nor are they working their muscles adequately. Worse still, they are setting themselves up for injury.

The more you can concentrate and focus on each repetition, the better your results will be. You may also want to keep an activity journal to track your aerobic activities as well as your strength training. In this you can record the weights that you use with each workout, as well as the number of repetitions and sets performed. This enables you to monitor your progress and usually helps to motivate you.

POWER CARDIO

If you have had any success in the past with high-intensity workouts, my guess is that the past few pages of this chapter may have frustrated you. It's hard to convince avid weightlifters and spinning aficionados that moderate-intensity workouts are the best way to burn fat. Most everyone has been trained that the harder you work out and the more you sweat, the more fat you shed. I've already discussed the reasoning for my moderate-intensity preference, but let me explain this a little further before going on.

High-intensity anaerobic workouts obviously have proven value. Not only that, but also studies in recent years have shown that these "power cardio" routines can be just as effective as longer, moderate-intensity workouts. It's no surprise, then, that the American public, with its usual "faster is better" mind-set, has adopted this as the preferred way to lose fat. However, after helping thousands of overweight and obese individuals successfully lose weight and keep it off, I believe I have enough credentials to speak on this matter. And to me, it comes down to staying the course.

Remember all the diets you've tried in the past? Remember all the New Year's Days you committed to joining the gym and working out more? What happened in each of these cases? Your commitment fizzled. Something got in the way and distracted you enough to veer you from your ultimate goal. It's the same way with being active. I believe the biggest obstacle for most obese individuals is not working out; it's adopting that activity as part of a lifestyle. And just as I've said throughout this book, if you can't do it for life, you won't do it for long!

Let me offer a suggestion for those who have exercised religiously in the past or who bore quickly with moderate-intensity workouts. Try varying it up once in a while with some high-intensity interval training (HIIT). Notice the word *interval*, however. This is simply alternating between brief, hard bursts of exercise and short stretches of lower-intensity exercise or rest. Various studies in recent years have proven this to be an effective way to improve not only overall cardiovascular health but also your ability to burn fat faster. One study at the University of Guelph in Ontario, Canada, found that following an interval training session with an hour of moderate cycling increased the amount of fat burned by 36 percent.[14]

> ### HIGH-INTENSITY INTERVAL TRAINING (HIIT)
>
> High-intensity interval training (HIIT) mixes high-intensity bursts of exercise with moderate-intensity recovery periods, usually for a period of less than twenty minutes. It is used mostly for individuals trying to lose weight.

My suggestion is to hold off on HIIT, regardless of your exercise past, until you've consistently done some moderate-intensity activity for several months. I'd rather see you be able to sustain your momentum for the long haul rather than have you burn out, not because of eating the wrong things, but simply because you wanted to sprint to the finish line faster.

PUTTING IT ALL TOGETHER

To lose weight, you can literally start your activity program on the right foot. Unless you are physically restricted, walking is the easiest way to stay active. All you need for equipment are some comfortable clothes and a good pair of walking shoes. It's a great way to enjoy the outdoors, and with a walking partner, you can even catch up on conversation while he or she keeps you accountable with your exercise. Change your walking routine periodically; go to a park or a hiking trail in order to have variety.

As the sidebar on this page states, it is also proven that monitoring your exercise yields better results.[15] An excellent way to monitor your walking during the day is by using a pedometer. (See Appendix H.) I urge all my patients to get one and track their step count during the day. Typically a person walks three thousand to five thousand steps a day. To stay fit, your goal should be around ten thousand steps, which is approximately five miles, but to lose weight, you should aim for between twelve thousand and fifteen thousand daily steps a day. Other ways to get your daily twelve-thousand-plus steps are by walking your dog, parking farther out in the parking lot when going shopping or at work, and taking the stairs instead of the elevator whenever possible.

KEEPING TRACK

Researchers say that self-monitoring devices such as a pedometer, heart rate monitor, or even a simple exercise journal can account for a 25 percent increase in successfully controlling your weight.[16] (See Appendix H.)

Before engaging in any activity, make sure that you have either eaten a meal two or three hours prior, or you have a healthy snack about thirty minutes to an hour beforehand. It is never good to work out when you are hungry because you may end up burning muscle protein as energy—which is very expensive fuel since losing muscle lowers your metabolic rate.

After you have gotten into the routine of regularly walking for approximately thirty minutes five to six days a week, or you're getting your twelve thousand steps a day on your pedometer, you can then begin strength training. Before your strengthening routine, always do a five-minute warm-up by walking on a treadmill or elliptical machine or riding a stationary bike at low intensity. This increases blood flow to your muscles and joints, prepares the muscles and joints for strengthening workouts, and significantly reduces the risk of injury.

Once you have warmed up, practice mindfulness as you do a twenty- to thirty-minute strengthening workout using free weights, machines, calisthenics, Pilates, or some other strengthening activity. This burns up much of the glycogen stored in the muscles and liver. Following this you will be ready for a thirty-minute aerobic workout, such as brisk walking on a treadmill, cycling, or using an elliptical machine or other cardio equipment. This aerobic session allows you to mainly burn fat.

When you are finished with both the strength and aerobic parts of your workout, cool down by doing a low-intensity aerobic activity for another five minutes just like your warm-up. You may also want to do some stretching after your cooldown.

I recommend you perform a strengthening program three to four days a week every other day for twenty to thirty minutes, along with an aerobic program five to six days each week for thirty minutes. Always remember to warm up before starting any activity and cool down at the end of the program. And keep things fun by periodically changing up your routine. By varying your activities every month or so, you can shock your muscles into new growth—which, as we know by now, means more fat burned.

For starters, simply begin walking for twenty minutes a day or for ten minutes twice a day. Walk slow enough that you can talk but fast enough that you can't sing. Remember, 94 percent of the "effective losers" of the National Weight Control Registry increased their activity, with walking the most reported form of activity.[17]

"Can Do" Points to Remember

1. Adults typically lose ½ to 1 pound of muscle each year after the age of twenty-five.

2. Your activity goal should be to stay within your target heart rate zone, which is where you'll burn the most fat.

3. If you are overweight or obese, working out at a higher intensity for long stretches may not only sabotage your ability to burn fat, but it may also increase cortisol levels, which can cause more belly fat to accumulate.

4. Moderate-intensity activity is usually walking slowly enough so that you can talk but fast enough so that you cannot sing.

5. As you increase your stamina, you can complement your moderate-intensity activities with strengthening activities and eventually high-intensity interval training.

21

SUPPLEMENTING YOUR WEIGHT LOSS

I HEARD A STORY recently of a four-year-old boy who, like most boys his age, loved to hang around his dad whenever something needed fixing around the house. He would watch his dad like a hawk, observing how he studied the problem, thought through the situation, and then resolved it in a matter of minutes. While sitting in his Sunday school class at church one week, the boy listened as his teacher shared about how God loved people so much that He sent His own Son to fix their natural brokenness. "Does anyone know how God could mend a broken soul?" the teacher asked. The boy quickly raised his hand and then proudly said, "My dad says you can fix *anything* with duct tape."

Too many people are just as naïve when it comes to fixing their weight problem. Instead of duct tape, they think a certain diet pill will do the trick, or that by downing the latest health drink a few times a day their extra pounds will somehow suddenly disappear. Many of these individuals are looking for a magic pill that will enable them to eat anything they want, never exercise, and yet lose weight.

Unfortunately, no such pill exists. Oh sure, amphetamines will appear to do the trick for a little while. They'll suppress appetite and accelerate metabolism, allowing you to lose weight for a time. But the adverse reactions can be extreme: insomnia, nervousness, palpitations, headaches, arrhythmias, angina, heart attack, stroke, hypertension, hostility, aggressive behavior, and addiction, to name a few. Amphetamines may also worsen depression and anxiety, and they can produce equally severe reactions as those I just listed when you stop taking them. In fact, one of the most common withdrawal responses among users is that they not only regain the weight they had lost, but they also generally gain even more weight than when they started.

SEARCHING FOR THE MAGIC BULLET

For years doctors, researchers, pharmaceutical companies, and nutritional companies have been on the hunt for The Pill to End All Diets. In the early

1990s, researchers believed they had finally found this magic bullet when they combined two appetite suppressants, phentermine and fenfluramine. This drug combo, known as fen-phen, was a hit and effectively suppressed appetite. Individuals who took fen-phen lost weight and kept it off as long as they continued on the medication. Studies revealed the stunning results: on average, most users lost almost 16 percent of their body weight in just eight months. That correlates to a 200-pound person, for example, losing an impressive 32 pounds in just eight months.

> **WILLING TO PAY**
>
> Sales of weight-loss drugs in the United States, Europe, and Japan reached $600 million in 2005 and are expected to surge worldwide to $2 billion by 2010.[2]

As you would expect, once this was discovered, weight-loss clinics sprung up across America, and many doctors began prescribing this miracle pill combo. But after only a few years of prescribing this, a tiny percentage of users began dying of an extremely rare disease called primary pulmonary hypertension (PPH). Three or four patients out of one hundred thousand were affected, and about half of those eventually required a heart-lung transplant in order to survive. To their credit, the drug companies immediately pulled the two fenfluramine drugs, Pondimin and its derivitive Redux, off the market. However, phentermine was found to be relatively safe.

A few years later, supplement companies once again believed they had found the magic pill combo by combining the herb ephedra with caffeine. This too formed a powerful formula that was able to turn down the appetite while burning fat. But over the years, both the effectiveness and the safety of ephedra have been called into question and remain highly controversial. Ephedra has been linked to severe side effects, including arrhythmias, heart attack, stroke, hypertension, psychosis, seizure, and even death. To show what a major concern this is, you only have to look at a single statistic from the National Institutes of Health: products containing ephedra comprise less than 1 percent of all dietary supplement sales, yet those products are responsible for an incredible *64 percent* of adverse reactions from dietary supplements.[1]

In 2004, the Food and Drug Administration (FDA) finally banned ephedra products in the United States due to safety concerns. However, the ban was quickly overturned. As of this book's printing, ephedra is legal in the United States, but its use is still controversial. A few ephedra-related herbs such as bitter orange (citrus aurantium) and country mallow are still on the market. Like ephedra, bitter orange supplements have also been linked to stroke, cardiac arrest, angina, heart attack, ventricular arrhythmias, and death. These

products are potentially lethal, and I do not recommend them unless under the direction of a knowledgeable physician who can regularly monitor you.

Among other herbs that should cause concern is aristolochia, which is found in some Chinese herbal weight-loss supplements and may not even be listed as an ingredient. Aristolochia is a known kidney toxin and carcinogen in humans. There are also products containing usnea (usnic acid), a lichen for weight loss that can cause severe liver toxicity. In addition, some Brazilian diet pills have been found to be contaminated with amphetamines and other prescription drugs.[3]

ALLI AND HYDROXYCUT SIDE EFFECTS

Alli, one of the most common over-the-counter diet pills, may cause bowel changes in its users. These changes, which result from undigested fat going through the digestive system, may include: gas with an oily discharge, loose stools or diarrhea, more frequent and urgent bowel movements, and hard-to-control bowel movements.

Hydroxycut products were recalled in May 2009 after reports of deadly liver failure and disease in individuals who took the products to lose weight. According to the *World Journal of Gastroenterology*, an ingredient in Hydroxycut from a fruit called *Garcinia cambogia* caused the liver disease and failure.[4]

MEANT TO SUPPLEMENT, NOT REPLACE

I hope you are beginning to understand that for every supposed magic weight-loss pill, potential dangerous side effects loom nearby. Unfortunately, these often remain undiscovered until thousands, if not millions, of hopeful dieters have used them—and a few of those have died. Let me remind you, the foundation for weight loss is simply a healthy dietary plan and a regular activity program. The main reason people are overweight or obese is because of increased calorie intake and decreased physical activity. It's certainly not because they failed to discover the latest product promising to instantly shed those extra pounds.

A weight-loss supplement is a nutritional product or herb intended to *assist* your healthy eating and activity plan with the ultimate goal of losing weight. A supplement comes alongside; it does not replace. Do not be deceived by crafty marketing schemes that promise otherwise. Most supplements for weight loss have no sound clinical research supporting their claims, and some are downright dangerous. It's important to realize that weight-loss and dietary supplements are not subject to the same standards as prescription drugs or medications sold over the counter. They can be marketed with only limited proof of safety or effectiveness.

However, there are a number of safe and fairly effective dietary supplements that look promising for weight loss. Each supplement has its own unique mechanism of action for weight loss, with some having more than one. I have categorized these beneficial and proven supplements into the following categories:

- Thermogenic agents (fat-burning agents)
- Appetite suppressants
- Supplements to increase satiety
- Supplements to improve insulin sensitivity
- Supplements to increase energy production

There are many causes of obesity; however, aging is one of the most common reasons. There is a decrease in energy expenditure associated with aging, which may cause 120–190 excess calories to be stored in the body every day, according to scientists. This may mean an extra 13–20 pounds of extra body fat a year.[5] Since there are many causes of obesity, I recommend adding a few safe nutritional supplements that work through different mechanisms such as thermogenic agents, natural appetite suppressants that increase satiety, supplements that increase insulin sensitivity, and energy products. In treating hypertension, heart disease, diabetes, and other diseases, doctors add different medications with different mechanisms of action because when they are combined, their action is synergetic and more powerful. We now have very safe natural supplements that work by different mechanisms in helping an individual lose weight. Combining these will usually increase their effectiveness.

> **GREEN IS GOOD**
>
> A study found that after three months of taking green tea extract, overall body weight went down by 4.6 percent while waist circumference decreased by 4.48 percent.[6]

THERMOGENIC (FAT-BURNING) AGENTS

The term *thermogenic* describes the body's natural means of raising its temperature to burn off more calories. More specifically, thermogenesis is the process of triggering the body to burn white body fat, which is the kind of fat we often accumulate in excess as we age—the kind we typically see in overweight or obese people. Thermogenic agents, then, are fat burners that help

to increase the rate of white body fat breakdown. Fortunately, most unsafe thermogenic agents have been pulled off the market.

Green tea

Green tea and green tea extract are my favorite weight-loss supplements. Green tea has been used for thousands of years in Asia as both a tea and an herbal medicine. It has two key ingredients, a catechin called epigallo-catechin gallate (EGCG) and caffeine, both of which lead to the release of more epinephrine, which then increases the metabolic rate. Ultimately, green tea promotes fat oxidation, which is fat burning. It also increases the rate at which you burn calories over a twenty-four-hour period.

An effective daily dose of EGCG is 90 milligrams or more, which can also be consumed by drinking three or four cups of green tea a day. Do not add sugar, honey, or artificial sweeteners to your tea; instead use the natural sweetener stevia.

Italian researchers created a green tea phytosome by combining green tea polyphenols with phospholipids, which caused a significant increase in the absorption of the polyphenols, including EGCG. A clinical trial involved one hundred significantly overweight subjects. Half the group received the green tea phytosome in a dose of two 150-milligram tablets daily. Both groups were placed on a reduced-calorie diet (1,850 calories a day for men; 1,350 calories a day for women). However, after forty-five days, the control group lost an average of 4 pounds and the green tea phytosome group lost an average of 13 pounds, which was triple the amount of the control group. After ninety days, the control group lost an average of 9.9 pounds, and the green tea group lost 30.1 pounds. There was a 10 percent decrease of waist circumference in the green tea phytosome group and a 5 percent reduction in the control group.[7] I recommend 100 milligrams of green tea phytosome three times a day. (See Appendix H.)

> ### BUT CAN IT CLEAN MY HOUSE?
>
> It's no wonder Chinese doctors have used green tea for centuries as a cure-all. Drinking green tea has not only been proven to help prevent cancer and help with rheumatoid arthritis, high cholesterol, cardiovascular disease, infection, and impaired immune function, but it can also help prevent tooth decay!

Fucoxanthin

Derived from various types of edible seaweed, this carotenoid was traditionally only known for its antioxidant powers. However, research in recent

years has uncovered another major benefit to fucoxanthin: losing weight. Although early studies were done exclusively on animals, causing many critics to discredit its effectiveness in burning human fat, recent studies involving people are beginning to change this. Evidence of one such study found that combining fucoxanthin and pomegranate seed oil significantly increases metabolism. After sixteen weeks, researchers reported that those using the combination supplement had lost 15 pounds, compared to the average of 3 pounds lost by those taking a placebo.[8]

As we age, our metabolic rate naturally decreases, which prompts more storage of white body fat. Most people automatically turn to diets to solve this problem. But what is often overlooked is that aging brings about a decline in our *resting* metabolic rate, meaning that the white body fat we naturally store is no longer burned as quickly while we are sedentary. For this reason, fucoxanthin appears to be a good supplement that can increase resting energy, decrease abdominal and liver fat storage, and ultimately reduce your overall body weight.[9] A commonly recommended dose of fucoxanthin is 5 milligrams three times a day. You can find this supplement in most health food stores.

Appetite Suppressants

These supplements generally act on the central nervous system to decrease appetite or create a sensation of satiety or fullness. Although some medications in this category include risk-prone phenylpropanolamine (found in products such as Dexatrim), I have found a few safe, natural supplements that are extremely effective appetite suppressants.

L-tryptophan and 5-HTP

L-tryptophan and 5-hydroxytryptophan (commonly known as 5-HTP) are amino acids that help to manufacture serotonin. As we learned in the early chapters of this book, serotonin assists in controlling carbohydrate and sugar cravings. L-tryptophan and 5-HTP also function like natural antidepressants. If you are taking migraine medications called triptans or SSRI (selective serotonin reuptake inhibitors) antidepressants, you should talk with your physician before taking either L-tryptophan or 5-HTP. The typical dosage of L-tryptophan is 500 to 2,000 milligrams at bedtime; for 5-HTP the dose is typically 50 to 100 milligrams three times a day. I prefer 5-HTP for most of my patients. (See Appendix H.)

THE PROGRAM

L-tyrosine, N-acetyl L-tyrosine, and L-phenylalanine

L-tyrosine, N-acetyl L-tyrosine, and L-phenylalanine are naturally occurring amino acids found in numerous protein foods, including cottage cheese, turkey, and chicken. They help to raise norepinephrine and dopamine levels in the brain, which then helps to decrease appetite, cravings, and improve your mood. (SAM-e is another amino acid that helps raise norepinephrine and dopamine levels.) Doses of L-tyrosine, N-acetyl L-tyrosine, and L-phenylalanine may range from 500 to 2,000 milligrams a day (and sometimes higher), but they should be taken on an empty stomach. I prefer N-acetyl L-tyrosine for most of my patients since it is even better absorbed than L-tyrosine or L-phenylalanine. My patients typically start with 500 milligrams of L-tyrosine thirty minutes before breakfast and thirty minutes before lunch. (See Appendix H.) I do not recommend taking any of these supplements in the late afternoon because it may interfere with sleep.

> ## WHAT'S THE POINT IF A PILL CAN DO IT?
>
> Marketing researchers have found that the more proven a drug is to be effective at shedding pounds, the more lax the efforts of the user at continuing to eat well and exercise. Those who take prescription or over-the-counter diet pills are more likely to engage in eating junk food and living a sedentary lifestyle.[11]

SUPPLEMENTS TO INCREASE SATIETY

Fiber supplements and foods high in fiber increase satiety by using several different mechanisms. Fiber slows the passage of food through the digestive tract, decreases the absorption of sugars and starches into the stomach, and expands and fills up the stomach—which obviously turns down the appetite. Although the American Heart Association and the National Cancer Institute recommend 30 grams or more of fiber each day, the average American only consumes between 12 to 17 grams a day.[10]

> ## FIBER AWAY!
>
> In addition to PGX, another great fiber for weight loss is glucomannan, made from the Asian root konjac. Glucomannan is five times more effective in lowering cholesterol compared to other fibers such as psyllium, oat fiber, or guar gum. Because it expands to ten times its original size when placed in water, it is a great supplement to take before a meal to reduce your appetite as it expands in your stomach.

Soluble fiber

The two main types of fiber are soluble and insoluble fiber. Insoluble fibers are

important for the GI tract and help to relieve constipation and gas. They increase the size of the stool, improve stool transit time, and help to sweep the colon clean. Soluble fiber, on the other hand, helps with weight loss by increasing satiety. It actually acts similar to a sponge, binding toxins, lowering cholesterol and triglycerides, and stabilizing blood sugar levels. Soluble fibers are found in such foods as oat bran, oats, flaxseeds, barley, legumes, beans, lentils, peas, seeds, fruits, and vegetables.

A little fiber goes a long way when it comes to losing weight. One study found that consuming an extra 14 grams of soluble fiber each day for only two days was associated with a 10 percent decrease in caloric intake.[12] Soluble fiber supplements also significantly increase post-meal satisfaction and should be taken before each meal to assist in weight loss.

Many people shy away from fiber because of gas, diarrhea, or other bowel disturbances that occur when it is first taken. However, most of these are purely related to the initial amounts being excessive. To avoid these side effects, start with a low dose of soluble fiber (one capsule of PGX fiber) taken before each meal, and slowly increase the dose (to two to four capsules) over two to three weeks. As your body adjusts to the increased fiber intake, the side effects will usually disappear. Also, by combining soluble fiber with insoluble fiber, these side effects are often lessened considerably.

Taking soluble fiber before meals helps you feel satisfied sooner and usually decreases the amount of calories consumed. One study showed that 7 grams of psyllium (another fiber supplement) before a meal decreased hunger and food intake while stabilizing blood sugar and insulin levels. In fact, special fiber blends such as

PGX Fiber

PGX is short for PolyGlycoPlex and is a unique blend of highly viscous fibers that act synergistically to create a much higher level of viscosity than the individual fibers alone. The viscosity is the gelling property. PGX absorbs hundreds of times its weight in water over one to two hours and expands in the digestive tract, creating a thick gelatinous material. It creates a feeling of fullness, stabilizes the blood sugar and insulin levels, and stabilizes appetite hormones. PGX lowers blood sugar after eating by about 20 percent and lowers insulin secretions by about 40 percent. Researchers have found that higher doses of PGX can decrease appetite significantly. PGX also has fewer gastrointestinal side effects than other viscous dietary fibers. However, start slowly or you may develop gas. It works similar to gastric banding.

Read More About It

Please refer to my book *The New Bible Cure for Diabetes* for more information.

glucomannan, xanthan, and alginate (PGX) appear to be even more effective than taking a single type of soluble fiber. In another study, participants took six PGX capsules before every meal. By the end of the three-week study, those taking the PGX had decreased their body fat by 2.8 percent.[13] Therefore, a blend of different soluble fiber appears to be even more effective than most single types of soluble fiber. (See Appendix H.)

The fiber that I prefer for my weight-loss patients is PGX fiber. I start them with one capsule with 8–16 ounces of water before each meal and snack, and then gradually increase the dose to two to four capsules until the appetite is controlled. However, it is most important to take with the evening meal and evening snack. (See Appendix H.)

SUPPLEMENTS TO IMPROVE INSULIN RESISTANCE

Approximately one-quarter of the adult population in the United States has metabolic syndrome, the underlying cause of which is insulin resistance. As we've touched on throughout this book, high insulin levels can lead to obesity, especially truncal obesity or belly fat, as well as a host of other diseases. The key to overcoming insulin resistance is choosing low-glycemic foods, exercising to lose belly fat, and resensitizing the cells to insulin with supplements. The following supplements help to resensitize cells to insulin.

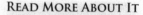
READ MORE ABOUT IT

For more information on insulin resistance and supplements to combat it, please refer to *The New Bible Cure for Diabetes.*

Irvingia gabonensis

Irvingia grows in the jungles of Cameroon in Africa. It appears to be able to reverse leptin resistance by lowering levels of C-reactive protein, an inflammatory mediator. In a double-blind study, 102 overweight participants received either 150 milligrams of Irvingia or a placebo twice a day for ten weeks. At the end of the ten weeks, the Irvingia group lost an average of 28 pounds and the placebo group just 1 pound. They also lost 6.7 inches from their waistline and decreased their total body fat by 18.4 percent. The Irvingia group also had a 26 percent reduction of total cholesterol, a 27 percent decrease in LDL, a 32 percent decrease in fasting

SUGAR DOWN

Cinnamon, omega-3 fats, chromium, vitamin D, and lipoic acid can all promote healthy glucose metabolism, which helps to lower blood sugar.

blood sugar, and the CRP fell by 52 percent.[14] Irvingia also has an inhibitory effect on an enzyme produced in fat cells that helps convert blood sugar to triglycerides (fat). Research has shown that Irvingia stimulates the expression of the adiponectin gene in the fat cells. Adiponectin plays an important role in normal metabolism. The recommended dose is 150 milligrams of standardized Irvingia extract two times a day. (See Appendix H.)

READ MORE ABOUT IT

Other supplements that improve insulin resistance, such as chromium, cinnamon, lipoic acid, vitamin D, and omega 3 fats, are disucssed in detail in my book *The New Bible Cure for Diabetes.*

SUPPLEMENTS TO INCREASE ENERGY PRODUCTION

L-carnitine

L-carnitine is an amino acid that functions as a transporter of energy by shuttling fatty acids into the mitochondria, which are the energy factories in our cells. These fatty acids are then burned as energy. In essence, L-carnitine helps us to turn food into energy. Humans synthesize very little carnitine, so we may need to supplement from outside sources. This applies especially to obese and older individuals, both of whom typically have lower levels of carnitine than those within the average-weight segment. As you might expect, individuals with insufficient carnitine have greater difficulty burning their fat for energy.

Milk, meat, fish, and cheese are good sources of L-carnitine, while mutton and lamb are also rich in the amino acid. In supplement form, I recommend combining L-carnitine with lipoic acid, coenzyme Q_{10}, and omega-3 fats to increase energy production. One form of carnitine, acetyl-L-carnitine, is also able to cross the blood brain barrier and increase the energy of brain cells. This has numerous neuroprotective benefits and helps to increase neurotransmitters in the brain. It also protects brain cells from the effects of stress.

Overall, I recommend a combination of L-carnitine and acetyl-L-carnitine to be taken with fish oil, coenzyme Q_{10}, and lipoic acid. Start by taking 500 milligrams a day of both L-carnitine and acetyl-L-carnitine, and if needed, gradually work up to 2 grams a day. It may take up to 4 grams a day for obese patients to notice the increased energy provided by these supplements. Yet by increasing your energy, you will be more likely to exercise regularly and burn more fat. The best time to take your carnitine supplements is in the morning and in the early afternoon (before 3:00 p.m.) on an empty stomach. Any later and this supplement can impair your sleep. You can find these supplements at most health food stores.

Also, green tea supplements as well as N-acetyl L-tyrosine help to increase your energy.

OTHER COMMON SUPPLEMENTS TO ASSIST WITH WEIGHT LOSS

Calcium

Both children and adults with a low calcium intake are more likely to gain weight or be overweight or obese when compared to individuals with a higher calcium intake. Dairy products, such as plain low-fat yogurt and kefir, that provide a total calcium intake of 800 to 1,200 milligrams a day help to lower body fat, increase muscle mass, and ultimately help with weight loss. However, it's interesting to note that taking calcium supplements alone does not appear to help with weight loss.

The Hoodia controversy

Hoodia is a South African plant similar to a cactus that may help to suppress the appetite. It was initially used by African tribe leaders to enable them to go on long journeys without getting hungry, and various sources cite thousands of years' worth of Bushman history to verify its effectiveness. Although these tribal hunters obviously have not conducted scientific studies to prove Hoodia as an effective appetite suppressant, one clinical study in 2001 by a company called Phytopharm found individuals who consumed the plant ate 1,000 fewer calories a day than those who didn't take Hoodia.[15] One of the company's researchers, Richard Dixey, MD, explained that Hoodia contains a molecule that is 10,000 times more active than glucose.[16]

There's a catch, however: when news broke about this supposed miracle supplement, dozens, if not hundreds, of companies began marketing bottles of Hoodia—without having any actual Hoodia in their products. The result was that more Hoodia was "produced" in a single year than in all of African history—which is unlikely, to say the least. Even today, it's possible that much of what's sold in the United States either contains ineffective Hoodia variations or no Hoodia at all.

IN SUMMARY

As you can see, there are some questionable products on the market, but there are also a variety of safe and effective over-the-counter dietary supplements for weight loss. Some people may find that incorporating a combination of these

into their eating and activity plans works wonders. Others may not need to take any supplements. Most of my overweight and obese patients in the past have found that at least drinking green tea or taking green tea phytosome, certain amino acids such as 5-HTP and N-acetyl L-tyrosine, PGX fiber supplements before each meal and snack (especially the evening meal and snack), and Irvingia helped them shed the pounds. There are many other supplements touted for weight loss; however, I have found the ones listed in this chapter to be more effective and very safe.

If you continue to have problems with controlling your appetite, or if you struggle with specific food cravings, decreased energy, or insulin resistance, you will likely require one or more of the supplements we covered in this chapter. The same goes if you do not feel full or satisfied after a meal, or if you have low hormone levels. I will remind you again, however, that a supplement is just that—a supplement. You will not find a magic pill or easy-fix to a situation that is probably years in the making—namely, your excess weight. The good news is that you don't have to be duped anymore by a wonder-working, "as seen on TV," flab-busting promise. Armed with the proper eating and activity plans, you can do this—*successfully*—for life!

"CAN DO" POINTS TO REMEMBER

1. No magic pill, herb, or medicine for weight loss exists. You will always need to follow a healthy lifestyle, including healthy food choices and a regular activity program.

2. A weight-loss supplement is a nutritional product or herb intended to *assist*—not replace—your healthy eating and activity plan with the ultimate goal of losing weight.

3. Green tea helps promote fat-burning.

4. L-tryptophan, 5-HTP, and N-acetyl L-tyrosine may help control food cravings.

5. The average American only consumes between 12 and 17 grams of fiber a day, which is about half the recommended amount.

6. L-carnitine can increase energy production and may help your body burn fat.

SECTION IV

WHEN WEIGHT LOSS STALLS OR STOPS

22

WHAT'S KEEPING YOU FROM LOSING WEIGHT? TAKE THE TEST AND FIND OUT!

YOU'VE BEEN THERE: For the first few weeks, the pounds seem to drop off like never before. Your eating plan isn't too hard, you are exercising well, and you feel invigorated and energized. And then it hits: the dreaded plateau. First, your weight loss hits what you think is a "momentary" standstill. Then the days turn into weeks, and your momentum seems to evaporate. Finally, discouragement settles in, and within a few weeks you've abandoned ship

Before I go any further, let me remind you that this is completely normal. Plateaus are a part of losing weight. In fact, after helping thousands of patients, I have yet to find one who, in trying to lose a significant amount of weight, did not at some point reach a plateau. I understand that these apparent holding patterns can cause you to feel discouraged, disappointed, and frustrated.

However, the following test, which has been broken into several questionnaires, will help you to determine if there are any underlying conditions in your body that are interfering with your best efforts to lose weight. I encourage you to take every questionnaire that follows as there may be more than one weight-loss saboteur for you to tackle. Some questionnaires have similar questions as symptoms may overlap. Even though you may have many of the symptoms of a particular disorder, a lab test is more definitive than the results of a questionnaire. Therefore I encourage you to follow up with a knowledgeable physician for the appropriate lab tests. (See Appendix H to find a knowledgeable physician.)

After completing each questionnaire, please read chapter 23 to find out what you can do to begin to overcome your roadblocks to weight loss. For even more complete information, go to www.thecandodiet.com and complete the same questionnaires that appear in this book. You will receive immediate results online and be directed to more than ten chapters' worth of advice addressing those specific roadblocks that we simply could not fit in this book.

Neurotransmitter Deficiency Questionnaires

Norepinephrine deficiency

	YES	NO
1. Do you feel hungry throughout most of the day?	☐	☐
2. Do you have an insatiable appetite or eat large meals?	☐	☐
3. Do you not know when to stop eating?	☐	☐
4. Do you never really feel full or satisfied even after eating?	☐	☐
5. Can you eat almost anything in sight?	☐	☐
6. Do you feel out of control, especially with your appetite?	☐	☐
7. Do you think about food most of the time?	☐	☐
8. Do you crave starches (breads and pastas) rather than sweets or junk food?	☐	☐
9. Do you have or have you even been diagnosed with ADD or ADHD?	☐	☐
10. Are you especially hungry in the late afternoon and evening?	☐	☐
11. Are you always tired, run-down, or chronically fatigued?	☐	☐
12. Do you have low energy levels?	☐	☐
13. Are you too tired to exercise?	☐	☐
14. Do you feel down, depressed, or just blah?	☐	☐
15. Do you wake up tired?	☐	☐
16. Is it difficult for you to get going in the morning?	☐	☐
17. Are you exhausted in the afternoon or need an afternoon nap?	☐	☐
18. Do you have problems focusing, concentrating, or staying alert?	☐	☐
19. Are you easily distracted?	☐	☐
20. Are you mentally sluggish?	☐	☐
21. Do you have a hard time finishing or starting a project or task?	☐	☐
22. Do you have problems getting motivated?	☐	☐

Points for each "yes" answer:

- Questions 1–7: 5 points each   Subtotal_____
- Questions 8–22: 2 points each   Subtotal_____

Total_____

SCORE:

- 0–10: Unlikely you have norepinephrine deficiency
- 11–19: Mild norepinephrine deficiency
- 20–29: Moderate norepinephrine deficiency
- 30+: Severe norepinephrine deficiency

NEUROTRANSMITTER DEFICIENCY QUESTIONNAIRES

Serotonin deficiency   YES NO

1. Do you crave sweets or starches in the afternoon and evening? ☐ ☐
2. Do you crave chocolate, or do you find chocolate irresistible at times? ☐ ☐
3. Do you eat when you are stressed, anxious, lonely, depressed, angry, or experiencing any other distressing emotion? ☐ ☐
4. Do you think about food constantly? ☐ ☐
5. Are you a compulsive eater, or are you obsessed with food? ☐ ☐
6. Do you find yourself eating, snacking, or munching unconsciously? ☐ ☐
7. Do you eat when you are not hungry? ☐ ☐
8. Do you binge on foods or eat massive quantities of food at one time? ☐ ☐
9. Do you wake up in the middle of the night and eat? ☐ ☐
10. Do you eat unconsciously and wonder why afterward? ☐ ☐
11. Do you eat such large quantities of food that you get nauseated? ☐ ☐
12. Are you depressed, irritable, frustrated, or moody? ☐ ☐
13. Do you suffer from insomnia regularly? ☐ ☐
14. Do you find it difficult to fall back asleep when you are awakened? ☐ ☐
15. Are you tired or just don't have enough energy to exercise? ☐ ☐
16. Do you have problems relaxing? ☐ ☐
17. Do you have generalized anxiety, panic attacks, bulimia, phobias, or obsessive-compulsive disorder, or are you just nervous or anxious? ☐ ☐
18. Do you have migraine headaches? ☐ ☐
19. Do you have irritable bowel syndrome? ☐ ☐
20. Women, do you have PMS? ☐ ☐
21. Do sugar cravings increase dramatically at the time of your period? ☐ ☐

Points for each "yes" answer:

- Questions 1–8: 5 points each   Subtotal_____
- Questions 9–21: 2 points each   Subtotal_____
                                                            Total_____

SCORE:

- 0–10: Unlikely you have serotonin deficiency
- 11–19: Mild serotonin deficiency
- 20–29: Moderate serotonin deficiency
- 30+: Severe serotonin deficiency

NEUROTRANSMITTER DEFICIENCY QUESTIONNAIRES

Dopamine deficiency
                                                                    YES NO

1. Do you regularly crave salty foods or fatty foods such as steak, hamburgers, bacon, sausage, salami, pepperoni, or a meat lover's pizza? ☐ ☐
2. Do you regularly crave salty starches such as french fries, potato chips, corn chips, pretzels, popcorn, or crackers? ☐ ☐
3. Do you feel depressed or down, or do you lack an interest in life? ☐ ☐
4. Do you find it difficult to enjoy life or to get motivated? ☐ ☐
5. Are you or have you ever been addicted to alcohol, cigarettes, drugs, gambling, sex, or food? Or do you have an addictive personality? ☐ ☐
6. Do you have a strong family history of addictions? ☐ ☐
7. Do you have sexual problems such as delayed orgasm or an inability to have an orgasm? ☐ ☐
8. Do you have a decreased sex drive? ☐ ☐
9. Are you tired, or do you have a significant loss of energy? ☐ ☐
10. Are you mentally sluggish? ☐ ☐
11. Do you drink coffee or caffeinated beverages to keep you going? ☐ ☐
12. Are you a procrastinator? ☐ ☐
13. Are you forgetful, or do you fail to listen to or follow instructions? ☐ ☐
14. Do you regularly isolate yourself from others? ☐ ☐
15. Do you have an inability to handle stress? ☐ ☐
16. Do you have episodes of low blood sugar with light-headedness, irritability, extreme hunger, and cloudy thinking? ☐ ☐
17. Do you get excessive amounts of sleep and still awaken tired? ☐ ☐
18. Do you regularly have mood swings? ☐ ☐
19. Are you easily angered, irritated, or frustrated? ☐ ☐
20. Do you rarely get excited about anything? ☐ ☐
21. Do you need medication to cope with or forget your problems? ☐ ☐

Points for each "yes" answer:
- Questions 1–5: 5 points each   Subtotal_____
- Questions 6–21: 2 points each   Subtotal_____
                                        Total_____

SCORE:
- 0–10: Unlikely you have dopamine deficiency
- 11–19: Mild dopamine deficiency
- 20–29: Moderate dopamine deficiency
- 30+: Severe dopamine deficiency

See Appendix H for neuroscience testing if you have a neurotransmitter deficiency.

FOOD ADDICTIONS QUESTIONNAIRE

	YES	NO
1. After bingeing on foods, do you purge later with vomiting, laxatives, or other methods?	☐	☐
2. Do you have obsessive thoughts about food?	☐	☐
3. Do you binge on food?	☐	☐
4. Do you eat to relieve stress or worry?	☐	☐
5. Do you continue to eat even though you are full?	☐	☐
6. Do you feel guilty or ashamed after you eat?	☐	☐
7. Do you eat alone or in secret?	☐	☐
8. Do you hide food or stash it away so that you can eat it when no one is watching?	☐	☐
9. Do you never refuse food when it is available even though you are not hungry?	☐	☐
10. Do you eat such a large amount of food that you feel sick?	☐	☐
11. Do you eat at a fast pace so that you can eat more?	☐	☐
12. After dieting and losing weight, do you binge on food?	☐	☐
13. Do you eat when you are not hungry?	☐	☐
14. Do you eat differently while in front of others than you do when you are alone?	☐	☐
15. Do you eat foods that you know are harmful to you?	☐	☐

Points for each "yes" answer:

- Questions 1–3: 5 points each   Subtotal_____
- Questions 4–15: 2 points each   Subtotal_____

Total_____

SCORE:

- 0–4: Unlikely you have a food addiction
- 5+: Likely you have a food addiction

Metabolically Compromised Questionnaire

	YES	NO
1. Have you followed more than one fad diet for a few months or longer?	☐	☐
2. Have you lost weight and regained the weight on more than two occasions (yo-yo dieting)?	☐	☐
3. Do you take steroids such as prednisone on a regular basis?	☐	☐
4. Do you take antipsychotic medications?	☐	☐
5. Do you take lithium?	☐	☐
6. Do you take insulin?	☐	☐
7. Did you start gaining weight when you stopped smoking?	☐	☐
8. Do you take antidepressants?	☐	☐
9. Do you take heartburn medication?	☐	☐
10. Do you take high blood pressure medication?	☐	☐
11. Do you take antihistamines for allergies?	☐	☐
12. Do you use diabetic medication?	☐	☐

Points for each "yes" answer:

- Questions 1–2: 10 points each   Subtotal_____
- Questions 3–7: 5 points each   Subtotal_____
- Questions 8–12: 2 points each   Subtotal_____

Total_____

SCORE:

- 0–4: Unlikely you are metabolically compromised
- 5–10: Mildly metabolically compromised
- 11–19: Moderately metabolically compromised
- 20+: Severely metabolically compromised

CHRONIC STRESS QUESTIONNAIRES

	YES	NO
1. Are you in serious financial debt?	☐	☐
2. Are you feeling overwhelmed on your job, or is it too stressful?	☐	☐
3. Is your marriage too stressful, or are you going through a divorce?	☐	☐
4. Do you suffer from anxiety, depression, or nervousness?	☐	☐
5. Do you have any legal problems or IRS problems?	☐	☐
6. Do you have frequent problems sleeping or insomnia?	☐	☐
7. Do you frequently argue with your spouse?	☐	☐
8. Do you have frequent arguments or disagreements with your children?	☐	☐
9. Do you have too many obligations?	☐	☐
10. Do you have a child in rebellion?	☐	☐
11. Are you too busy?	☐	☐
12. Are you easily upset, frustrated, or irritated?	☐	☐
13. Do you have problems saying no to the requests of others?	☐	☐
14. Are your neck and shoulder muscles frequently tight?	☐	☐
15. Do you grind your teeth at night or suffer from TMJ?	☐	☐
16. Do you suffer from irritable bowel syndrome?	☐	☐
17. Are you a compulsive eater?	☐	☐
18. Do you have a critical attitude?	☐	☐
19. Are you easily angered?	☐	☐
20. Have you lost your sense of humor, or do you rarely laugh?	☐	☐
21. Are you forgetful, or do you have problems thinking clearly?	☐	☐
22. Are you always running late?	☐	☐
23. Do you frequently drive in heavy traffic?	☐	☐

Points for each "yes" answer:

- Questions 1–5: 5 points each   Subtotal_____
- Questions 6–23: 2 points each   Subtotal_____

Total_____

SCORE:

- 0–10: Unlikely you are overly stressed
- 11–19: Mildly overstressed
- 20–29: Moderately overstressed
- 30+: Severely overstressed

Chronic Stress Questionnaires

Adrenal fatigue

	YES	NO
1. Are you chronically fatigued?	☐	☐
2. Do you crave salt or salty foods?	☐	☐
3. Do you get light-headed when you stand up rapidly?	☐	☐
4. Do you have regular bouts of hypoglycemia (low blood sugar)?	☐	☐
5. Are you so lethargic that even the simplest chores become a major challenge?	☐	☐
6. Are you most fatigued in the early morning and again in the afternoon between 3:00 p.m. and 5:00 p.m.?	☐	☐
7. Do you feel better around 6:00 p.m. and get another boost of energy at 11:00 p.m.?	☐	☐
8. Is your best sleep between 7:00 a.m. and 9:00 a.m.?	☐	☐
9. Do you need one or more cups of coffee or some other stimulant to get going in the morning?	☐	☐
10. Do you have a reduced ability to withstand emotional pressure?	☐	☐
11. Do you lack stamina?	☐	☐
12. Do you have problems either sleeping or getting up in the morning?	☐	☐
13. Do you need to lie down and rest after a stressful event?	☐	☐
14. Do you have allergies, sensitivities, asthma, or eczema?	☐	☐
15. Do you have problems concentrating, especially before lunch?	☐	☐
16. Are you easily confused?	☐	☐
17. Do you get frequent colds or infections?	☐	☐
18. Are you chronically nervous or suffer from anxiety?	☐	☐
19. Do you often feel apathetic?	☐	☐
20. Has your sex drive diminished?	☐	☐
21. Do you suffer from insomnia?	☐	☐

Points for each "yes" answer:

- Questions 1–8: 5 points each   Subtotal_____
- Questions 9–21: 2 points each   Subtotal_____

    Total_____

SCORE:

- 0–10: Unlikely you have adrenal fatigue
- 11–19: Mild adrenal fatigue
- 20–29: Moderate adrenal fatigue
- 30+: Severe adrenal fatigue

HORMONAL IMBALANCE QUESTIONNAIRES

Estrogen deficiency (for women only)	YES	NO
1. Do you have vaginal dryness?	☐	☐
2. Do you have more wrinkles than the average person your age?	☐	☐
3. Have you noticed a decrease in breast size?	☐	☐
4. Do you have droopy or sagging breasts?	☐	☐
5. Do you have hot flashes or night sweats?	☐	☐
6. Have your menstrual periods stopped?	☐	☐
7. Is your skin thinner?	☐	☐
8. Do you have a hollow face?	☐	☐
9. Do you have osteopenia or osteoporosis?	☐	☐
10. Is intercourse painful?	☐	☐
11. Are you moody and irritable?	☐	☐
12. Do you have a menopot (potbelly)?	☐	☐
13. Do you have stress incontinence?	☐	☐
14. Do you have decreased sex drive?	☐	☐
15. Do you have decreased memory?	☐	☐
16. Do you have elevated cholesterol?	☐	☐
17. Do you have frequent urinary tract infections?	☐	☐
18. Do you have high blood pressure?	☐	☐
19. Do you have acne or oily skin?	☐	☐
20. Have you noticed a decrease in creativity?	☐	☐
21. Do you have insomnia?	☐	☐
22. Have you noticed a decrease in fine motor skills?	☐	☐
23. Are you depressed or anxious?	☐	☐
24. Are you tired or unmotivated?	☐	☐
25. Do you have dry or dehydrated skin?	☐	☐

Points for each "yes" answer:
- Questions 1–6: 5 points each   Subtotal_____
- Questions 7–25: 2 points each   Subtotal_____

Total_____

SCORE:
- 0–10: Unlikely you have estrogen deficiency
- 11–19: Mild estrogen deficiency
- 20–29: Moderate estrogen deficiency
- 30+: Severe estrogen deficiency

Hormonal Imbalance Questionnaires

Estrogen dominance (too much estrogen; for women only)   YES NO

1. Do you have fibrocystic breasts? ☐ ☐
2. Do you have uterine fibroids? ☐ ☐
3. Do your breasts become swollen? ☐ ☐
4. Do you have heavy periods? ☐ ☐
5. Do you have weight gain, especially in your hips, thighs, and abdomen? ☐ ☐
6. Do you take birth control pills or oral estrogen? ☐ ☐
7. Do you take equine estrogen (Premarin)? ☐ ☐
8. Do you regularly eat fatty cuts of meat, whole-fat dairy, and/or grains? ☐ ☐
9. Do you often experience abdominal bloating? ☐ ☐
10. Do you have mood swings and irritability? ☐ ☐
11. Do you have insomnia? ☐ ☐
12. Do you have anxiety or panic attacks? ☐ ☐
13. Have you had uterine cancer? ☐ ☐
14. Do you regularly get headaches? ☐ ☐
15. Do you have water retention? ☐ ☐
16. Do you have a decreased sex drive? ☐ ☐
17. Are you depressed? ☐ ☐
18. Are you easily agitated? ☐ ☐
19. Have you had cervical dysplasia? ☐ ☐
20. Have you had breast cancer (estrogen receptor positive)? ☐ ☐

Points for each "yes" answer:
- Questions 1–7: 5 points each   Subtotal_____
- Questions 8–20: 2 points each   Subtotal_____
                                  Total_____

SCORE:
- 0–10: Unlikely you have estrogen dominance
- 11–19: Mild estrogen dominance
- 20–29: Moderate estrogen dominance
- 30+: Severe estrogen dominance

HORMONAL IMBALANCE QUESTIONNAIRES

Progesterone deficiency (for women only)   YES NO

1. Do you have very heavy menstrual periods or irregular periods? ☐ ☐
2. Do you have PMS? ☐ ☐
3. Do you have significant premenstrual bloating? ☐ ☐
4. Are you irritable, aggressive, or have mood swings, especially prior to your menstrual periods? ☐ ☐
5. Do you have polycystic ovary syndrome? ☐ ☐
6. Do you take synthetic progesterone (progestins) or birth control pills? ☐ ☐
7. Did you have postpartum depression? ☐ ☐
8. Do you have anxiety or depression? ☐ ☐
9. Do have mood swings or irritability? ☐ ☐
10. Do you have osteoporosis or osteopenia? ☐ ☐
11. Do you have insomnia? ☐ ☐
12. Do you have bouts of excessive anger or outbursts of rage? ☐ ☐
13. Do you have panic attacks? ☐ ☐
14. Do you have an increased sensitivity to pain? ☐ ☐
15. Do you have a reddish face? ☐ ☐
16. Do you get swollen breasts? ☐ ☐
17. Do you get swollen feet and ankles? ☐ ☐
18. Do you have increased abdominal fat? ☐ ☐
19. Do you get a bloated abdomen? ☐ ☐
20. Do you get a swollen or puffy face? ☐ ☐
21. Do you have muscle tension? ☐ ☐

Points for each "yes" answer:

- Questions 1–6: 5 points each   Subtotal_____
- Questions 7–21: 2 points each   Subtotal_____
                                        Total_____

SCORE:

- 0–10: Unlikely you have progesterone deficiency
- 11–19: Mild progesterone deficiency
- 20–29: Moderate progesterone deficiency
- 30+: Severe progesterone deficiency

Hormonal Imbalance Questionnaires

Testosterone deficiency (for men and women)	YES	NO
1. Do you have a decrease in muscle size, strength, or tone?	☐	☐
2. Do you have a decreased sex drive?	☐	☐
3. Do you have thin skin or poor elasticity in your skin?	☐	☐
4. Do you have a decreased amount of pubic hair or axillary hair?	☐	☐
5. Have you developed thin lips, sagging cheeks, or droopy eyelids?	☐	☐
6. Have you lost muscle mass in your arms and legs and gained fat all over your body?	☐	☐
7. Have you become grumpy, irritable, or angry?	☐	☐
8. Are you tired, or do you suffer from decreased stamina?	☐	☐
9. Do you have decreased flexibility or increased stiffness?	☐	☐
10. Do you get frequent muscle and joint aches or neck and back pain?	☐	☐
11. Have you noticed a decrease in competitiveness?	☐	☐
12. Are you depressed or apathetic?	☐	☐
13. Has your interest in hobbies or things you once enjoyed decreased?	☐	☐
14. Are you more forgetful?	☐	☐
15. Do you feel burned out?	☐	☐
16. Have you noticed a decrease in mental sharpness?	☐	☐
17. Are you less motivated or less confident?	☐	☐
18. Do you get light-headed, dizzy, or experience ringing in the ears?	☐	☐
19. Do you have type 2 diabetes, obesity, hypertension, high cholesterol, prostate problems, or asthma?	☐	☐

Additional questions for men only

	YES	NO
20. Have you noticed a decrease in spontaneous early morning erections?	☐	☐
21. Do you have problems maintaining a full erection?	☐	☐
22. Do you have increased fat in the breast area or hips?	☐	☐

Points for each "yes" answer:

- Questions 1–6, 20–22: 5 points each   Subtotal_____
- Questions 7–19: 2 points each   Subtotal_____

Total_____

SCORE:

- 0–10: Unlikely you have testosterone deficiency
- 11–19: Mild testosterone deficiency
- 20–29: Moderate testosterone deficiency
- 30+: Severe testosterone deficiency

HORMONAL IMBALANCE QUESTIONNAIRES

Human growth hormone deficiency (for men and women)   YES NO

1. Has your body prematurely aged? ☐ ☐
2. Do you have a flabby, droopy abdomen? ☐ ☐
3. Do you have sagging triceps? ☐ ☐
4. Do you have decreased muscle size? ☐ ☐
5. Are you feeble, or do you feel like you have aged rapidly? ☐ ☐
6. Do you have sagging inner thighs? ☐ ☐
7. Do you have sagging back muscles? ☐ ☐
8. Do you have decreased muscle strength? ☐ ☐
9. Do you have decreased lean body mass? ☐ ☐
10. Do you have thin skin? ☐ ☐
11. Do you have droopy eyelids, sagging cheeks, thin lips, and wrinkly skin? ☐ ☐
12. Do you have decreased stamina? ☐ ☐
13. Are you obese, with fat replacing the muscles in your arms, legs, and hips? ☐ ☐
14. Have you lost thickness in the soles of your feet? ☐ ☐
15. Do you tend to be depressed? ☐ ☐
16. Do you lack self-confidence? ☐ ☐
17. Do you need a lot of sleep (nine hours or more)? ☐ ☐
18. Do you have a decreased appetite for meat? ☐ ☐
19. Are you chronically exhausted? ☐ ☐
20. Do you have cold intolerance? ☐ ☐

Points for each "yes" answer:
- Questions 1–9: 5 points each   Subtotal_____
- Questions 10–20: 2 points each   Subtotal_____

Total_____

SCORE:
- 0–10: Unlikely you have human growth hormone deficiency
- 11–19: Mild human growth hormone deficiency
- 20–29: Moderate human growth hormone deficiency
- 30+: Severe human growth hormone deficiency

INSULIN RESISTANCE QUESTIONNAIRE

YES NO

1. Is your waist measurement greater than 40 inches for a man or greater than 35 inches for a woman (measured around the belly button)? ☐ ☐
2. Is your fasting blood sugar greater than 100 mg/dL?* ☐ ☐
3. Is your serum HDL less than 40 mg/dL for a man and less than 50 mg/dL for a woman?* ☐ ☐
4. Is your blood pressure greater than 130/85 mmHg, or are you taking medication for your blood pressure?* ☐ ☐
5. Is your fasting serum triglyceride level greater than 150 mg/dL?* ☐ ☐
6. Are you unable to lose weight even when following a low-calorie diet, exercising regularly, and controlling food cravings? ☐ ☐
7. Do you regularly eat sugary foods, breads, crackers, pasta, potatoes, rice, corn, or other starches? ☐ ☐
8. Do you have a potbelly? ☐ ☐
9. Do you have a hard time losing belly fat? ☐ ☐
10. Have you been diagnosed with polycystic ovary syndrome? ☐ ☐
11. Women, did you have gestational diabetes? ☐ ☐
12. Are you Native American, African American, or Hispanic? ☐ ☐
13. Do you have regular episodes of low blood sugar (i.e., shakiness or cloudy thinking that goes away with eating)? ☐ ☐
14. Do you have acanthosis (darkened skin) on your neck, beneath your breasts, or in your armpits that is warty or mossy-like? ☐ ☐
15. Do you regularly drink alcohol? ☐ ☐
16. Do you get little to no regular exercise or physical activity? ☐ ☐
17. Do you have burning feet? ☐ ☐
18. Does your blood pressure fluctuate dramatically at various times? ☐ ☐

Points for each "yes" answer:
- Questions 1–5: 5 points each   Subtotal_____
- Questions 6–18: 2 points each   Subtotal_____
                                    Total_____

SCORE:
- 0–10: Unlikely you have insulin resistance
- 11–19: Mild insulin resistance
- 20–29: Moderate insulin resistance
- 30+: Severe insulin resistance

* If you don't know the answers to questions 2 through 5 but answered yes to most of the remaining questions, it is still possible that you have insulin resistance, and I encourage you to visit your doctor.

Low Thyroid Questionnaire

	YES	NO
1. Do you regularly have a low body temperature, cold hands, and cold feet?	☐	☐
2. Have you lost the outer third of your eyebrows?	☐	☐
3. Do you have swollen eyelids?	☐	☐
4. Are you cold when others feel warm?	☐	☐
5. Do you have rough, dry skin, especially on your elbows?	☐	☐
6. Are you regularly constipated?	☐	☐
7. Are you unable to lose weight even with proper diet and exercise?	☐	☐
8. Do you have yellowing of your palms and soles?	☐	☐
9. Are you depressed?	☐	☐
10. Are you forgetful, or do you feel like you are in a fog?	☐	☐
11. Is your hair coarse, dry, brittle, or breaking?	☐	☐
12. Are you sluggish, fatigued, or lethargic?	☐	☐
13. Do you have swollen legs, hands, and feet?	☐	☐
14. Do you have a hoarse, husky voice?	☐	☐
15. Do you have carpal tunnel syndrome?	☐	☐
16. Do you have a puffy face?	☐	☐
17. Do you have brittle nails?	☐	☐
18. Do you move slowly and think slowly?	☐	☐
19. Do you have stiffness or aches and pains in various joints?	☐	☐
20. Does your tongue feel swollen?	☐	☐

Points for each "yes" answer:

- Questions 1–6: 5 points each   Subtotal_____
- Questions 7–20: 2 points each   Subtotal_____

Total_____

SCORE:

- 0–10: Unlikely you have low thyroid
- 11–19: Symptoms of mildly low thyroid
- 20–29: Symptoms of moderately low thyroid
- 30+: Symptoms of severely low thyroid

Inflammation Questionnaire

YES NO

1. Is your waist measurement greater than 40 inches for a man or greater than 35 inches for a woman (measured around the belly button)? ☐ ☐
2. Do you eat fried foods on a regular basis? ☐ ☐
3. Is your hs C-reactive protein (CRP) level greater than 1.0 mg/dL?* ☐ ☐
4. Do you have a disease associated with inflammation, including:

Coronary artery disease	☐ ☐	Inflammatory bowel disease	☐ ☐
Allergies	☐ ☐	Hepatitis	☐ ☐
Diabetes	☐ ☐	Celiac disease	☐ ☐
Metabolic syndrome	☐ ☐	Cancer	☐ ☐
An autoimmune disease	☐ ☐	HIV	☐ ☐
Arthritis	☐ ☐	Chronic viral or bacterial	
Eczema or psoriasis	☐ ☐	infection	☐ ☐

5. Do you consume large amounts of salad dressing or corn, sunflower, soybean, or cottonseed oil? ☐ ☐
6. Do you regularly eat margarine, peanut butter, cake icing, shortening, etc.? ☐ ☐
7. Do you regularly eat large portions of corn-fed beef? ☐ ☐
8. Do you regularly eat eggs, pork, red meat, or shellfish? ☐ ☐
9. Do you drink sodas daily or frequently eat sugary foods? ☐ ☐
10. Do you regularly eat white bread, white rice, potatoes, pasta, crackers, bagels, pretzels, or chips? ☐ ☐
11. Do you regularly eat popcorn, corn chips, or other forms of corn? ☐ ☐
12. Do you regularly eat fried fish? ☐ ☐
13. Do you rarely eat fruits or veggies? ☐ ☐
14. Do you have joint aches or muscle aches on a regular basis? ☐ ☐
15. Is your nose stuffy or runny much of the time? ☐ ☐
16. Do you have chronic sinusitis or frequent colds, or flu? ☐ ☐
17. Do you smoke cigarettes or abuse drugs? ☐ ☐
18. Do you tend to get rashes? ☐ ☐

Points for each "yes" answer:

- Questions 1–8: 5 points each (for each inflammatory disease in question 4, add another 5 points) Subtotal_____
- Questions 9–18: 2 points each Subtotal_____

Total_____

SCORE:

- 0–10: Unlikely your weight gain is due to inflammation
- 11–19: Mild inflammation
- 20+: Moderate inflammation

---

* If you don't know the answer to this question but answered yes to most of the remaining questions, you may still be suffering from inflammation, and I encourage you to visit your doctor.

DELAYED FOOD SENSITIVITIES QUESTIONNAIRE

	YES	NO
1. Have you gained weight, and no diet seems to work?	☐	☐
2. Do you have chronic postnasal drip with thick mucus?	☐	☐
3. Do you commonly develop canker sores in your mouth?	☐	☐
4. Have you been diagnosed with chronic sinusitis?	☐	☐
5. Do you have chronic bad breath or halitosis?	☐	☐
6. Do you have nasal or sinus polyps?	☐	☐
7. Have you been diagnosed with eczema?	☐	☐
8. Do you have urticaria or hives from time to time?	☐	☐
9. Have you been diagnosed with irritable bowel syndrome?	☐	☐
10. Do you have frequent heartburn or acid reflux?	☐	☐
11. Have you been diagnosed with Crohn's disease or ulcerative colitis?	☐	☐
12. Do you have a history of migraine or cluster headaches?	☐	☐
13. Have you been diagnosed with chronic fatigue syndrome and/or fibromyalgia?	☐	☐
14. Have you been diagnosed with ADD, ADHD, or autism?	☐	☐
15. Do you have a history of PMS? (women only)	☐	☐
16. Do you have recurrent vaginal itching or discharge? (women only)	☐	☐
17. Have you been diagnosed with degenerative arthritis?	☐	☐
18. Have you been diagnosed with mitral valve prolapse?	☐	☐
19. Do you experience fatigue after meals?	☐	☐
20. Do you have frequent bloating and gas after eating?	☐	☐

Points for each "yes" answer:

- Questions 1–20: 2 points each   Total: _____

SCORE:

- 0–4: Unlikely you have a delayed food sensitivity
- 4+: Likely you have a delayed food sensitivity

Altered GI Ecology (or Imbalanced Gut or GI Flora) Questionnaire

	YES	NO
1. Have you ever taken antibiotics for a month or longer?	☐	☐
2. Have you taken a broad-spectrum antibiotic three or more times a year?	☐	☐
3. Have you had at least one annual round of a broad-spectrum antibiotic for a couple of years?	☐	☐
4. Do you ever feel like an airhead after eating sugar, bread, or pasta?	☐	☐
5. Have you ever had oral thrush?	☐	☐
6. Have you ever had yeast vaginitis?	☐	☐
7. Have you taken prednisone or cortisone for longer than two weeks?	☐	☐
8. Have you taken birth control pills longer than two years?	☐	☐
9. Have you ever had fungal skin problems (athlete's foot, ringworm, jock itch, or nail fungus)?	☐	☐
10. Do you crave sugar?	☐	☐
11. Do you crave breads or pasta?	☐	☐
12. Do you crave alcohol or cheese?	☐	☐
13. Are you intolerant to perfumes, fragrances, or chemical odors?	☐	☐
14. Do you have regular bouts of abdominal bloating and gas?	☐	☐
15. Do you have vaginal itching or discharge?	☐	☐
16. Do you have regular abdominal pain, constipation, or diarrhea?	☐	☐
17. Do you have food sensitivities or food intolerances?	☐	☐
18. Do you have rectal itching?	☐	☐
19. Are your symptoms of abdominal bloating and gas worse when you eat aged cheese, drink alcohol, or have soy sauce?	☐	☐
20. Have you taken chemotherapy medications for cancer?	☐	☐

Points for each "yes" answer:
- Questions 1–2: 10 points each   Subtotal_____
- Questions 3–8: 5 points each   Subtotal_____
- Questions 9–20: 2 points each   Subtotal_____

Total_____

SCORE:
- 0–9: Unlikely you have altered GI ecology or imbalanced gut flora
- 10–19: Mild symptoms of imbalanced gut flora
- 20–29: Moderate symptoms of imbalanced gut flora
- 30+: Severe symptoms of imbalanced gut flora

DEPRESSION QUESTIONNAIRE

	YES	NO
1. Do you think about dying a lot?	☐	☐
2. Do you usually feel depressed, dejected, and blue?	☐	☐
3. Do you have frequent crying spells?	☐	☐
4. Do you not enjoy the things you used to enjoy?	☐	☐
5. Do you feel your friends and family would be better off if you were dead?	☐	☐
6. Is it very difficult for you to make decisions?	☐	☐
7. Do you have no hope for the future?	☐	☐
8. Do you have little to no sex drive?	☐	☐
9. Do you have problems sleeping each night?	☐	☐
10. Do you awaken in the early morning and find it very difficult to fall back asleep?	☐	☐
11. Are you very fatigued and run down?	☐	☐
12. Do you have no appetite?	☐	☐
13. Do you want to eat all the time?	☐	☐
14. Is your mind confused and you are unable to concentrate?	☐	☐
15. Do you find it very difficult to do the things you used to do?	☐	☐
16. Are you usually irritable and grumpy?	☐	☐
17. Is your life empty?	☐	☐
18. Do you feel worthless?	☐	☐
19. Do you feel worse in the morning and don't want to get out of bed?	☐	☐
20. Do you move and think slower than usual?	☐	☐

Points for each "yes" answer:

- Questions 1–5: 5 points each   Subtotal_____
- Questions 6–20: 2 points each   Subtotal_____

                                                   Total_____

SCORE

- 0–10: Unlikely you have depression
- 11–19: Mild depression
- 20–25: Moderate depression
- 26+: Severe depression

23

WHEN WEIGHT LOSS STALLS OR STOPS

Y OUR ANSWERS TO the questionnaires in the last chapter should have helped you to pinpoint one or several underlying physical conditions that may be causing your weight-loss efforts to stall. But as you'll discover in this final chapter of the book, there are several ways you can overcome whatever has prompted your plateau. This chapter covers each plateau briefly. For more in-depth explanations and advice on the following causes of weight-loss plateaus, please go to www.thecandodiet.com.

THE PROLONGED PLATEAU

When my patients reach a prolonged plateau—typically a month or longer—with no weight loss, I will often have them come into my office with their food diary and exercise journal. I review what they've recorded and discuss their food and beverage choices, as well as portion sizes and snacks, to determine if they are eating the wrong types of foods or consuming too many calories or too many carbohydrates late in the day. I also make sure that they are not consuming complex carbohydrates, even low-glycemic complex carbs, after 6:00 p.m., and I discuss their meal planning. I then look at their activity journal to see what kind of activities or exercises they are doing on a regular basis. If they haven't yet calculated their optimum fat-burning heart rate range, I'll help them do this and also encourage them to start a muscle-strengthening program. Most patients get significantly better results when they work with a certified personal trainer for at least a month or longer. This not only helps them get on a structured strengthening program catered to their needs, but it also allows them to learn proper lifting techniques. For the aerobic program, I will usually make sure they are exercising in their fat-burning zone and help them calculate their ideal heart rate for burning fat. I make sure they are able to talk while exercising, and increase their exercise time to forty-five minutes to an hour. I also encourage them to exercise six days a week. And if patients are well conditioned, I may place them on high-intensity interval training (HIIT).

By following these simple suggestions, most people will break through their prolonged plateau. For others, it's a matter of meal planning, rotating their low-glycemic complex carbohydrates (which I will discuss shortly), and eating every three to three and a half hours. In these cases, I help my patients accurately calculate their basal metabolic rate and adjust their meals and snacks accordingly, and I make sure that they are daily choosing proper portion sizes of low-glycemic foods. Consuming either too many fats or too many starches can often lead to a plateau, and again, someone trying to lose weight must eat every three to three and a half hours. I also often find that patients need to rotate their complex low-glycemic carbohydrates.

RESETTING A SLUGGISH METABOLISM AND/OR MEAL PLANNING

I have learned over the years from patients who are bodybuilders the importance of rotating complex low-glycemic carbohdrates for those with a sluggish metabolism or those who plateau. The key lies in the timing of eating carbs and rotating the low-glycemic carbs. For weight loss, I do not recommend eating any complex carbs for dinner or for the evening snack, but only for breakfast, midmorning snack, lunch, and midafternoon snack. Examples of complex low-glycemic carbs include sweet potatoes, whole-grain pasta cooked al dente, brown or wild rice, beans, peas, lentils, Ezekiel 4:9 bread, double-fiber breads, certain cereals, and regular, steel-cut, and high-fiber instant oatmeal. Two slices of double-fiber bread have 40 grams of complex carbs. One cup of brown rice has approximately 40 grams of carbs; ½ cup steel-cut oatmeal has 54 grams of carbs. One packet of high-fiber instant oatmeal has 34 grams of carbs and 10 grams of fiber, and so on.

The key to breaking through a plateau is to vary the amount of carbohydrates taken in daily by a simple method that in turn usually helps to reset the metabolic rate. Here is a simple example of rotating complex low-glycemic carbohydrates (men usually start with 200 grams of low-glycemic carbs, with women usually starting with 150 grams of low-glycemic carbs):

- Day 1: 200 grams of complex low-glycemic carbs—75 grams for breakfast; 25 grams for midmorning or three hours after breakfast; 75 grams for lunch; 25 grams for midafternoon snack or three hours after lunch; 0 grams for dinner; and 0 grams for late-night snack

- Day 2: 150 grams of complex low-glycemic carbs—50 grams for breakfast; 25 grams for midmorning or three hours after breakfast; 50 grams for lunch; 25 grams for midafternoon snack or three hours after lunch; 0 grams for dinner; and 0 grams for late-night snack

- Day 3: 150 grams of complex low-glycemic carbs—50 grams for breakfast; 25 grams for midmorning or three hours after breakfast; 50 grams for lunch; 25 grams for midafternoon snack or three hours after lunch; 0 grams for dinner; and 0 grams for late-night snack

- Day 4: 125 grams of complex low-glycemic carbs—40 grams for breakfast; 20–22 grams for midmorning or three hours after breakfast; 40 grams for lunch; 20–22 grams for midafternoon snack or three hours after lunch; 0 grams for dinner; and 0 grams for late-night snack

- Day 5: 100 grams of complex low-glycemic carbs—30 grams for breakfast; 20 grams for midmorning or three hours after breakfast; 30 grams for lunch; 20 grams for midafternoon snack or three hours after lunch; 0 grams for dinner; and 0 grams for late-night snack

- Day 6: 50 grams of complex low-glycemic carbs—20 grams for breakfast; 5 grams for midmorning or three hours after breakfast; 20 grams for lunch; 5 grams for midafternoon snack or three hours after lunch; 0 grams for dinner; and 0 grams for late-night snack

- Day 7: 50 grams of complex low-glycemic carbs—20 grams for breakfast; 5 grams for midmorning or three hours after breakfast; 20 grams for lunch; 5 grams for midafternoon snack or three hours after lunch; 0 grams for dinner; and 0 grams for late-night snack

- Day 8: The cycle starts all over again with 200 grams of complex low-glycemic carbs for this day.

  Females: 1,800 calories (never below 1,400)
  Males: 2,200 calories (never below 1,600)
  See Appendix H for information on contacting Lee Vierson for meal planning.

The reality is, however, that even after following these suggestions, some individuals will still be stuck on a weight-loss plateau. These individuals usually fall into the category of the metabolically compromised.

Metabolically Compromised

If you are metabolically compromised, it essentially means you have a low metabolic rate, have difficulty losing weight, and tend to plateau often. My hope is that most of you reading this don't fall into this category, but sadly, my experience and statistics tell me you might. For those who are sure you're metabolically compromised, the simple questionnaires in the previous chapter should have helped you to determine which category or categories of the metabolically compromised you fall into. After practicing medicine for more than twenty-five years, I have found that people who plateau for a prolonged period tend to fall into one or more of the following metabolically compromised categories.

- Chronic stress
- Insulin resistance
- Neurotransmitter imbalance
- Food addiction
- Hormonal imbalance and aging
- Low thyroid function
- Inflammation
- Delayed food sensitivities
- Altered GI ecology
- Excessive fad and yo-yo dieting
- Depression
- Medications or smoking cessation

I encourage you to visit www.thecandodiet.com, where I address each of these categories in extensive detail. The site also includes a questionnaire similar to those in the previous chapter to help you assess whether you have the specific medical condition addressed that could be preventing you from losing weight. If you are stuck in a rut due to one of these conditions, my hope is that the information contained in this chapter and on the Web site will be the impetus to regaining your momentum.

In some cases, you may need to take a medication, a hormone, a supplement, or have certain tests such as a test for delayed food sensitivities to overcome your condition. Make an appointment with your primary care physician to order the recommended diagnostic tests. Some individuals may need to see a bariatric specialist or a board-certified anti-aging physician since most regular physicians are not adequately trained to deal with some of these conditions. (To find a bariatric physician near you, visit www.bariatricnetwork.org; to locate a board-certified anti-aging physician in your area, check out www.worldhealth.net.)

CHRONIC STRESS

There are two major types of stress: major life-event stress (death of a spouse or family member, divorce, job termination, and so forth) and daily life stress (such as finances, traffic, arguments, job stress, relationship stress). Both types can cause weight gain for different reasons. However, the daily life stressors tend to cause the most weight gain due to chronically raising a person's cortisol levels.

READ MORE ABOUT IT

I discuss more about stress in my books *Stress Less, The Bible Cure for Stress,* and *Deadly Emotions.*

When your cortisol and adrenaline levels are chronically elevated, this causes stored sugar (known as glycogen) to be released from the muscles and liver into the bloodstream. It also causes the release of fat into the bloodstream to be used as energy. But since Americans are not using the fats and sugar to "fight or flee," they are being stored as fat. Fat and sugar, as you know, are great when they are immediately burned for energy, but they cause weight gain when they are stored. Unfortunately, the latter happens more frequently in society today because our stressors are increasingly psychological and decreasingly physical. Remember how I mentioned the redefinition of stress? This has literally changed the shape of our nation. Since more individuals are emotionally and psychologically stressed, there are naturally more obese people.

Back in the "old days" when our stress response was physical, we would run or fight, which would burn off the sugars and fats released into our bloodstream. Now that most of our stress is psychological, we do not run or fight but simply stew in our own stress juices. Instead of burning sugars and fats, we actually release more insulin, which causes even more fat to be stored. It's a relatively simple equation: when cortisol levels rise, insulin levels also rise. Chronic stress raises cortisol, which then raises insulin levels. The two work together as the "dynamic duo" of weight gain.

How ugly is this two-headed beast? Let me mention just a few of the ways one of these elements—cortisol—triggers the problem of gaining weight.

Chronically elevated cortisol levels make your body less sensitive to leptin, the hormone that tells your brain you are full. These high cortisol levels also stimulate the appetite, making you extremely hungry. At the same time, cortisol promotes the release of neuropeptide Y, a chemical in the brain that triggers the body to crave carbohydrates. So far, that's three negatives each coming from a different angle. Not good.

We'll deal with insulin later in this chapter.

When you face a physical stressor such as being attacked, your fight-or-flight response suppresses the appetite during the event. But following the traumatic occurrence, the raised cortisol levels will actually induce an increased appetite. The same is true for psychological stress; after the trauma, your cortisol levels rise. Instead of helping you burn fat, these high cortisol levels cause your metabolic rate to slow down. And if you are regularly stressed, your testosterone and DHEA levels also dwindle. Both of these valuable hormones not only assist in building muscle and burning fat but also help you cope with

stress. To make matters worse, cortisol is the only hormone in the body that actually increases as you age.

Foods and beverages that raise cortisol

Although skipping meals is one of the prime offenders for causing raised cortisol levels, several foods and drinks prompt the same response in the body. Sugars, desserts, sodas, high-glycemic starches, and alcoholic beverages can raise both cortisol and insulin levels. Foods high in sugar spike the blood sugar, which in turn usually causes the pancreas to secrete too much insulin. This may also trigger hypoglycemia or low blood sugar. When this happens, the brain sends a signal to the adrenal glands to increase cortisol levels, which raises the blood sugar. Skipping meals also raises cortisol levels, which is why I emphasize to my patients to eat every three to three and a half hours.

Caffeine will also raise cortisol levels. Only 200 milligrams of caffeine, which is equivalent to one and a half to two cups of coffee, can raise cortisol levels by 30 percent within just one hour. Now imagine what a Starbucks grande coffee with 330 milligrams of caffeine can do to your cortisol level! Sodas high in both caffeine and sugar are a double whammy at raising cortisol levels. Foods that you are allergic or sensitive to can raise cortisol levels as well, as can herbal stimulants such as guarana, bitter orange, and country mallow. Excessive intake of chocolate can also raise your cortisol levels.

If you are stuck in obesity and deal with chronic stress, I believe you can break free and live a healthier life. It may be as simple as incorporating a few of the everyday practical tips to reduce stress, or it may require several stress-reduction techniques along with adaptogenic herbs. But know that you do not have to follow the crowd toward the obesity epidemic in this country. You can turn off a stressful, overweight lifestyle and turn on a healthy, energetic, trimmed-down you.

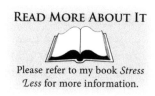

READ MORE ABOUT IT

Please refer to my book *Stress Less* for more information.

You may also be suffering from adrenal fatigue. Visit the Web site www .thecandodiet.com for more information on adrenal fatigue.

INSULIN RESISTANCE

Insulin resistance occurs when the body's cells and tissues no longer respond normally to insulin. To understand this condition better, we first need to know about the various functions of insulin. A hormone secreted by the pancreas,

insulin's primary function is regulating blood sugar levels throughout the body by lowering blood sugar when it is elevated.

Think of insulin as a key that opens the door to each cell so that sugar can enter into that cell. Much of the food you eat is first converted to sugar and then arrives at the door of a cell in the form of blood sugar. When your insulin is functioning effectively, it figuratively unlocks the door by binding to the insulin receptors on the surface of the cell. These receptors let the sugar in, upon which it is then used to produce energy or build tissue.

When you have insulin resistance, however, the door's locks—those insulin receptors on the surface of the cells—do not function properly and figuratively become rusty. Normally, sugars and highly refined, high-glycemic carbohydrates convert to glucose and rapidly raise the blood sugar. The pancreas responds just as quickly by releasing large amounts of insulin to lower the blood sugar. This can go on for years without a person developing obesity, prediabetes, or type 2 diabetes. But after continuously eating these kinds of foods, a person's cells can eventually become more resistant to insulin in the same way that a lock can begin to rust. As the blood sugar continues to rise, the pancreas keeps churning out even more insulin to lower the blood sugar and drive the sugar inside the cells. These elevated insulin levels then program the body for even more fat storage, especially in the abdominal area. The higher the insulin levels in the blood, the greater the chance of storing belly fat—which, unfortunately, is the hardest fat to lose.

There are varying degrees of insulin resistance. To discover the extent of insulin resistance, have your physician perform a fasting blood sugar (FBS) test. This test, which measures your blood glucose level, is usually done in the morning while fasting, but it can be administered anytime after not eating anything for at least eight hours. If your FBS is greater than or equal to 100 mg/dL, you have insulin resistance and prediabetes.

Reversing insulin resistance

The most important ways to reverse insulin resistance are by choosing low-glycemic foods instead of moderate- or high-glycemic foods, as well as exercising to lose belly fat. Avoid sugars, sugary foods, and refined carbohydrates such as white bread, white rice, instant and regular potatoes, chips, crackers, and the like. It is also crucial that you eat more vegetables (especially those high in soluble fiber) and natural foods. (Review chapters 6 and 7 for a refresher on the various foods that have low or high glycemic index values.)

I also recommend that you not drink sodas, alcohol, sugar-laden coffees, or even fruit juices. It is also important to avoid trans fats and to decrease

your consumption of salad dressings (with omega-6 oils), sauces, doughnuts, pastries, cake icing, and most fried foods, cooking oils, and (most) crackers. Excessive consumption of saturated fats can also lead to insulin resistance. This includes fatty meats such as sausage, bacon, hamburgers, pepperoni, and hot dogs, as well as dairy foods such as cheese, butter, and whole milk. In addition, large portion sizes can cause insulin resistance.

Regular exercise and supplements are also critical for reversing insulin resistance. (Insulin resistance is intricately related to many of the other factors we discuss in this book. To provide the foundation for overcoming insulin resistance, I advise you to review chapters 5, 6, 9, 11, and 20.)

Type 2 diabetics and people with significant belly fat may require more extreme measures since they are often severely metabolically compromised *and* severely insulin resistant. Please refer to www.thecandodiet.com and my book *The New Bible Cure for Diabetes* for my recommendations for people in this situation.

NEUROTRANSMITTER IMBALANCE

To understand how neurotransmitter imbalance affects weight loss, you have to begin with a basic knowledge of what certain neurotransmitters do. There are two main types of neurotransmitters: inhibitory and excitatory. The primary inhibitory neurotransmitter involved in weight loss and appetite control is serotonin, while the main excitatory neurotransmitters for losing weight are norepinephrine and dopamine.

I described the deficiencies of these three main neurotransmitters in chapter 3. Let's now delve into each one a little more deeply.

Norepinephrine

Low brain norepinephrine is the most common neurotransmitter deficiency that I see among obese patients. When you have low norepinephrine levels in the brain, you are prone to depression, whereas high levels can cause anxiety. As a dual-purpose hormone and neurotransmitter, norepinephrine also serves as a powerful stress hormone involved in the fight-or-flight stress response, along with its "sister hormone" epinephrine, better known as adrenaline. Both cause an increased blood flow to the brain that increases the brain's activity during a stressful experience, making a person more focused and alert.

This is the reason medical doctors prescribe Ritalin or Adderall to children with attention deficit disorder (ADD) or attention deficit hyperactivity disorder (ADHD). The temporary result, of course, is that these kids feel more

focused and alert while usually also being more calm. While on the medication, they may maintain a healthy weight—with some overweight children actually losing weight because of the common side effect of a decreased appetite. Sadly, however, the medicine may be slowly wearing away the norepinephrine in their brains. Over time, they may eventually be deficient and no better off. Without medication, they may experience more side effects as they grow older. Most will be even less alert and focused, while also having an increased appetite. Many will never feel full after meals and will not know when to stop eating. They will typically crave starches such as crackers, chips, breads, and pasta instead of sweets. All of this usually leads them to becoming overweight. And in addition, their low norepinephrine levels leave them feeling tired, exhausted, frustrated (from their inability to concentrate), and prone to feeling depressed.

Does this sound like you? You may have been diagnosed with ADD or ADHD as a child and took Ritalin, Adderall, or some other medication all the way through high school. If you stopped taking one of these, you've since realized that it did not fix your ADD or ADHD problems. Most likely, you still have low norepinephrine levels in your brain, and without the medication you are probably prone to weight gain. Maybe you've seen a doctor in recent years about your depression, and he placed you on Lexapro, Zoloft, Paxil, or some other antidepressant that caused you to gain even more weight. That has only left you more frustrated and stressed, which may have caused your norepinephrine levels to drop even lower.

Whether this describes your case or not, I hope you can still see the spiral effect this has on the millions of people who have never gotten to the neurochemical root of their weight problems. Fortunately, there is a way out of this abyss. Please visit www.thecandodiet.com to find out which natural supplements can restore this important

STARTING YOUNG

Of the 2.4 million children in the United States with ADHD,[1] 30 to 70 percent of them will continue to show symptoms in their adult years.[2]

neurotransmitter to adequate levels for weight loss. You can learn more about all of the neurotransmitters in this section at www.neurorelief.com.

Serotonin

Serotonin deficiency in the brain is the second-most common neurotransmitter deficiency that I see in obese patients in my practice. As the "feel good" neurotransmitter, serotonin is what gives you the sense of being happy, full, and sleepy after a large Thanksgiving dinner with turkey, dressing, creamed potatoes, corn, and lots of desserts. Approximately 95 percent of your sero-

tonin is located in your GI tract or your "gut brain," so it's no wonder that food intake has a close connection with the release of serotonin. When your brain is flooded with this neurotransmitter, satiety normally occurs. However, a lack of serotonin exhibits the exact opposite behavior, often producing carbohydrate, sugar, and chocolate cravings and bingeing that ultimately lead to excess body fat. In fact, recent studies suggest that regardless of what or how much they eat, obese individuals usually have an ongoing reduction in serotonin production that contributes to impaired satiety. This, in turn, leads to even more calories consumed because they never feel full.[3]

Besides weight gain, low levels of serotonin in the brain are also associated with depression, anxiety, insomnia, panic attacks, OCD, bulimia, phobias, irritable bowel syndrome, anger, migraine headaches, compulsive eating, cravings for sugar and chocolate, bingeing, PMS, irritability, and fibromyalgia.

Most patients with food addictions have serotonin deficiency and/or norepinephrine and dopamine deficiency. Unfortunately, the common story among individuals who have serotonin deficiency is that after seeing a medical doctor, they are placed on antidepressants, which then can cause even more weight gain and more sugar, chocolate, and carbohydrate cravings. After repeated bouts of this, these individuals typically gain even more weight and may feel hopeless and helpless, which may lead to depression. Does this sound like you? If so, most likely you are unaware of your low serotonin levels. For a list of the natural supplements I recommend to boost your serotonin levels, please visit www.thecandodiet.com.

> **LISTEN TO YOUR BRAIN**
>
> Although the brain contains only 2 to 3 percent of your overall serotonin, its supply of the neurotransmitter is what exclusively turns off your cravings for sugars and carbs. In other words, your brain is better suited to control your appetite than a full stomach.

Dopamine

The last neurotransmitter imbalance that I frequently see among obese individuals involves dopamine. Dopamine is the "pleasure neurotransmitter" that enables you to both feel and seek out pleasure. It differs from serotonin in how the brain distinguishes between the two. When your serotonin levels are low, you're susceptible to feeling depressed or anxious; when your dopamine levels are low, however, you are likely to do whatever it takes to get a "natural high." Many people call this "wanting an adrenaline rush" or "seeking out a thrill," when often they're referring to the natural good feeling you get from raised dopamine levels.

Part of your brain is purely dedicated to pleasure. This portion, known as the limbic lobe, houses every one of your drives, urges, and desires. As you might guess, it also contains and is strongly affected by dopamine. Many people inherit low dopamine levels, while others experience declining levels, especially later in life—usually from chronic stress. These individuals are more prone to developing an addiction involving drugs, alcohol, cigarettes, gambling, sex, food, or any other vice. They typically have addictive personalities and a strong family history of addictions (there is a strong genetic component to dopamine deficiency), and they are also prone to developing depression, irritability, and moodiness. They often feel down, dull, bored, and have an overall lack of interest in life. It is difficult for them to get motivated about anything, and they are usually unable to enjoy daily life. Ultimately, they just can't seem to get excited about anything.

Is it any wonder, then, why many of these people turn to drugs such as cocaine, methamphetamines, and other "uppers"? Cocaine is actually the most powerful substance known to raise dopamine levels. It, along with other uppers, raises their dopamine levels and gets them feeling excited about life. Because they rarely experience that feeling, it's easy for them to become addicted to the high. Others turn to other medications, including alcohol, marijuana, heroin, and other downers. Unlike the uppers, however, the result of these is often more irritability, moodiness, and depression.

Dopamine deficiency also is associated with weight gain and obesity. Many times, patients with low dopamine levels crave salty and fatty foods, salty starches, or a combination of these foods. I've had many patients who went most of the day craving such foods as bacon, steak, hamburgers, salami, pepperoni, sausage, and pizzas topped with various meats. At times, they also became almost obsessed over eating such salty starches as chips, pretzels, popcorn, french fries, and crackers.

SEXUAL SIDE EFFECTS

Individuals with dopamine deficiency often experience sexual problems such as delayed ejaculation or the inability to have an orgasm.

I strongly believe that if we do not correct these neurotransmitter deficiencies, we will continue to see more obesity-related diseases and food addictions simply because we failed to address the real problem for many obese individuals. If you suspect this section on neurotransmitters may apply to you, take the questionnaire online at www.thecandodiet.com, and you will be directed to more information about supplements and medications that can help balance these deficiencies. I encourage you to get tested to be sure you do indeed have a deficiency, and then talk to your doctor about the natural

supplements I recommend rather than taking antidepressants, which can cause weight gain. (To find a doctor about testing you for neurotransmitter deficiencies, go to www.neurorelief.com.) If you do, you will be on your way to finally tackling the *real* issues holding you back from losing weight.

FOOD ADDICTIONS

Like other addictions, food addictions are about loss of control. There are both physical and psychological reasons behind food addictions, and they are associated with other health conditions such as obesity, diabetes, stroke, high blood pressure, and heart attack. Food addictions also usually involve neurotransmitter imbalances, which I've just addressed.

If you took the questionnaire in the last chapter and think you may be dealing with an addiction to food, the good news is that recovery is possible. I recommend that you contact a professional who has been trained to counsel people with eating disorders such as food addiction. The following are general guidelines for the steps you will likely need to take during your treatment:

- Admit that you have a food addiction problem.
- Identify your trigger foods (the foods that cause cravings).
- Modify your eating habits, practice meal planning (with the guidance of your health-care professional), and eat every three to three and a half hours.
- Begin exercising.
- Check your neurotransmitter levels and complete the tests for neurotransmitters. (See www.neurorelief.com.)

There are different types of treatment programs (inpatient, outpatient, and others) that provide you with options that will best suit your individual needs. I provide more information on this subject at www.thecandodiet.com.

HORMONAL IMBALANCE AND AGING

The body's hormones are much like instruments in an orchestra. Each offers something unique and shares a distinct part in bettering the whole body. And each needs a conductor. When it comes to hormones, however, that role is filled by two parts of the brain: the hypothalamus and the pituitary. These two glands are maestros at controlling and manipulating the output of hormones from specific glands.

However, as we age—especially after we turn thirty-five—our hormonal

levels typically begin to drop. But the good news is that when properly conducted, your hormones can still play—regardless of your age—a key role in losing weight and keeping it off.

Estrogen

Estrogen has more than four hundred vital functions in the female body, some of which improve sleep, maintain muscle, increase the metabolic rate, and help to balance neurotransmitters in the brain (which in turn helps to reduce food cravings). Estrogen also improves insulin sensitivity, which helps patients who deal with insulin resistance. The bottom line: the correct amount of bioidentical estrogen helps you lose weight in many different ways.

The tricky part is that both extremes of estrogen levels (too much or too little) can lead to weight gain. Having too much estrogen (estrogen dominance) can especially lead to extra pounds in the abdomen, hips, thighs, and waist. Estrogen dominance may be caused by taking birth control pills or by synthetic hormone replacement therapy, which involves synthetic hormones that do not function the same as bioidentical ones. Estrogen dominance can also be caused by constipation, obesity, or an increased intake of xenoestrogens found in pesticides, herbicides, petrochemicals, and plastics.

Having too little estrogen creates problems as well. During menopause a woman's ovaries typically stop producing estrogen and progesterone. Common symptoms of menopause include hot flashes, night sweats, vaginal dryness, mood swings, irritability, hair loss, palpitations, lapses in memory, and weight gain. Menopause is also associated with an increased risk of heart disease, osteoporosis, obesity, memory loss, and insulin resistance. During this time women often begin developing a "menopot" or potbelly. Many menopausal women also experience various and severe food cravings because of low or fluctuating hormone levels. Similar to the cravings some women experience during pregnancy, these strong desires generally revolve around starches such as breads, pasta, and sweets—especially chocolate.

As you can imagine from these cravings, many women end up becoming overweight or obese during their menopause years. Depression also runs higher among these women, yet unfortunately most physicians' response is to prescribe an antidepressant. This only complicates the matter and typically leaves patients gaining even more weight. The truth is, most menopausal women simply need a bioidentical estrogen and progesterone found in a transdermal cream. Unfortunately, even taking estrogen in pill or capsule form can cause weight gain and further increase your cravings for carbohydrates. That is why I prescribe hormone replacement therapy in transdermal creams.

Progesterone

Decreased progesterone is associated with many symptoms, including mood swings, palpitations, insomnia, irritability, PMS, anxiety, depression, hair loss, decreased sex drive, and weight gain. Because there is such a wide range of symptoms, and because many of those symptoms are so common, many gynecologists or family physicians now routinely treat patients exhibiting these with an antidepressant. For instance, if a woman is experiencing irregular menstrual cycles, severe cramping, or excessive bleeding problems, it is normal for a doctor to prescribe synthetic progesterone or a birth control pill. However, *all* of these temporary solutions cause weight gain, which obviously complicates the problem.

Testosterone and women

Most physicians believe that testosterone is unimportant for women. They feel women only need to concentrate on their estrogen and progesterone levels. However, we now know that testosterone is just as crucial for women when it comes to controlling their weight, as this powerful hormone helps them increase muscle mass and strength as well as toning muscles. Testosterone also increases sex drive, physical stamina, and helps with overall weight loss.

Grumpy-old-man syndrome

General symptoms of low testosterone in men include a decrease in any or all of the following: sex drive, spontaneous early morning erections, mental acuity, competitiveness, muscle mass and tone, strength, and stamina. Along with these symptoms, men suffering from hypogonadism often experience grumpiness, irritability, anger, depression, loss of pubic and axillary hair, fatigue, and an overall feeling of being burned out.

It has been proven that obesity, diabetes, and high blood pressure all affect testosterone levels. A recent study of more than twenty-one hundred men age forty-five and older found that those with obesity were 2.4 times more likely as other men the same age to have hypogonadism. Those with type 2 diabetes were 2.1 times more likely, and those with hypertension were 1.8 times more likely to have low testosterone levels. In addition, men with elevated cholesterol, prostate disease, and asthma have increased chances of hypogonadism than healthy men.[4]

Growth hormone

Serving a variety of purposes in the body, this hormone is most evident in the childhood and adolescent years as we become taller. It stimulates both growth and cell reproduction, increases muscle mass, reduces body fat, helps

in controlling insulin and sugar levels, assists in retaining calcium throughout the body, along with many other functions. Therefore, when we lack growth hormone, our growth—as you'd expect by its very name—levels off. In general, the older we get, the less growth hormone we produce. Symptoms of low growth hormone include thin lips, droopy eyelids, sagging cheeks, loose skin folds under the chin, thin muscles, floppy triceps, a fat droopy abdomen, sagging back muscles, thin skin, and thin soles of the feet—all typical signs of getting old.

Balancing other hormones also helps to raise growth hormone levels. In males, it is important to equilibrate testosterone, and in females, the key balance is between estrogen, progesterone, testosterone, and thyroid. In addition, supplementing with melatonin at bedtime and getting adequate sleep can help to raise growth hormone levels.

A combination of amino acids, including arginine, ornithine, glutamine, lysine, glycine, leucine, isoleucine, and valine, can significantly boost growth hormone levels. There is a nanoliposomal amino acid complex called Secretropin, containing some of these amino acids in very low doses, that can be taken sublingually. This has been shown to be effective at increasing IGF-1 and IGFBP-3 levels, which indicate a rise in growth hormone. For patients with low growth hormone levels that do not respond to the above measures, I recommend growth hormone. To find a physician who can prescribe these supplements and growth hormone, go to www.worldhealth.net.

We have looked at four of the major players in the hormonal orchestra. When conducted properly, these hormones can play a key role in helping you burn fat and build muscle. In combination with proper nutrition and exercise, they create harmonious music—the way the body intended.

Unfortunately, some obese patients continue to face a cacophony within their bodies because they lack another hormone. No matter how in balance their estrogen, progesterone, testosterone, or growth hormone levels are, they still cannot lose weight. The reason—low thyroid levels—is what we will dive into next.

Low Thyroid Function

It's estimated that more than 5 percent of all Americans—around twenty-seven million people—suffer from a thyroid disorder.[5] Yet almost thirteen million of those individuals never even realize it. Why are so many people walking around unaware that they have a low thyroid? Many doctors mistake the symptoms of low thyroid for normal signs of aging, depression, chronic

fatigue, or obesity. And unfortunately, if these physicians rely solely on blood tests for a diagnosis, they can miss a major portion of low thyroid cases among patients.

Most doctors use the TSH blood test as the gold standard to diagnose hypothyroidism. TSH is a hormone that is produced in the pituitary gland. The main problem I have with the TSH test is that its range of what is considered "normal" is too wide. A normal blood level of TSH is 0.35 to 5.5 uIU/mL in most labs. However, I have found that many patients with a TSH of 2.5 to 5.0 who have many of the symptoms of low thyroid will respond very well to low doses of thyroid hormone. Some patients still have symptoms of low thyroid even with a TSH of 2.0. I believe the ranges of TSH may eventually be lowered to 0.5 to 2.5, partly because research indicates that individuals with TSH values greater than 2.0 have a significantly higher risk of developing hypothyroidism over the next twenty years.[6]

The two main hormones produced by the thyroid gland are thyroxine (T4) and triiodothyronine (T3). Most of the thyroid hormones in the body, or around 80 percent, is T4. T3 is the active form of thyroid hormone and is several times stronger than T4. It is also very important for weight loss. Eighty percent of the T3 in our bodies comes from the conversion of T4 to T3 in such organs and tissues as the kidneys, liver, and muscle. Both of these thyroid hormones gradually decline with age. Yet many obese people may show signs of a sluggish thyroid. I believe one of the main reasons for this is because some are poor converters of T4 to T3. After seeing hundreds of obese people in my practice struggle to convert T4 to T3, I have identified the following reasons for their poor conversion:

- The primary reason is chronic unremitting stress. I mentioned earlier that chronic stress elevates your cortisol levels, which then acts like a fat magnet and programs you for weight gain. Unfortunately, it also blocks (to a certain degree) the conversion of T4 to T3.
- Another reason why people are poor converters is because certain medications interfere with the conversion. These medications include birth control pills, estrogen, hormone replacement therapy, beta-blockers, chemotherapy, theophylline, lithium, and Dilantin. In addition, any oral estrogen or birth control pill simply increases thyroid-binding globulin and decreases the amount of thyroid hormone that is free and active.
- Another common cause of poor conversion is eating certain foods. Soy products are one of the main foods that decrease the conversion of T4

to T3. (That is why, if you haven't already noticed, I do not recommend any soy products on this program—shocking for a weight-loss plan, isn't it?)

- Excessive consumption of raw cruciferous vegetables such as cabbage, broccoli, cauliflower, and brussels sprouts can also decrease the conversion of T4 to T3. For those who eat an abundance of raw cruciferous vegetables (three or more servings a day), you may be sabotaging your weight loss by becoming a poor converter of T4 to T3. However, it should be noted that very rarely do I encounter patients eating excessive cruciferous veggies.

- Low-fat diets, low-carbohydrate diets, or low-protein diets will also make you a poor converter—just another reason why I hate diets. Additionally, excessive alcohol intake will make you a poor converter.

INFLAMMATION

The obesity and inflammation connection is cyclical in nature: obesity causes increased inflammation, and increased inflammation causes even more weight gain. Essentially, the more body fat you have—particularly belly fat—the more inflammation you generally have.

Belly fat

Most people think of fat tissue as being inactive tissue, but that is far from the truth. Fatty tissue or fat storage areas, such as belly fat, are active endocrine organs that produce numerous types of hormones. The more fat cells you have, the more estrogen, cortisol, and testosterone your body produces. When your fatty tissues are spewing out all these hormones—most likely raising your estrogen, testosterone, and cortisol levels—and producing tremendous inflammation in your body, there is only one result: weight gain.

Across the board, studies show that fat deposited in the abdominal area leads to the greatest amount of inflammation. Conversely, when you decrease your body's inflammatory response, you will also lower your weight as well as your waist size. To find out what foods can trigger inflammation and which ones help to control it, please refer to the information available at www.thecandodiet.com.

Food allergies and sensitivities

Food allergies are a typical inflammatory response that is often found on the pathway to obesity. The most common food allergies are caused by eggs, cow's

milk and other dairy products, peanuts, wheat (gluten), soy, tree nuts (almonds, cashews, pecans, walnuts, and so on), fish, shellfish, and seeds (sesame and sunflower seeds). An estimated forty to fifty million Americans have environmental allergies, but only 4 percent of all adults are allergic to foods or food additives. Among children under the age of three, this increases to 6 to 8 percent who have confirmed food allergies.[7]

FOOD ALLERGIES AND WEIGHT GAIN

Food allergies as well as food sensitivities can cause weight gain, bloating, and swelling in the hands, feet, ankles, abdomen, chin, and around the eyes. Much of the weight gained is fluid retention caused by inflammation and the release of certain hormones. In addition there is fermentation of foods, particularly carbohydrates, in the intestines that can result in a swollen, distended belly and gas production.

Symptoms of food allergies include hives; eczema; nausea; vomiting; diarrhea; stomach cramps; asthma; runny, stuffy, or itchy nose; sneezing; problems breathing; and anaphylaxis. These symptoms usually occur within minutes to a few hours after eating the offending food. Food allergies cause significant inflammation in the body and need to be identified and removed. However, I have found that many obese patients have delayed food sensitivities.

Delayed food sensitivities

The American Allergy and Immunology Association only allows immunoglobulin E (IgE) reactions to be called "allergy reactions." IgE food allergies produce symptoms such as tingling lips or tongue, swollen lips, wheezing, and so forth that generally occur within minutes to a few hours after eating a food.

GENETICALLY MODIFIED FOODS (GM FOODS OR GMOS)

Many food allergies are associated with genetically modified foods (GM foods). The four most commonly produced GM foods are: soy, corn, rapeseed (canola), and potatoes.[8]

However, there are three other very common allergy pathways that are not being addressed. Type II, III, and IV reactions are delayed food reactions where symptoms may not occur for hours to days after ingesting the food. These delayed allergy reactions are very common, but because it usually takes hours or days for symptoms to occur, patients and physicians often don't recognize them as the result of delayed food allergies.

Many cases of obesity and weight gain in which no diet works are due to these delayed food sensitivities. Other diseases commonly associated with delayed food sensitivities include migraine headaches, psoriasis, irritable

bowel syndrome, eczema, arthritis, chronic fatigue syndrome, ADD and ADHD, asthma, fibromyalgia, chronic sinusitis, colitis, Crohn's disease, acid reflux, autism, and rosacea. (For information about delayed food sensitivity testing, refer to Appendix H.)

Leaky gut

Delayed food sensitivities start in the intestinal tract when the lining of the GI tract becomes inflamed and hyperpermeable. When the intestinal tract develops an increase in permeability, some doctors have coined this as "leaky gut." What has happened is simply that the GI tract has become inflamed from numerous causes, such as intestinal infections (food poisoning; bacterial, parasitic, viral, and yeast infections), certain medications (aspirin, anti-inflammatory meds, antibiotics, and so on), or ingesting gut-irritating foods and beverages such as alcohol or hot spices.

The inflamed gut causes the tight junctions between mucosa cells in the small intestines to open, which then allows an increased absorption of partially digested proteins. Under normal circumstances, the GI tract only absorbs amino acids (not proteins), glucose, and short-chain fatty acids. However, with increased intestinal permeability, large food proteins, antigens, and toxins are absorbed into the body. The body then produces antibodies against harmless foods that we once enjoyed.

The body actually views these foods as invaders and forms antibodies to fight them. IgG antibodies and immune complexes are formed, which then may inflame and damage many different tissues and organs. This eventually leads to the diseases I mentioned above as well as the inability to lose weight. The most common delayed food sensitivities are dairy, gluten (wheat), eggs, peanuts, corn, soy, chocolate, fish, shellfish, and tree nuts (almonds, cashews, and walnuts).

Altered GI flora or dysbiosis

Although many bacteria are beneficial, some are potentially pathogenic, and others are full-fledged pathogens. Pathogenic bacteria often make toxins that can be absorbed back into the bloodstream. Bacterial enzymes can also convert bile into chemicals that promote the development of cancer.

READ MORE ABOUT IT

For more information, please read my book *The Bible Cure for Candida and Yeast Infections.*

The problem for most people is that because doctors are quick to pull the trigger on prescribing antibiotics, these patients' natural beneficial bacteria levels become imbalanced. When we use

antibiotics for too long or too frequently, it can create an overabundance of pathogenic bacteria and yeast. These upset the natural balance in the large intestines by killing off many of the beneficial bacteria, which can then allow more of the pathogenic bacteria and yeast to grow unrestrained. Under normal circumstances, massive amounts of bacteria coexist with significantly less colonies of yeast. The excessive number of beneficial bacteria prevents the yeast from enlarging their territory. However, frequent or prolonged use of antibiotics destroys much of the beneficial bacteria and does no harm to the yeast, allowing them to grow unhindered. This, in turn, can lead to chronic inflammation of the GI tract, food cravings, certain food sensitivities, increased intestinal permeability, and almost always weight gain.

THE HCG DIET/ SIMEON'S PROTOCOL

The HCG Diet is based on Dr. A. T. W. Simeon's book Pounds & Inches: A New Approach to Obesity and was previously only available in weight-loss clinics. But the diet is now available online, and I've had many people ask me about it. During the course of this extremely low-calorie diet, people are given supplements of human chorionic gonadotropin (hCG), a polypeptide hormone produced by the human placenta and assumed to improve the metabolic rate. You are born with enough hCG to last your entire life, but the supplements are given because the chemicals in many American foods are believed to remove hCG from your body. There are potential side effects. I have personally treated people who developed gallstones after being on this diet; therefore, I only recommend people attempt this diet under direct supervision of a doctor. Unfortunately this is a very low-calorie diet, and most people regain their weight.

DEPRESSION

Depression has a way of making you feel isolated and trapped, with no light at the end of the tunnel. This is another reason why many dieters who plateau eventually give up and gain their weight back. Once they hit a snag that turns from temporary to seemingly permanent, they give in to depression when nothing they do seems to work. This isn't just feeling blue or down on occasion, but it is actual clinical depression in which you cannot control your pessimistic mood or helpless, hopeless thoughts.

Although clinical depression has many symptoms, there are even more factors that can lead to it. The list is extensive to say the least. Genetics can play a major role in causing depression, as can any past traumatic experiences. Chronic illnesses such as cardiovascular disease, cancer, multiple sclerosis, Parkinson's disease, and other chronic degenerative diseases are commonly

associated with depression. The mental disorder can also be a side effect of certain medications such as prednisone and other steroids or birth control pills.

Depression may be a delayed response to various traumatic life experiences such as divorce, a loved one's death, loss of a job, or rape. And, of course, depression may be due to a variety of physical and physiological factors: chemical imbalance in the brain, a lack of sleep, head trauma, chronic pain, hormonal imbalance, and excessive chronic stress, to name a few.

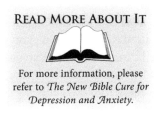

READ MORE ABOUT IT

For more information, please refer to *The New Bible Cure for Depression and Anxiety.*

Sometimes balancing neurotransmitters with targeted amino acid therapy is enough to help someone out of depression. Yet often when dealing with clinical depression (especially severe cases), psychological treatment is just as important. It is often essential to combine balancing neurotransmitters with what is called cognitive behavioral therapy, which helps an individual identify any distortional thought patterns and replace them with rational ones.

Similar to cognitive behavioral therapy, reframing involves a person shifting his focus away from his present point of view so that he can see another person or situation from a new perspective. One of the most powerful aspects of reframing comes when you opt to see things from *God's* perspective. Scriptural reframing replaces our grief, sorrows, pains, fears, worries, and failures with God's promises. There are more than seven thousand promises of God in the Bible, and each one is like a blank check waiting to be used.

DIETING, MEDICATIONS, AND SMOKING

So far in this final chapter of the book, I have discussed many factors that affect the metabolic rate, including lack of exercise, skipping meals, chronic stress, insulin resistance, neurotransmitter imbalance, hormone imbalance, low thyroid, delayed food sensitivities, inflammation, and so forth. If you visit www.thecandodiet.com, you can access more information on each of these health issues. My hope is that through the summaries of information I've included in this chapter, you have identified what may be causing a plateau in your weight-loss efforts—and by taking the questionnaire and following the advice I've provided online, you are about to find a solution that will take you to the next level.

However, some people do not fall into any of the categories we have addressed yet are still metabolically compromised. As I've already alluded to,

for many of these people there is a strong genetic component for obesity that can include having a sluggish metabolic rate.

What happens if you are still not covered, so to speak? What are you to do when none of the aforementioned conditions matches your current struggle? I want to address a trio of additional issues that may have left you metabolically compromised. While each has its own unique challenges, each is also relatively simple to identify. In fact, I imagine some of these may come across as "no-brainers." Yet my twenty-five-plus years of experience tell me it is often the seemingly "little" things that people often neglect to consider when they have hit a weight-loss plateau. Again, I hope this chapter can pinpoint one of these roadblocks for you, and that as a result, you put the information available on our Web site to use and change your approach in order to get your metabolic rate restored back to normal.

Fad dieting and yo-yo dieting

In chapter 5, I discussed how fad dieting lowers the metabolic rate. It doesn't matter whether you are on the latest fad diet, are a regular yo-yo dieter, or both: dieting can damage your metabolism. The typical woman dieting in the United States aims for the dieting "magic threshold," eating fewer than 1,500 calories a day. This is already 300 fewer calories than the World Health Organization's definition of a starvation diet. Not only are these women starving themselves for no reason, but they're also eroding their metabolism—which has the exact opposite long-term result than what they are after.

When a typical diet drops your total calorie intake below your resting metabolic rate (the minimum number of calories required to keep your metabolism running efficiently each day), your body then responds by slowing down your metabolic rate even more. This is a protective mechanism that keeps you from true starvation. However, most dieters are unknowingly triggering the starvation response in their bodies.

In addition, when you follow the average diet, you almost always lose muscle mass. Your brain requires sugar, yet when you consume an inadequate amount of calories to be converted to sugar, your body sacrifices muscle tissue in order to convert that to sugar. You are then burning the most expensive fuel in the body and lowering your metabolic rate in the process. Sure, you may lose weight on a diet, just as most people do. Yet what you may not realize is that about half of the weight you've lost is fat and the other half is usually muscle. This is yet another reason diets don't work long term: once you return to eating your favorite foods, you typically start to gain your

weight back rapidly—yet each time your metabolic rate has been taken down yet another notch.

To add to the bad news, the weight that you then gain back is practically all fat. Every time you diet, you continue to lose more muscle and regain more fat. Eventually, you get stuck in metabolic limbo and usually become frustrated, discouraged, and metabolically compromised.

My advice to you is the same that I have offered since the first page of this book: stop following all of the other dieting advice out there! Whether it's one of the big-name diets that seem to come in and out of fashion every few years or the latest Hollywood diet that only includes coffee and cucumbers, it won't work. Trust me, you'll do much better once you hop off the diet train. Read the information on page 242 on how to reset a sluggish metabolism and eat the proper ratio of protein, fats, and low-glycemic carbs every three to three and a half hours.

As you follow the exercise and strengthening parts of the "I Can Do This" program, you can slowly regain the muscle tissue lost. It may take some time, but the good news is that all is not lost. Remember, this muscle tissue is essential to losing more weight even faster, because muscle cells burn about seventy times more calories than fat cells.

Sometimes, however, exercise is simply not enough. It's possible you may need hormone therapy, especially if you are hormone deficient. Or it may be that you are metabolically compromised because of three other issues I'm about to address: medications, smoking cessation, and depression.

Medications that cause weight gain

Many prescription and over-the-counter medications can stop or stall weight loss, while still others can cause weight gain. Although there is no official count of how many medications actually cause weight gain, experts estimate the figure among everyday drugs to be at least fifty, and probably more. It is certainly high enough to have affected many of the patients I have helped lose weight. Can you imagine their frustration when they followed a nutritional and dietary program to the letter and exercised and strength-trained five to six days a week, yet never lost weight—and some even gained weight? Of course you can—you may be experiencing the same frustration!

That is why prior to seeing patients I always ask what prescriptions and over-the-counter medications they are taking. Many of the most common medications have weight gain as a potential side effect. Let's look at some of the most common offenders of this. (Keep in mind that just because your

particular medication is not mentioned, it doesn't necessarily mean that it still cannot cause weight gain or stall your weight-loss efforts.)

- Oral and injectable steroids: Steroids include prednisone, Medrol Dosepak, dexamethasone, cortisone, hydrocortisone, Kenalog, and Depo-Medrol. In addition, steroid inhalers for asthma and nasal steroids for allergies can occasionally cause weight gain.
- Antidepressants: The older tricyclic antidepressants such as Elavil and Tofranil are notorious for causing significant weight gain. Many of the SSRI antidepressants such as Zoloft, Lexapro, and Paxil commonly cause weight gain, as do many of the other newer anti-depressants. It should be noted, however, that Wellbutrin typically does not cause weight gain.
- Antipsychotic medications: Both Zyprexa and Seroquel are associated with weight gain. In addition, lithium for bipolar disorder is commonly associated with adding pounds.
- Anticonvulsant medications: Depakote commonly causes weight gain.
- Heartburn medications: Nexium, Prilosec, and Prevacid can all cause weight gain.
- High blood pressure medications: These medications include beta-blockers (e.g., Inderal, atenolol), calcium channel blockers (e.g., verapamil), diuretics (e.g., HCTZ), and alpha-blockers (e.g., Cardura), and can all cause weight gain.
- Antihistamines: Both prescription and over-the-counter antihistamines such as Benadryl and Zyrtec can prompt weight gain. These medications are commonly used for allergies.
- Insulin and insulin-stimulating medications: I have noticed that whenever diabetic patients start on insulin, they always gain weight. The patients who use insulin pumps seem to fair better. Medications that increase insulin tend to also cause weight gain. However, metformin and Byetta are often associated with weight loss.

> ## ARTIFICIAL CIGARETTES
>
> For many smokers, smoking is more than just a "nicotine fix." It is an ritual involving all the senses, including the senses of touch and taste. Holding a cigarette in the hand, putting it in the mouth, puffing it…these are all part of the ritual of smoking, just as much as the nicotine.
>
> Quitting smoking can be just as much quitting the ritual as the nicotine withdrawal. There are now artificial cigarettes to help smokers make the transition from smoker to nonsmoker more easily.

Realize that these medications do not have the same effect on all people. However, if you have noticed weight gain after starting one of these medications, either consider asking your physician to switch you to a different class of medication or consider a natural alternative.

Smoking cessation

There is one last group among the metabolically compromised, and it is made up of individuals who stop smoking. The average weight gain in individuals who stop smoking is between 11 and 13 pounds.[9] Women tend to gain slightly more weight than men. Typically, smokers will gain weight after they stop smoking—often within the first two years—even if they do not eat more. One of the reasons for this is that nicotine raises the metabolic rate slightly. When people quit smoking, their metabolic rate decreases, but their sense of taste and smell improves, which makes food more appealing.

Ex-smokers also tend to use snacking as a substitute for smoking. Most of the weight gain that occurs in individuals who stop smoking occurs in the first six months after quitting. The best way to prevent this weight gain is to follow the healthy food plan and snack plan outlined in the "I Can Do This" program, in addition to regularly exercising. You should also drink green tea throughout the day (sweetened with stevia if needed). Most people who have quit smoking want to keep something in their mouth, so to avoid this being a comfort food, try sugar-free chewing gum sweetened with xylitol and not aspartame.

TRUE WELLNESS

As a Christian physician, I believe all healing starts with a relationship with Jesus Christ. I'm not talking about a religion; it starts with a real relationship with Him. The bridge to true peace is only through Him. If this is something you want and have never asked for, receiving it is incredibly simple. It starts with praying a simple prayer like this one:

> *Lord Jesus, I believe that You are the Son of God and that You died for my sins. I also believe that You were raised from the dead and are alive and well. Now I want to know You as my Savior and Lord. I ask You to forgive my sins and change my heart so that I can live with You eternally. Thank You for Your peace. Help me to walk with You so that I can begin to know You as my best friend and my Lord. Amen.*

If you prayed that prayer for the first time, let me be the first to both congratulate you and welcome you into a new life. Trust me, you will never be the

same! I also encourage you to find others who have prayed a similar prayer and are living out a daily relationship with Jesus Christ. As any recovering addict or depressed person knows, it's important to surround yourself with those who are on the same journey. And as Christians, we are all linked by the same narrow road we travel. Get involved with a church or ministry that will help as you continue toward wholeness. For the entirety of this book, we've dealt with bettering your body. I pray you can couple this with a spiritual wellness that comes only through Jesus Christ.

If you have any of these symptoms listed in this chapter, please complete the questionnaire online at www.thecandodiet.com, which will then direct you to more information and my treatment recommendations for each specific roadblock we've discussed in this chapter. I also encourage you to talk to your health care professional about the various tests and natural therapies I've recommended.

APPENDIX A

WEIGHT-LOSS CONTRACT

I, _____ [print your name], hereby commit to Dr. Colbert's "I Can Do This" diet.

- I commit to strictly following this program for four weeks as directed without cheating.
- I commit to a regular activity schedule of walking for twenty to thirty minutes at least five days a week. This can be increased to a brisk walk as tolerated.
- I commit to maintaining a daily food and exercise/activity diary.
- I commit to practice portion control.
- I commit to visualizing myself at my ideal weight.
- My family is committed to my weight-loss goals.
- I commit to removing all junk food, foods high in sugar content, addictive foods, or foods I crave from my cabinets, refrigerator, freezer, and house.
- I commit to having an accountability partner.
- I commit to eating three meals a day and two snacks, and no longer eating complex carbs after 6:00 p.m.
- I commit to eating breakfast like a king, lunch like a prince, and dinner like a pauper.
- I commit to saying to myself every day, "I forgive myself, accept myself, and love myself," even if I cheat or fall.

I understand that failure to comply may sabotage my weight-loss goals. I agree to adhere to all of the above commitments in order to achieve weight loss.

Your signature: _____ Date: _____

Witness's signature: _____

Note: You can print a copy of this contract at www.thecandodiet.com.

APPENDIX B

GOD'S PROMISES FOR WEIGHT LOSS

Scripture Promise	Confession
"Where there is no vision, the people perish" (Proverbs 29:18, KJV).	I envision myself weighing _____ [goal weight].
"Write the vision and make it plain on tablets" (Habakkuk 2:2).	I have a picture of myself at my goal weight on my refrigerator and bathroom mirror, and by faith I look like the picture.
"Yet in all these things we are more than conquerors through Him who loved us" (Romans 8:37).	I am a conqueror and have successfully lost weight. By faith I see myself at my goal weight.
"Do you not know that you are the temple of God and that the Spirit of God dwells in you? If anyone defiles the temple of God, God will destroy him. For the temple of God is holy, which temple you are" (1 Corinthians 3:16–17).	I am the temple of God, and I refuse to pollute my temple by eating junk food and sugary foods.
"Or do you not know that your body is the temple of the Holy Spirit who is in you, whom you have from God, and you are not your own? For you were bought at a price; therefore glorify God in your body and in your spirit, which are God's" (1 Corinthians 6:19–20).	I am bought by the blood of Jesus, and my body belongs to Him. I will glorify Him in my body by choosing the proper foods.
"No temptation has overtaken you except such as is common to man; but God is faithful, who will not allow you to be tempted beyond what you are able, but with the temptation will also make the way of escape, that you may be able to bear it" (1 Corinthians 10:13).	The Holy Spirit enables me to overcome all food temptations as I abide in Him and He abides in me.
"Now thanks be to God who always leads us in triumph in Christ" (2 Corinthians 2:14).	I will triumph and reach my goal weight because God always causes me to triumph.
"For we are His workmanship, created in Christ Jesus for good works" (Ephesians 2:10).	I am His workmanship, and my weight and shape are being transformed into a picture of health.

Scripture Promise	Confession
"Being confident of this very thing, that He who has begun a good work in you will complete it until the day of Jesus Christ" (Philippians 1:6).	I commit to following this program, and when my willpower is weak, the Holy Spirit makes me strong. I started this program, and I will finish it and succeed.
"I can do all things through Christ who strengthens me" (Philippians 4:13).	Christ strengthens me and enables me to choose the right foods and to resist food temptations.
"He who is in you is greater than he who is in the world" (1 John 4:4).	The Holy Spirit dwells within me and comforts me; no longer will I allow food to be my comforter.
"Now this is the confidence that we have in Him, that if we ask anything according to His will, He hears us. And if we know that He hears us, whatever we ask, we know that we have the petitions that we have asked of Him" (1 John 5:14–15).	It is God's will that I be at a healthy weight. He promises to answer this prayer.

Note: You can print a copy of these promises at www.thecandodiet.com.

APPENDIX C

AFFIRMATIONS FOR WEIGHT LOSS

Repeat these confessions aloud with conviction, one to three times a day or more.

1. I weigh _____ pounds [desired weight] by faith.
2. I see myself weighing _____ pounds [desired weight].
3. I promise to no longer use food to soothe hurts and emotional pains, including grief, fear, anxiety, depression, and so forth.
4. I refuse to pollute my body by eating junk food, sugar, fried foods, and any other food that is unhealthy.
5. I promise to do aerobic exercises such as walk or cycle five days a week.
6. I promise to lift weights or perform callisthenic exercises two or three times a week.
7. I want to lose weight and keep it off.
8. I deserve to lose weight and keep it off.
9. Losing weight is good for me.
10. Losing weight is good for others.
11. It is safe for me to lose weight.
12. I will do all things necessary to lose weight and keep it off.
13. I will give my body what it needs and not what it craves.
14. I promise to eat three meals a day, including breakfast, and a healthy midafternoon snack.
15. I promise to practice portion control.
16. I love myself so much that I choose to develop new dietary habits, practice portion control, exercise regularly, and eat three healthy, balanced meals a day, a healthy midafternoon snack, and a healthy beverage.

17. I forgive myself for gaining weight and for every negative decision, action, or reaction I have made.

18. I promise to clean all high-calorie and junk food out of my cabinets, refrigerator, and freezer.

19. I promise to change bad dietary and lifestyle habits to healthy dietary and lifestyle habits.

20. I promise today that no longer will food be my comforter.

Note: You can print a copy of these affirmations at www.thecandodiet.com.

APPENDIX D

RECOMMENDATIONS AT A GLANCE

Before giving you a week's worth of sample meals, allow me to quickly recap what I feel are very important recommendations to keep in mind on the "Can Do" diet.

General recommendations

- Remember, eat every three to three and a half hours to keep blood sugar levels stable. If you eat at different times than the schedule shown on the following pages, it's fine. Just be sure to eat either a meal or snack every three to three and a half hours and to have your evening snack.
- For meals, choose a protein, a carb, and a fat (but make sure you go "carb free" and low fat after 6:00 p.m.)
- For morning snacks, the easiest thing to do is choose a piece of fruit from the approved fruits on pages 159–160, but you may also choose from the afternoon snacks in the sample menus in Appendix F or the approved snacks on page 281 if you prefer. Take two to three PGX fiber capsules with 16 ounces of water before or after your snack.
- For afternoon snacks, choose any of the approved snacks from page 281 or a "mini-meal" consisting of a half-serving of protein, a half-serving of carbs, and a half-serving of fat. (See pages 174–175 for examples of a "mini-meal.") Take one Serotonin Max if craving sugar or carbs. Take two to three PGX fiber capsules with 16 ounces of water before or after your snack.
- For evening snacks, choose any of the approved snacks from page 281 or a "mini-meal" (but leave out the carbs and fats).
- It's best to drink green, white, or regular tea with your snacks, except for your evening snack.
- Serving size for protein is typically 2–4 ounces for women and 3–6 ounces for men. (If you need to eat more protein, you can increase the amounts to 6 ounces for women and 8 ounces for men, but only with your evening meal.)
- Limit red meat intake to 18 ounces or less per week.
- All soups should be broth based, not cream based.

- Himalayan or Celtic sea salt is preferred over regular table salt (in small amounts, less than 1 teaspoon a day).
- If you are gluten sensitive, you can easily substitute millet bread for Ezekiel 4:9 bread or other types of breads I've recommended in this book.
- If desired, you may sweeten foods and beverages with stevia or Just Like Sugar. It is best to avoid artificial sweeteners such as Nutra-Sweet and Splenda.
- You may add a small amount of organic skim milk to your coffee, if desired
- If organic foods are too expensive, one option is to at least choose organic options for your meat or the foods you consume most often. If you aren't able to buy organic at all, simply choose very lean cuts of meat, peel the skin off of poultry, thoroughly wash fruits and vegetables that cannot be peeled, and choose skim milk or 1 percent dairy products. (However, organic is the best choice; range fed is also a good choice. For meats, Maverick Ranch or Applegate Farms are good choices. I recommend getting prepackaged nitrate-, nitrite-free turkey breast, chicken breast, ham, or lean roast beef slices, which are available.)
- In the sample menus (Appendix F), I recommend large salads for a majority of the lunches and dinners. If you are getting tired of eating salad at both meals, you can save the salad for your evening meal.
- If you choose to make your smoothies with coconut milk, be sure that it contains only 80 calories per cup. (So Delicious is one brand that meets this criterion.) You may have to purchase it from the health food store; coconut milk sold at your local supermarket may be much higher in calories and can sabotage your weight-loss goals.

Recommended appliances (all are optional)

To save time on cooking and preparing meals, I recommend:

- George Foreman Next Grilleration Grill
- Vegetable steamer
- Blender
- Toaster
- Convection oven

Recommended nutritional supplements (all are optional)

You will experience weight loss without taking these supplements, but to help you feel full longer, fight cravings, and lose weight faster, I recommend:

- PGX fiber, to help you feel full longer: Start with one capsule at the beginning of each meal. Slowly work up to two to four capsules with each meal until desired feeling of fullness is achieved. It is best taken with 16 ounces of water, except for evening snack. Use only 8 ounces of water with your evening snack since 16 ounces may interfere with sleep.*
- Serotonin Max, to help with food cravings: Take one capsule with your midafternoon snack and with your evening meal or evening snack (if craving sugars or carbs).
- Irvingia, to help burn fat faster: Take one capsule twice a day.
- Green Tea Elite with EGCG, to help burn fat faster: Take one capsule three times a day.

Recommended protein powders and protein bars (all are optional)

I do not recommend soy-based protein. I recommend banana- or vanilla-flavored protein powder; this can also be added to oatmeal or cereal.

- Whey isolate—examples: Isopure Whey Protein or Jay Robb Whey Protein (available from health food stores), Energy First Whey Protein (available from health food stores, www.energyfirst.com, or 1-888-88-ENERGY)
- Undenatured whey protein—examples: Warrior Milk (available from www.defensenutrition.com), Immunplex (available from www.immunesupport.com), Physicians' Protein Complex (available from www.drcolbert.com)
- Vegetarian protein powder—examples: Life's Basics Protein (available from health food stores or www.drcolbert.com), Pure Encapsulations PureLean (available from www.drcolbert.com)
- Rice protein—examples: Nutrabiotics (available from health food stores)
- Jay Robb Coconut or Fudge Brownie Jay Bar (available from health food stores, 1-877-JayRobb, or www.jayrobb.com) (Men may have a full bar, and women may have ½ or ⅔ bar)

---

* If you can only afford one supplement, this is the most important one. The most critical times to take it are before your afternoon snack, evening meal, and evening snack.

- NuGo Gluten Free Chocolate Crunch Bar (available from health food stores, 1-888-421-2032, or www.nugonutrition.com)
- Nutiva Hemp Chocolate Bar (available from www.drcolbert.com)
- FitSmart Bar (available from health food stores)

Recommended fiber bars (all are optional)

These are the serotonin-boosting fiber bars I recommend. Please refer to page 179 for other serotonin-boosting snacks.

- Fiber One: Oats & Chocolate, Oats & Peanut Butter, Oats & Caramel, Oats & Strawberry, Oats & Apple Streusel, Chocolate Mocha (You should take one Serotonin Max midafternoon in conjunction with your high fiber bar IF you are craving sugars and carbs.)

DR. COLBERT'S "CAN DO" SALAD DRESSING

¼ cup organic extra-virgin olive oil

¾ cup balsamic vinaigrette (or other vinegar if preferred)

Juice of ½–1 lemon or lime

¼ cup cilantro leaves (optional)

1–2 garlic cloves, pressed (or as many as desired for taste)

Salt and pepper to taste (Himalayan sea salt is preferred)

Mix all ingredients and transfer to a spritzer bottle. Makes 1 cup, which should last three months refrigerated.

DR. COLBERT'S "CAN DO" SMOOTHIE

If you feel you are too busy to eat breakfast, here's an extremely easy recipe for a kefir and fruit smoothie that takes only two minutes. Combine the following ingredients in a blender for a snack:

8 oz. organic skim milk, low-fat kefir, coconut kefir, or coconut milk* (midmorning or midafternoon snack only; for evening snack, use 4 oz. water and 4 oz. milk or kefir)

½ frozen banana or ¼ cup frozen blueberries or raspberries (omit for evening snack)

1–2 Tbsp. ground flaxseeds (omit for evening snack)

1 scoop of chocolate-, vanilla-, or banana-flavored whey protein powder (I prefer PureLean or Life's Basics Plant Protein powder)

* Make sure that the coconut milk has only 80 calories per cup.

Note: You can find more recipes like these at www.thecandodiet.com.

DR. COLBERT'S APPROVED "CAN DO" FOODS

SNACKS

Crackers and cheese (combine serving of a healthy cracker with serving of a fat-free cheese)

Crackers
- Garlic Roasted Triscuit—1 ounce (7 crackers)
- Herb Garden Triscuit—1 ounce (7 crackers)
- Wheat Thins Fiber Selects—1 ounce (13 crackers)
- Rice Bran (Healthy Way)—1 ounce (7 crackers)
- Triscuit Deli-Style Rye Crackers—1 ounce (7 crackers)

Cheese
- Cheddar sharp, fat-free (Kraft Singles)—two slices, 3/4 ounce each
- American cheese, fat-free (Kraft Single)—two slices, 3/4 ounce each
- Cottage cheese, nonfat (Breakstone)—1/2 cup
- Mozzarella, nonfat (Kraft Singles)—two slices, 3/4 ounce each
- Swiss cheese, nonfat (Kraft Singles)—two slices, 3/4 ounce each

Kefir and fruit (blend plain low-fat kefir with fruit)
- Lifeway Organic kefir, low-fat plain—8 ounces
- One medium apple

Cheese, fruit, and nuts
- Two slices of fat-free cheese with one medium apple and five to ten pecans, walnuts, or almonds

Protein powder
- 1/2 cup organic skim milk mixed with one-half scoop of Life's Basics or PureLean protein powder

Mini-meal
- Remember, every meal can be cut down to a snack-size portion; left-overs from dinner make for an excellent snack the next day.

FROZEN ENTRÉES (FOR LUNCH ONLY)

- Stouffer's Lean Cuisine Grilled Chicken Teriyaki
- Stouffer's Lean Cuisine Steak, Cheddar and Mushroom Panini
- Stouffer's Lean Cuisine Café Classics Shrimp Alfredo
- Stouffer's Lean Cuisine Café Classics Steak Tips Portabella
- Stouffer's Lean Cuisine Café Classics Sesame Chicken
- Stouffer's Lean Cuisine Spa Cuisine Classics Butternut Squash Ravioli
- Weight Watchers Smart Ones Chicken Parmesan
- Weight Watchers Smart Ones Sante Fe Style Rice and Beans
- Kashi Chicken Pasta Pomodoro
- Kashi Black Bean Mango
- Kashi Chicken Florentine
- Kashi Garden Vegetable Pasta
- Birds Eye Voila! Pesto Chicken Primavera
- Healthy Choice Chicken Fettuccini Alfredo
- Healthy Choice Sesame Chicken
- Healthy Choice Café Steamers Creamy Dill Salmon
- Healthy Choice Café Steamers Roasted Beef Merlot
- Healthy Choice All Natural Entrées Pumpkin Squash Ravioli
- Healthy Choice Café Steamers Five-Spice Beef and Vegetables
- Marie Callender's Salisbury Steak Dinner

EATING OUT AT SUBWAY (BREAKFAST AND LUNCH ONLY)

Breakfast subs (women, remove one piece of bread)
- Six-inch Wheat with Ham and Egg
- Six-inch Wheat with Steak and Egg
- Six-inch Wheat with Veggies and Egg
- Six-inch Wheat Western Style with Egg

Regular subs (be sure to load up on veggies; women, remove one piece of bread)
- Roasted Chicken Breast
- Chicken Teriyaki
- Ham with Honey Mustard
- Roast Beef
- Subway Club

- Turkey Breast
- Turkey Breast with Ham
- Veggie Delight

Double meat subs (men only)
- Roasted Chicken Breast
- Chicken Teriyaki
- Ham
- Roast Beef
- Subway Club
- Turkey Breast
- Turkey Breast with Ham
- Wraps
- Turkey Breast

EATING OUT AT CHICK-FIL-A (LUNCH ONLY)

Cool wraps
- Char-Grilled Chicken
- Chicken Caesar
- Spicy Chicken

Chicken sandwiches (women, remove one piece of bun)
- Char-Grilled
- Char-Grilled Club (no sauce)
- Chicken Salad

EATING OUT AT BOSTON MARKET

Meats
- Garlic Rotisserie Chicken (1/4 dark or 1/4 white, no skin)
- Tuscan Rotisserie Chicken (1/4 spicy white, no skin)

Other entrées
- Honey Glazed Ham
- Rotisserie Turkey

Vegetables
- Green Bean Casserole (one serving)
- Green Beans (one serving)
- Sautéed Spinach (one serving)

APPENDIX F

SAMPLE MENUS FOR ONE WEEK

If you don't want to have to think at all about what to eat while you're losing weight on Dr. Colbert's "I Can Do This" diet, this section of the book was created for you! I've done all the calculating and thinking to make it as easy as possible for you to follow the program and start losing weight. Simply follow these menus for a week, and visit www.thecandodiet.com for additional weekly menu plans that have been created for you.

But keep in mind that these are only samples. If any food item on the following menus does not agree with your taste or budget, you can substitute it with any of the recommended foods I listed for you in chapter 16. Also, I think you'll find it very helpful to refer to Appendix D and use the general guidelines for the "Can Do" diet that have been recapped for you. This will help insure that you stick with the "Can Do" game plan when making your substitutions.

Also remember the times are suggestions only. You don't have to get up and eat at 6:00 a.m. if this is not your normal routine. The key is to make sure you eat a meal or snack at least every three to three and a half hours and that you eat your evening snack.

Monday	
Breakfast: 6:00 a.m	2–3 PGX fiber capsules with 16 oz. water (optional) Quaker Oats Cinnamon High-Fiber Instant Oatmeal (½–1 cup for women; 1 cup for men) ¼ cup berries Handful of almonds (approximately 10) Dr. Colbert's "Can Do" Smoothie (recipe on page 280) 1 cup green tea or coffee
Midmorning snack: 9:00 a.m.	2–3 PGX fiber capsules with 16 oz. water (optional) Granny Smith apple
Lunch: 12:00 p.m.	2–3 PGX fiber capsules with 16 oz. water (optional) Grilled skinless chicken breast (2–4 oz. for women; 3–6 oz. for men) Brown rice (½ cup for women; 1 cup for men) Steamed vegetables (as much as desired) seasoned with small amount of salt, if desired 1 cup green tea, water, sparkling water, or unsweetened iced tea with lemon or lime
Midafternoon snack: 3:00 p.m.	2–3 PGX fiber capsules with 16 oz. water (optional) 6 Wheat Thin Fiber Selects crackers with 2 slices of reduced-fat cheese, 2 Tbsp. fat-free Philadelphia Cream Cheese, Laughing Cow Light cheese, or ½ cup nonfat plain cottage cheese Serotonin Max, if craving sugar or carbs (optional)
Dinner: 6:00 p.m.	2–3 PGX fiber capsules with 16 oz. water (optional) Large salad made of romaine lettuce or other salad greens, sliced cucumber, chopped tomato, and salad spritzer dressing or Dr. Colbert's "Can Do" Salad Dressing (recipe on page 280) 96/4 Extra-lean beef (96/4 means 4 percent fat content) seasoned with Mrs. Dash, small amount of salt, or pepper, if desired (2–6 oz. for women; 3–8 oz. for men) Steamed broccoli (as much as desired) seasoned with small amount of salt, if desired Bowl of broth-based bean or vegetable soup (optional) 1 cup green or white tea, sparkling water, water, or unsweetened iced tea with lemon or lime
Evening snack: 9:00 p.m.	2–3 PGX fiber capsules with 8 oz. water (optional) You can substitute the suggested snack with one "cheat" snack from page 176 if you are craving ice cream or chocolate. Lettuce wrap with chicken, onions, peppers, and other veggies, seasoned to taste Serotonin Max, if craving sugar or carbs (optional)

Tuesday	
Breakfast: 6:00 a.m.	2–3 PGX fiber capsules with 16 oz. water (optional) 2–3 eggs, poached, scrambled, or fried; 1 yolk and 3 egg whites; or Egg Beaters 2–3 oz. Canadian bacon Toasted Ezekiel 4:9 bread (1–2 slices for women; 2 slices for men) with 1 pat (½ tsp.) of organic butter or Smart Balance per slice ½ cup of fruit 1 cup green tea or coffee
Midmorning snack: 9:00 a.m.	2–3 PGX fiber capsules with 16 oz. water (optional) Banana (not overly ripened)
Lunch: 12:00 p.m.	2–3 PGX fiber capsules with 16 oz. water (optional) Salmon (wild-caught preferred) (2–4 oz for women; 3–6 oz. for men) Steamed asparagus (as much as desired) with lemon pepper Small red or new potatoes* (½ cup, or tennis ball for women; 1–2 tennis balls for men) with 1 tsp. of organic butter or Smart Balance. Large salad with plenty of colorful vegetables and salad spritzer dressing or Dr. Colbert's "Can Do" Salad Dressing (recipe on page 280) 1 cup green tea, sparkling water, water, or unsweetened iced tea with lemon or lime
Midafternoon snack: 3:00 p.m.	2–3 PGX fiber capsules with 16 oz. water (optional) Fiber bar (if craving sugar or carbs) or protein bar Serotonin Max, if craving sugar or carbs (optional)
Dinner: 6:00 p.m.	2–3 PGX fiber capsules with 16 oz. water (optional) Large salad with plenty of colorful vegetables and salad spritzer dressing or Dr. Colbert's "Can Do" Salad Dressing (recipe on page 280) Bowl of Campbell's Select Harvest Minestrone Soup or other broth-based soup Grilled turkey breast (2–6 oz. for women; 3–8 oz. for men) As many green veggies as you like (broccoli, asparagus, green beans, etc.) seasoned with garlic, lemon pepper, or small amount of salt, if desired 1 cup green or white tea, sparkling water, water, or unsweetened iced tea with lemon or lime
Evening snack: 9:00 p.m.	2–3 PGX fiber capsules with 8 oz. water (optional) You can substitute the suggested snack with one "cheat" snack from page 176, if you are craving ice cream or chocolate. Salad with 1–2 oz. chicken, turkey, or tuna (tongol) Serotonin Max, if craving sugar or carbs (optional)

* Boiled new potatoes have a glycemic index of 56, so although they aren't quite low-glycemic (GI = 55 or less), they are a better choice than baked potatoes (GI = 83) or mashed potatoes (GI = 73)

Wednesday	
Breakfast: 6:00 a.m.	2–3 PGX fiber capsules with 16 oz. water (optional) 1 cup Fiber One or other cereal (see page 159) with 4–8 oz. skim or 1 percent milk; topped with ¼ cup of fruit and 10 nuts (almonds, walnuts, or pecans) 2–3 oz. turkey bacon or turkey sausage (squeeze sausage between two napkins to remove fat) 1 cup green tea or coffee
Midmorning snack: 9:00 a.m.	2–3 PGX fiber capsules with 16 oz. water (optional) Tangerine
Lunch: 12:00 p.m.	2–3 PGX fiber capsules with 16 oz. water (optional) Large salad with plenty of colorful vegetables and salad spritzer dressing or Dr. Colbert's "Can Do" Salad Dressing (recipe on page 280) Tuna sandwich: 2–6 oz. tongol tuna topped with 1 Tbsp. of Vegenaise, Smart Balance Light Mayonnaise, or grape seed oil mayonnaise, sliced tomato, and romaine lettuce. Serve on 1 to 2 slices of toasted Ezekiel 4:9 bread ¼ cup of fruit 1 cup green or white tea, sparkling water, water, or unsweetened iced tea with lemon or lime
Midafternoon snack: 3:00 p.m.	2–3 PGX fiber capsules with 16 oz. water (optional) 6 oz. plain low-fat or nonfat yogurt or kefir blended with 1 medium apple to make a smoothie Serotonin Max, if craving sugar or carbs (optional)
Dinner: 6:00 p.m.	2–3 PGX fiber capsules with 16 oz. water (optional) Roast beef: rub extra-lean roast beef with minced garlic, dredge in arrowroot, brown in extra-virgin olive oil, and cook in a slow cooker with 2 cups of water and 2 packs of Lipton onion soup mix; add two chopped onions. Cook according to slow cooker directions. Green beans, broccoli, or other green vegetable (as much as desired) seasoned with lemon pepper, garlic, or small amount of salt, if desired Large salad with plenty of colorful vegetables and salad spritzer dressing or Dr. Colbert's "Can Do" Salad Dressing (recipe on page 280) 1 cup green tea, sparkling water, water, or unsweetened iced tea with lemon or lime
Evening snack: 9:00 p.m.	2–3 PGX fiber capsules with 8 oz. water (optional) You can substitute the suggested snack with one "cheat" snack from page 176 if you are craving ice cream or chocolate. Bowl of broth-based vegetable soup with chicken or beef Serotonin Max, if craving sugar or carbs (optional)

Thursday	
Breakfast: 6:00 a.m.	2–3 PGX fiber capsules with 16 oz. water (optional French toast: Beat 2 eggs; add 1 tsp. pure vanilla extract and ½ tsp. cinnamon and mix well. Dip Ezekiel 4:9 bread or other high-fiber bread (1–2 slices for women; 2 slices for men) in egg mixture, and brown on both sides in skillet sprayed with olive oil spray; top with ¼–½ cup of strawberries or fruit of your choice and 10 ground pecans or walnuts. Protein powder (1–2 scoops) mixed with 8 oz. of skim milk, coconut milk, or low-fat plain or coconut kefir (option: dilute the skim milk, coconut milk, or kefir by reducing it to 4 oz. and combining with 4 oz. of filtered water or spring water) 1 cup green tea or coffee
Midmorning snack: 9:00 a.m.	2–3 PGX fiber capsules with 16 oz. water (optional) Pear
Lunch: 12:00 p.m.	2–3 PGX fiber capsules with 16 oz. water (optional) Large salad with plenty of colorful vegetables and salad spritzer dressing or Dr. Colbert's "Can Do" Salad Dressing (recipe on page 280) Grilled wild tilapia (2–4 oz. for women; 3–6 oz. for men) Baked sweet potato (size of 1 tennis ball for women; size of 1–2 tennis balls for men) with 1 teaspoon of organic butter or Smart Balance 1 Tbsp. hummus with cucumber slices 1 cup green tea, sparkling water, water, or unsweetened iced tea with lemon or lime
Midafternoon snack: 3:00 p.m.	2–3 PGX fiber capsules with 16 oz. water (optional) Dr. Colbert's "Can Do" Smoothie (page 280) or protein powder (1–2 scoops) mixed with 8 oz. of skim milk, coconut milk, or coconut kefir (option: dilute the skim milk, coconut milk, or kefir by reducing it to 4 oz. and combining with 4 oz. of filtered water or spring water) Serotonin Max, if craving sugar or carbs (optional)
Dinner: 6:00 p.m.	2–3 PGX fiber capsules with 16 oz. water (optional) Large salad with plenty of colorful veggies and salad spritzer dressing or Dr. Colbert's "Can Do" Salad Dressing (recipe on page 280) Filet mignon steak (2–6 oz. for women; 3–8 oz. for men) seasoned with garlic, salt, pepper, or other seasonings, if desired Broccoli or other green vegetables (as much as desired) with 1 tsp. of organic butter or Smart Balance Bowl of broth-based vegetable soup 1 cup green tea, sparkling water, water, or unsweetened iced tea with lemon or lime
Evening snack: 9:00 p.m.	2–3 PGX fiber capsules with 8 oz. water (optional) You can substitute the suggested snack with one "cheat" snack from page 176 if you are craving ice cream or chocolate. Lettuce wrap with chicken, onions, peppers and other veggies, seasoned to taste Serotonin Max, if craving sugar or carbs (optional)

Friday	
Breakfast: 6:00 a.m.	2–3 PGX fiber capsules with 16 oz. water (optional) Sara Lee Heart Healthy Whole-Wheat Bagel—or millet bagel or toast, if gluten sensitive (½–1 bagel or 1–2 slices of bread for women; whole bagel or 2 slices of bread for men) 1–2 Tbsp. fat-free Philadelphia Cream Cheese 6 oz. plain nonfat yogurt or kefir with ¼–½ cup of organic berries and 10 chopped almonds or pecans 1 cup green tea or coffee
Midmorning snack: 9:00 a.m.	2–3 PGX fiber capsules with 16 oz. water (optional) Orange
Lunch: 12:00 p.m.	2–3 PGX fiber capsules with 16 oz. water (optional) Roast beef sandwich: extra-lean roast beef (2–4 oz. for women; 3–6 oz. for men), 1 slice of low-fat Swiss or mozzarella cheese, 1–2 slices of tomato, lettuce, 1 Tbsp. Smart Balance Light Mayonnaise or mustard; serve on Ezekiel 4:9 or other high-fiber bread (1–2 slices for women: 2 slices for men) Large salad with plenty of colorful vegetables and salad spritzer dressing or Dr. Colbert's "Can Do" Salad Dressing (recipe on page 280) Bowl of Campbell's Select Harvest Southwest Vegetable Soup or other broth-based bean or vegetable soup 1 cup green tea, sparkling water, water, or unsweetened iced tea with lemon or lime
Midafternoon snack: 3:00 p.m.	2–3 PGX fiber capsules with 16 oz. water (optional) Fiber bar (if craving sugar or carbs) or protein bar Serotonin Max, if craving sugar or carbs (optional)
Dinner: 6:00 p.m.	2–3 PGX fiber capsules with 16 oz. water (optional) Broth-based vegetable soup Wild Alaskan salmon with the juice of 1 lemon or lime Steamed broccoli (as much as desired) seasoned with salt if desired Salad made from romaine lettuce or other salad greens, chopped tomato, sliced cucumber, and salad spritzer dressing or Dr. Colbert's "Can Do" Salad Dressing (recipe on page 280) 1 cup green or white tea, sparkling water, water, or unsweetened iced tea with lemon or lime
Evening snack: 9:00 p.m.	2–3 PGX fiber capsules with 8 oz. water (optional) You can substitute the suggested snack with one "cheat" snack from page 176 if you are craving ice cream or chocolate. Protein powder (1–2 scoops) mixed with 8 oz. of skim milk, coconut milk, or low-fat plain or coconut kefir (option: dilute the skim milk, coconut milk, or kefir by reducing it to 4 oz. and combining with 4 oz. of filtered water or spring water) Serotonin Max, if craving sugar or carbs (optional)

Saturday	
Breakfast: 6:00 a.m.	2–3 PGX fiber capsules with 16 oz. water (optional) 1 cup Kashi Vive or Fiber One cereal with 4–8 oz. skim or 1% milk ¼–½ cup nonfat cottage cheese with ½ cup blueberries 1 cup green tea or coffee
Midmorning snack: 9:00 a.m.	2–3 PGX fiber capsules with 16 oz. water (optional) Grapefruit
Lunch: 12:00 p.m.	2–3 PGX fiber capsules with 16 oz. water (optional) Caesar salad: 1 cup romaine lettuce, 2–3 tsp. low-fat Parmesan cheese, and low-fat Caesar salad spritzer dressing Smoked turkey melt: Smoked turkey (2–4 oz. for women; 3–6 oz. for men) topped with 1 Tbsp. Vegenaise, Smart Balance Light Mayonnaise, or grape seed oil mayonnaise, sliced tomato and cucumbers, and lettuce. Serve on toasted Ezekiel 4:9 bread (1 slice for women; 2 slices for men); may add 1 wedge of Laughing Cow Light cheese for women; 1–2 wedges for men and melt over sandwich in sandwich maker or toaster oven (optional) 1 cup green tea, sparkling water, water, or unsweetened iced tea with lemon or lime
Midafternoon snack: 3:00 p.m.	2–3 PGX fiber capsules with 16 oz. water (optional) 6 oz. plain low-fat or nonfat yogurt or kefir blended with 1 medium pear, apple or berries to make a smoothie Serotonin Max, if craving sugar or carbs (optional)
Dinner: 6:00 p.m.	2–3 PGX fiber capsules with 16 oz. water (optional) Large salad made with romaine, spinach, or other greens, with plenty of colorful veggies, and salad spritzer or Dr. Colbert's "Can Do" Salad Dressing (recipe on page 280) Grilled shrimp (2–6 oz. for women; 3–8 oz. for men): coat shrimp with olive oil and season with Mrs. Dash, garlic, salt, lemon pepper, or other seasoning, if desired, and grill 2–3 minutes per side; squeeze lemon juice on shrimp just before removing from grill Grilled asparagus (as much as desired), seasoned to taste and grilled alongside shrimp Campbell's Select Harvest Tomato with Basil Soup 1 cup green tea, sparkling water, water, or unsweetened iced tea with lemon or lime
Evening snack: 9:00 p.m.	2–3 PGX fiber capsules with 8 oz. water (optional) You can substitute the suggested snack with one "cheat" snack from page 176 if you are craving ice cream or chocolate. Salad with 1–2 oz. turkey, chicken, salmon, or tongol tuna Serotonin Max, if craving sugar or carbs (optional)

Sunday	
Breakfast: 6:00 a.m.	2–3 PGX fiber capsules with 16 oz. water (optional) Omelet made from 2–3 eggs, or 1 egg yolk and 2–3 egg whites, or Egg Beaters; tomatoes; onions; mushrooms; or any other vegetables desired. Spray Pam or Smart Balance Butter Burst in skillet used for omelet (may use 1 wedge of Laughing Cow Light cheese for women; 1–2 wedges for men) Toasted Ezekiel 4:9 bread or double-fiber bread (1 slice for women; 2 slices for men) with 1 pat (½ tsp.) of organic butter or Smart Balance ¼–½ cup of fruit Handful of pecans (approximately 10) 1 cup green tea or coffee
Midmorning snack: 9:00 a.m.	2–3 PGX fiber capsules with 16 oz. water (optional) Granny Smith apple
Lunch: 12:00 p.m.	2–3 PGX fiber capsules with 16 oz. water (optional) Large salad with plenty of colorful vegetables and salad spritzer dressing or Dr. Colbert's "Can Do" Salad Dressing (recipe on page 280) Spaghetti with meat sauce: Cook 4 oz. (size of tennis ball) for women or 1 cup (size of 2 tennis balls) for men of whole-wheat spaghetti (not thin spaghetti or angel hair) according to package instructions for al dente; in skillet, brown 2–6 oz. browned, extra-lean ground beef with chopped onion, roasted minced garlic, Mrs. Dash Italian Blend seasoning mix, granulated garlic, salt, and pepper; add browned meat and onion to Classico or Newman's Own Tomato and Basil Pasta Sauce in saucepan and heat through; serve over pasta (½–1 cup for women; 1 cup for men). Bowl of broth-based bean or vegetable soup 1 cup green tea, sparkling water, water, or unsweetened iced tea with lemon or lime
Midafternoon snack: 3:00 p.m.	2–3 PGX fiber capsules with 16 oz. water (optional) 6–7 Wheat Thin Fiber Select crackers with 2 wedges Laughing Cow Light cheese Serotonin Max, if craving sugar or carbs (optional)
Dinner: 6:00 p.m.	2–3 PGX fiber capsules with 16 oz. water (optional) Large salad made with romaine, spinach, or other greens, with plenty of colorful veggies, and salad spritzer Barbecue pork chops: Coat lean pork chops (2–6 oz. for women; 3–8 oz. for men) with 1–2 Tbsp. of barbecue sauce and grill on both sides Cole slaw (1 cup): shred half a head of cabbage and mix with 1–2 Tbsp. Smart Balance Light Mayonnaise, ½ cup apple cider vinegar, 1 Tbsp. celery seed, and 1 grated carrot Bowl of broth-based bean or vegetable soup 1 cup green tea, sparkling water, water, or unsweetened iced tea with lemon or lime
Evening snack: 9:00 p.m.	2–3 PGX fiber capsules with 8 oz. water (optional) You can substitute the suggested snack with one "cheat" snack from page 176 if you are craving ice cream or chocolate. Protein powder (1–2 scoops) mixed with 8 oz. of skim milk, coconut milk, or coconut kefir Serotonin Max, if craving sugar or carbs (optional)

APPENDIX G

BODY MASS INDEX CHART

BODY MASS INDEX FOR ADULTS TABLE[1]

	Normal						Overweight					Obese									
BMI	19	20	21	22	23	24	25	26	27	28	29	30	31	32	33	34	35	36	37	38	39
Height (inches)	Body Weight (pounds)																				
58	91	96	100	105	110	115	119	124	129	134	138	143	148	153	158	162	167	172	177	181	186
59	94	99	104	109	114	119	124	128	133	138	143	148	153	158	163	168	173	178	183	188	193
60	97	102	107	112	118	123	128	133	138	143	148	153	158	163	168	174	179	184	189	194	199
61	100	106	111	116	122	127	132	137	143	148	153	158	164	169	174	180	185	190	195	201	206
62	104	109	115	120	126	131	136	142	147	153	158	164	169	175	180	186	191	196	202	207	213
63	107	113	118	124	130	135	141	146	152	158	163	169	175	180	186	191	197	203	208	214	220
64	110	116	122	128	134	140	145	151	157	163	169	174	180	186	192	197	204	209	215	221	227
65	114	120	126	132	138	144	150	156	162	168	174	180	186	192	198	204	210	216	222	228	234
66	118	124	130	136	142	148	155	161	167	173	179	186	192	198	204	210	216	223	229	235	241
67	121	127	134	140	146	153	159	166	172	178	185	191	198	204	211	217	223	230	236	242	249
68	125	131	138	144	151	158	164	171	177	184	190	197	203	210	216	223	230	236	243	249	256
69	128	135	142	149	155	162	169	176	182	189	196	203	209	216	223	230	236	243	250	257	263
70	132	139	146	153	160	167	174	181	188	195	202	209	216	222	229	236	243	250	257	264	271
71	136	143	150	157	165	172	179	186	193	200	208	215	222	229	236	243	250	257	265	272	279
72	140	147	154	162	169	177	184	191	199	206	213	221	228	235	242	250	258	265	272	279	287
73	144	151	159	166	174	182	189	197	204	212	219	227	235	242	250	257	265	272	280	288	295
74	148	155	163	171	179	186	194	202	210	218	225	233	241	249	256	264	272	280	287	295	303
75	152	160	168	176	184	192	200	208	216	224	232	240	248	256	264	272	279	287	295	303	311
76	156	164	172	180	189	197	205	213	221	230	238	246	254	263	271	279	287	295	304	312	320

	Extreme Obesity														
BMI	40	41	42	43	44	45	46	47	48	49	50	51	52	53	54
Height (inches)	Body Weight (pounds)														
58	191	196	201	205	210	215	220	224	229	234	239	244	248	253	258
59	198	203	208	212	217	222	227	232	237	242	247	252	257	262	267
60	204	209	215	220	225	230	235	240	245	250	255	261	266	271	276
61	211	217	222	227	232	238	243	248	254	259	264	269	275	280	285
62	218	224	229	235	240	246	251	256	262	267	273	278	284	289	295
63	225	231	237	242	248	254	259	265	270	278	282	287	293	299	304
64	232	238	244	250	256	262	267	273	279	285	291	296	302	308	314
65	240	246	252	258	264	270	276	282	288	294	300	306	312	318	324
66	247	253	260	266	272	278	284	291	297	303	309	315	322	328	334
67	255	261	268	274	280	287	293	299	306	312	319	325	331	338	344
68	262	269	276	282	289	295	302	308	315	322	328	335	341	348	354
69	270	277	284	291	297	304	311	318	324	331	338	345	351	358	365
70	278	285	292	299	306	313	320	327	334	341	348	355	362	369	376
71	286	293	301	308	315	322	329	338	343	351	358	365	372	379	386
72	294	302	309	316	324	331	338	346	353	361	368	375	383	390	397
73	302	310	318	325	333	340	348	355	363	371	378	386	393	401	408
74	311	319	326	334	342	350	358	365	373	381	389	396	404	412	420
75	319	327	335	343	351	359	367	375	383	391	399	407	415	423	431
76	328	336	344	353	361	369	377	385	394	402	410	418	426	435	443

BMI Categories

- Underweight = < 18.5
- Normal weight = 18.5–24.9
- Overweight = 25–29.9
- Obesity = BMI of 30 or greater

Note: You can also find at BMI calculator at www.thecandodiet.com.

APPENDIX H

RECOMMENDED PRODUCTS
AND RESOURCES

These are products mentioned throughout this book that are offered through Dr. Colbert's Divine Health Wellness Center.

Divine Health Nutritional Products
1908 Boothe Circle
Longwood, FL 32750
Phone: (407) 331-7007
Web site: www.drcolbert.com
E-mail: info@drcolbert.com

Maintenance nutritional supplements
Divine Health Living Multivitamin
Divine Health Multivitamin
Divine Health Living Omega
Divine Health Omega Pure

Supplements for weight loss
PGX fiber
Green Tea Elite (phytosome)
Irvingia with Green Tea

Amino acids to curb food cravings
Serotonin Max
N-Acetyl L-Tyrosine
5-HTP

Recommended natural sweeteners
Just Like Sugar
Liquid stevia
Truvia (can be purchased at your local supermarket)

Supplements for stress
Divine Health Stress Manager
Divine Health Relora Plus
Stress Relief drops
L-theanine

Exercise aids
Pedometer

Protein powders
PureLean, organic vanilla or chocolate
Life's Basics Protein
Divine Health Living Protein

Snack bars
Nutiva Hemp Seed Bar
Tempo Chocolate Mint snack bar (200 calories, 9.5g fiber, gluten-free). Order at www.drcolbert.com.

Chocolate
Belgium Dark Chocolate with Acai berry and blueberry

Digestion
Divine Health Digestive Enzyme with HCL

The following individuals and labs are also available to help you with your weight-loss goals:

- Amber Yoars, Amberly Healthy Living: For assistance with healthy shopping as well as meal preparation in the Central Florida area. Call 407-376-5179 or e-mail amberlyonline@gmail.com.
- Lee Viersen, Certified Personal Training: Can also assist with healthy shopping as well as personal training in the Central Florida area. Call 407-435-7059.
- Sage Medical Lab, for delayed food allergy testing. Visit their Web site at www.sagemedlab.com.
- Neuroscience: www.neurorelief.com
- Knowledgeable doctors in bioidentical hormone replacement (make sure they are board certified in antiaging): www.worldhealth.net

NOTES

INTRODUCTION

1. Barbara Hansen of the University of South Florida during a question-and-answer time at the Symposium, Obesity and Mortality: Controversy, Research, and Public Policy, American Association for the Advancement of Science (AAAS) National Conference, St. Louis, MO, February 17, 2006. The other panelists in attendance, representing a broad range of opinion, concurred or did not challenge her assessment. They were Katherine Flegal of the Centers for Disease Control and Prevention, and the National Center for Health Statistics; Frank Hu of Harvard University; William Harlan of the National Institute of Mental Health; and Mitch Gail of the National Cancer Institute.

2. ScienceDaily.com, "Dieting Does Not Work, Researchers Report," April 5, 2007, http://www.sciencedaily.com/releases/2007/04/070404162428.htm (accessed September 15, 2009).

1—THE OBESITY EPIDEMIC: WHAT WE'RE UP AGAINST

1. Wikipedia, s.v. "Super Size Me," http://en.wikipedia.org/wiki/Supersize_me (accessed September 15, 2009).

2. Associated Press, "Obesity Rates in U.S. Leveling Off," November 28, 2007, http://www.msnbc.msn.com/id/22007477/ (accessed September 15, 2009).

3. National Center for Health Statistics, *Health, United States, 2007* (Hyattsville, MD: U.S. Government Printing Office, 2007), 40–42.

4. A. Mokdad et al., "Actual Causes of Death in the United States, 2000," *Journal of the American Medical Association* 291 (2004): 1238–1245.

5. Reuters, "Smoking Rate Stalled at 21 percent, CDC Says," November 8, 2007, http://www.msnbc.msn.com/id/21694180/ (accessed February 17, 2008).

6. Associated Press, "Obesity Rates in U.S. Leveling Off."

7. Centers for Disease Control and Prevention, "Defining Overweight and Obesity," http://www.cdc.gov/nccdphp/dnpa/obesity/defining.htm (accessed September 15, 2009).

8. Gabriel I. Uwaifo, "Obesity," eMedicine.com, May 21, 2009, http://emedicine.medscape.com/article/123702-overview (accessed September 15, 2009).

9. HealthVideo.com, "Super-Sized Meals Are No Bargain," June 21, 2006, http://www.healthvideo.com/article.php?id=338&category=Heart+Health (accessed September 15, 2009).

10. National Institutes of Health: National Institute of Diabetes, Digestive and Kidney Diseases. "Statistics Related to Overweight and Obesity: Economic Costs Related to Overweight and Obesity," http://www.win.niddk.nih.gov/statistics/index.htm (accessed February 17, 2008).

11. Michael S. Rosenwald, "Why America Has to Be Fat," *Washington Post*, January 22, 2006: F01.

12. World Cancer Research Fund/American Institute for Cancer, *Food, Nutrition, Physical Activity, and the Prevention of Cancer: A Global Perspective* (Washington DC: 2007).

13. ScienceDaily.com, "Breast Cancer More Aggressive in Obese Women, Study Suggests," March 18, 2008, http://www.sciencedaily.com/releases/2008/03/080314085045.htm (accessed September 15, 2009).

14. Jason A. Efstathiou et al., "Obesity and Mortality in Men With Locally Advanced Prostate Cancer: Analysis of RTOG 85–31," *Cancer* 110, no. 12 (2007): 2691–2699.

15. Maigeng Zhou et al., "Body Mass Index, Blood Pressure, and Mortality From Stroke," *Stroke* 39 (2008): 753–759.

16. Eric Schlosser, *Fast Food Nation* (New York: Houghton Mifflin, 2001), 3, 242.

17. Centers for Disease Control and Prevention, "Childhood Overweight and Obesity," http://www.cdc.gov/obesity/childhood/index.html (accessed October 30, 2009).

18. Centers for Disease Control and Prevention, "National Diabetes Fact Sheet," http://www.cdc.gov/diabetes/pubs/estimates.html (accessed July 28, 2009).

19. United States Department of Health and Human Services, "The Problem of Overweight in Children and Adolescents," http://www.surgeongeneral.gov/topics/obesity/calltoaction/fact_adolescents.htm (accessed September 15, 2009).

20. Woodruff Health Sciences Center, "Excess Fat Puts Patients With Type 2 Diabetes at Greater Risk," March 26, 2009, http://whsc.emory.edu/home/news/releases/2009/03/excess-fat-puts-diabetic-patients-at-risk.html (accessed September 15, 2009).

21. ScienceDaily.com, "Obesity Increases Cancer Risk, Analysis of Hundreds of Studies Shows," February 18, 2008, http://www.sciencedaily.com/releases/2008/02/080217211802.htm (accessed September 15, 2009).

22. TheHealthierLife.com, "GERD: Obesity Can Increase Your Risk of Acid Reflux Disease," March 29, 2006, http://www.thehealthierlife.co.uk/natural-health-articles/digestive-problems/gerd-obesity-increase-risk-00212.html (accessed September 15, 2009).

23. Frank Mangano, "The Obesity-Hypertension Connection: Your Weight May Be Putting You at Risk," NaturalNews.com, July 27, 2009, http://www.naturalnews.com/026702_blood_blood_pressure_overweight.html (accessed September 15, 2009).

24. Michael F. Jacobson, *Liquid Candy: How Soft Drinks Are Harming Americans' Health* (Washington DC: Center for Science in the Public Interest, 2005), 8–11.

25. Rod Taylor, "The Beanie Factor," *Brandweek*, June 16, 1997.

26. Dan Morse, "School Cafeterias Are Enrolling as Fast-Food Franchisees," *Wall Street Journal*, July 28, 1998.

27. McDonalds.ca, "FAQs," http://www.mcdonalds.ca/en/aboutus/faq.aspx (accessed September 15, 2009).

28. A. J. Stunkard et al., "An Adoption Study of Human Obesity," *New England Journal of Medicine* 314, no. 4 (1986): 193–198.

29. National Institutes of Health, "What Causes Overweight and Obesity?" http://www.nhlbi.nih.gov/health/dci/Diseases/obe/obe_causes.html (accessed September 15, 2009).

30. Pamela Peeke, *Fight Fat After Forty* (New York: Viking, 2000), 58.

31. Eric Hübler, "The Fittest and Fattest Cities in America," MensFitness.com, http://www.mensfitness.com/city_rankings/463 (accessed September 15, 2009).

2—The Seven Habits of Highly Effective Losers

1. NWCR.ws, "The National Weight Control Registry," http://www.nwcr.ws (accessed September 15, 2009).

2. NWCR.ws, "NWCR Facts," http://www.nwcr.ws/Research/default.htm (accessed September 15, 2009).

3. *Consumer Reports*, "The Truth About Dieting," June 2002, 26–31.

4. Jeff S. Volek and Richard D. Feinman, "Carbohydrate Restriction Improves the Features of Metabolic Syndrome," *Nutrition & Metabolism* 2 (2005): 31.

5. David D. Gutterman et al., "Benefit of Low-Fat Over Low-Carbohydrate Diet on Endothelial Health in Obesity," *Hypertension* 51 (2008): 376–382.

6. Joseph Carroll, "Six in 10 Americans Have Tried to Lose Weight," Gallup.com, August 16, 2005, http://www.gallup.com/poll/17890/Six-Americans-Attempted-Lose-Weight.aspx (accessed September 15, 2009).

7. David Zinczenko with Matt Goulding, *Eat This, Not That!* (New York: Rodale, 2008), xii.

8. John Consoli, "Nielsen: TV Viewing Grows," MediaWeek, September 21, 2006 http://www.mediaweek.com/mw/news/recent_display.jsp?vnu_content_id=1003154980 (accessed September 15, 2009).

9. Zinczenko, *Eat This, Not That!* 283.

10. Kate M. Jackson, "0 Is the New 8," *Boston Globe,* May 5, 2006, http://www.boston .com/news/nation/articles/2006/05/05/0_is_the_new_8/ (accessed September 15, 2009).

11. Diane Berry, "An Emerging Model of Behavior Change in Women Maintaining Weight Loss," *Nursing Science Quarterly* 17, no. 4 (2004): 242–252.

12. Nanci Hellmich, "Weight War Can Be Never-Ending," *USA Today,* October 16, 2005, http://www.usatoday.com/news/health/2005-10-16-weight-war-remedies_x.htm (accessed September 15, 2009).

13. NWCR.ws, "NWCR Facts."

14. Sarah E. Lowery et al., "Body Image, Self-Esteem, and Health-Related Behaviors Among Male and Female First-Year College Students," *Journal of College Student Development* 46, no. 6 (2005): 612–623.

15. Linda J. Koenig and Erika L. Wasserman, "Body Image and Dieting Failure in College Men and Women: Examining Links Between Depression and Eating Problems," *Sex Roles: A Journal of Research* 32, no. 3–4 (1995): 225–249.

16. J. Ogden, "The Correlates of Long-Term Weight Loss: A Group Comparison Study of Obesity," *International Journal of Obesity* 24, no. 8 (2000): 1018–1025.

3—Hunger vs. Appetite

1. *Webster's New World College Dictionary,* 4th ed., s.v. "hunger," "appetite."

2. Bartley G. Hoebel, "Feeding and Self-Stimulation," *Annals of the New York Academy of Sciences* 157, no. 2 (1969): 758–778.

3. Ibid.

4. MSN Encarta, "Serotonin," http://encarta.msn.com/encyclopedia_761553105 /serotonin.html (accessed September 16, 2009).

5. S. Nishizawa et al., "Differences Between Males and Females in Rates of Serotonin Synthesis in Human Brain," *Proceedings of the National Academy of Sciences USA* 94 (1997): 5308–5313.

4—Irresistible Foods

1. C. H. Gilhooly et al., "Food Cravings and Energy Regulation: The Characteristics of Craved Foods and Their Relationship With Eating Behaviors and Weight Change During Six Months of Dietary Energy Restriction," *International Journal of Obesity* 31 (2007): 1849–1858.

2. Brian Wansink et al., "Exploring Comfort Food Preferences Across Age and Gender," *Physiology & Behavior* 79 (2003): 739–747.

3. M. T. McGuire et al., "Behavioral Strategies of Individuals Who Have Maintained Long-Term Weight Losses," *Obesity Research* 7, no. 4 (1999): 334–41.

5—How Metabolism Works

1. Barbara Bushman and Janice Clark-Young, *Action Plan for Menopause* (Champaign, IL: American College of Sports Medicine, 2005), 68–70.

2. Ibid.

3. *Webster's New World College Dictionary,* 4th ed., s.v. "metabolism."

4. ShapeFit.com, "Basal Metabolic Rate—BMR," http://www.shapefit.com/basal-metabolic -rate.html (accessed October 2, 2009).

5. Jim Harvey, "Measuring BMR in the Pulmonary Lab," *FOCUS: Journal for Respiratory Care and Sleep Medicine* (July 1, 2006), http://www.thefreelibrary.com/ Measuring+BMR+in+the+Pulmonary+lab.-a0186218061 (accessed September 22, 2009).

6. Uwaifo, "Obesity."

7. James Levine et al., "Interindividual Variation in Posture Allocation: Possible Role in Human Obesity," *Science* 307, no. 5709 (2005): 584–586.

8. Centers for Disease Control and Prevention, "Genomics Resources: Obesity and Genetics," http://www.cdc.gov/genomics/resources/diseases/obesity/obesedit.htm (accessed September 16, 2009).

9. Lawrence C. Wood et al., *Your Thyroid, A Home Reference* (New York: Ballantine Books, 1995).

10. Karilee Halo Shames et al., "The Thyroid Dance: Nursing Approaches to Autoimmune Low Thyroid," *AWHONN Lifelines* 6, no. 1 (2002): 52–59.

6—The Glycemic Index and Glycemic Load

1. MrBreakfast.com, "The Early Days of Breakfast Cereal," http://www.mrbreakfast .com/article.asp?articleid=13 (accessed September 16, 2009).

2. BestDietTips.com, "Glycemic Index List of Foods," http://www.bestdiettips .com/content/view/219/53/ (accessed September 16, 2009).

7—Carbohydrates: A Case of the Tortoise and the Hare

1. U.S. Department of Health and Human Services, *Dietary Guidelines for Americans, 2005*, 6th ed., (Washington DC: U.S. Government Printing Office, 2005).

2. Zinczenko, *Eat This, Not That!* 12.

3. Neal Barnard, *Breaking the Food Seduction* (New York: St. Martin's Press, 2003), 32.

4. WholeGrainsCouncil.org, "Whole Grains Stamp," http://www.wholegrainscouncil .org/whole-grain-stamp (accessed September 16, 2009).

5. Institute of Medicine, *Dietary Reference Intakes for Energy, Carbohydrate, Fiber, Fat, Fatty Acids, Cholesterol, Protein, and Amino Acids.* (Washington DC: The National Academies Press, 2002).

6. Nancy C. Howarth et al., "Dietary Fat and Fiber Are Associated With Excess Weight in Young and Middle-Aged U.S. Adults," *Journal of the American Dietetic Association* 105, no. 9 (2005): 1365–1372.

7. Center for Science in the Public Interest, "Sugar Intake Hit All-Time High in 1999," May 18, 2000, http://www.cspinet.org/new/sugar_limit.html (accessed September 16, 2009).

8. Becky Hand, "The Hunt for Hidden Sugar: How Much of the Sweet Stuff Is Hiding Your Foods?" BabyFit.com, http://www.babyfit.com/articles.asp?id=685 (accessed September 16, 2009).

9. Center for Science in the Public Interest, "Sugar Intake Hit All-Time High in 1999."

10. Ibid.

11. Splenda.com, "Splenda No-Calorie Sweetener FAQs," http://www.splenda.com /page.jhtml?id=splenda/faqs/nocalorie.inc#q0 (accessed September 16, 2009).

12. Sally Fallon Morell and Rami Nagel, "Worse Than We Thought: The Lowdown on High-Fructose Corn Syrup and Agave 'Nectar,'" *Wise Traditions*, Spring 2009, 44–51, http://www.westonaprice.org/modernfood/HFCSAgave.pdf (accessed October 22, 2009).

8—The Power of Protein

1. Walter C. Willett, "Eat, Drink, and Be Healthy," http://www.motherearthnews .com/Real-Food/2004-12-01/Be-Particular-About-Your-Protein.aspx (accessed September 16, 2009).

2. Institute of Medicine, *Dietary Reference Intakes for Energy, Carbohydrate, Fiber, Fat, Fatty Acids, Cholesterol, Protein, and Amino Acids* (Washington DC: National Academy of Sciences, 2002), 6.

3. P. Lemon, "Is Increased Dietary Protein Necessary or Beneficial for Individuals With a Physically Active Lifestyle?" *Nutrition Reviews* 54 (1996): S169–S175.

4. M. D. Brown et al., "Promotion of Prostatic Metastatic Migration Towards Human Bone Marrow Stoma by Omega 6 and Its Inhibition by Omega 3 PUFAs," *British Journal of Cancer* 94 (2006): 842–853.

5. D. Feskanich et al., "Protein Consumption and Bone Fractures in Women," *American Journal of Epidemiology* 143 (1996): 472–479.

6. LifeintheUSA.com, "Beef in America," http://www.lifeintheusa.com/food/beef.htm (accessed September 17, 2009).

7. Bryan Walsh, "Getting Real About the High Price of Cheap Food," *TIME*, August 21, 2009, http://www.time.com/time/health/article/0,8599,1917458,00.html (accessed October 15, 2009).

8. American College of Obstetricians and Gynecologists, "Nutrition During Pregnancy," June 2008, http://www.acog.org/publications/patient_education/bp001.cfm (accessed September 17, 2009).

9. Lynn R. Goldman et al., "American Academy of Pediatrics: Technical Report: Mercury in the Enfironment: Implications for Pediatricians," *Pediatrics* 108, no. 1 (July 2001): 197–205.

10. DoleNutrition.com, "Bean Scene," February 13, 2006, http://www.dole.com/LiveRight/Prevention/PreventionDetails/tabid/837/Default.aspx?contentid=4293 (accessed September 17, 2009).

11. Kate Murphy, "The Dark Side of Soy," BusinessWeek.com, December 18, 2000, http://www.businessweek.com/2000/00_51/b3712218.htm (accessed September 17, 2009).

12. Gabriel Cousens, MD, *There Is a Cure for Diabetes* (Berkeley, CA: North Atlantic Books, 2008), 179–182.

9—Fats That Make You Fat and Fats That Make You Lean

1. USDA Center for Nutrition Policy and Promotion, "Is Total Fat Consumption Really Decreasing?" *Nutrition Insights* 5 (1998).

2. Crisco.com, "Our History," http://www.crisco.com/About_Crisco/History.aspx (accessed September 17, 2009).

3. Associated Press, "Crisco Drops Trans Fats From Shortening Formula," MSNBC.com, January 25, 2007, http://www.msnbc.msn.com/id/16795455/ (accessed September 17, 2009).

4. Feskanich, "Protein Consumption and Bone Fractures in Women."

5. Electronic Code of Federal Regulations, "Title 21: Food and Drugs; 101.9 Nutrition Labeling of Food," http://ecfr.gpoaccess.gov/cgi/t/text/text-idx?c=ecfr&sid=77734a162c4f7ddd997233b4d623c029&rgn=div8&view=text&node=21:2.0.1.1.2.1.1.6&idno=21 (accessed September 17, 2009).

6. University of Dayton Research Institute, "Olive Oil, Lower Temperatures Less Toxic in Frying," *UDRI News*, September 2003, http://www.udri.udayton.edu/News/news0903.htm (accessed September 17, 2009).

7. American Heart Association, "Step I, Step II and TLC Diets," http://www.americanheart.org/presenter.jhtml?identifier=4764 (accessed September 17, 2009).

8. Anthony Kane, "Omega-3 Fatty Acids and Depression," ConsumerHealthDigest.com, http://www.consumerhealthdigest.com/omegafattyacids.htm (accessed September 17, 2009).

9. Walsh, "Getting Real About the High Price of Cheap Food."

10. Ancel Keys, *Seven Countries: A Multivariate Analysis of Death and Coronary Heart Disease* (Boston: Harvard University Press, 1980).

11. Tinker Ready, "Dueling Diets," *Harvard Public Health Review* (Fall 2004); Elizabeth Somer, MA, RD, "Pass the Olive Oil," April 30, 2001, http://greekfamilyoil.weebly.com/should-i-consume-olive-oil-if-im-trying-to-lose-weight.html (accessed September 17, 2009).

12. Walsh, "Getting Real About the High Price of Cheap Food."

10—Beverages: Are You Drinking Yourself Obese?

1. American Beverage Association, "What America Drinks," viewed at http://improveyourhealthwithwater.info/a1/whatamericadrinks.pdf (accessed September 17, 2009).

2. Ibid.

3. Judith Valentine, "Soft Drinks: America's Other Drinking Problem," http://www.westonaprice.org/modernfood/soft.html (accessed September 17, 2009).

4. Daniel DeNoon, "Drink More Diet Soda, Gain More Weight?" WebMD.com, June 13, 2005, http://www.webmd.com/diet/news/20050613/drink-more-diet-soda-gain-more-weight (accessed September 17, 2009).

5. Pamela L. Lutsey et al., "Dietary Intake and the Development of Metabolic Syndrome," *Circulation* 117 (2008): 754–761.

6. Jacobson, *Liquid Candy: How Soft Drinks Are Harming Americans' Health.*

7. Ibid.

8. Centers for Disease Control and Prevention, "Overweight and Obesity," http://www.cdc.gov/nccdphp/dnpa/obesity/ (accessed September 17, 2009).

9. Ramachandran Vasan, "Soft Drink Consumption and Risk of Developing Cardiometabolic Risk Factors and the Metabolic Syndrome in Middle-Aged Adults in the Community," *Circulation* 116 (2007): 480–488.

10. Jacobson, *Liquid Candy: How Soft Drinks Are Harming Americans' Health.*

11. Starbucks.com, "Starbucks Beverages," http://www.starbucks.com/retail/nutrition_beverages.asp (accessed September 17, 2009).

12. Zinczenko, *Eat This, Not That!* 258.

13. MayoClinic.com, "Caffeine: How Much Is Too Much?" http://www.mayoclinic.com/health/caffeine/NU00600 (accessed September 17, 2009).

14. Calorie Count, "Calories in Energy Drink: Gatorade Performance Series," http://caloriecount.about.com/calories-gatorade-energy-drink-i88302 (accessed September 17, 2009).

15. John Tesh, *Intelligence for Your Life* (Nashville: Thomas Nelson, 2008), 121.

16. Health4YouOnline.com, "Dehydration—the Benefits of Drinking Water," http://www.health4youonline.com/article_dehydration.htm (accessed September 17, 2009).

17. Susanna C. Larsson and Alicja Wolk, "Tea Consumption and Ovarian Cancer Risk in a Population-Based Cohort," *Archives of Internal Medicine* 165, no. 22 (December 12, 2005): http://archinte.ama-assn.org/cgi/content/full/165/22/2683 (accessed September 30, 2009).

18. Abdul G. Dulloo et al., "Efficacy of a Green Tea Extract Rich in Catechin Polyphenols and Caffeine in Increasing 24-h Energy Expenditure and Fat Oxidation in Humans," *American Journal of Clinical Nutrition* 70, no. 6 (December 1999): 1040–1045.

19. Jukka Hintakka et al., "Daily Tea Drinking Is Associated With a Low Level of Depressive Symptoms in the Finnish General Population," *European Journal of Epidemiology* 20, no. 4 (2005): 359–363.

20. Yerba Mate Association of the Americas, "FAQs: What Are the Health Benefits of Yerba Mate?" http://www.yerbamateassociation.org/index.php?p=faq#101 (accessed September 17, 2009).

11—PORTION SIZES

1. H. Weisel et al., "Discrepancy Between Self-Reported and Actual Caloric Intake and Exercise in Obese Subjects," *New England Journal of Medicine* 327, no. 27 (1992): 1893–1898.

2. Jaime Schwartz and Carol Byrd-Bredbenner, "Portion Distortion: Typical Portion Sizes Selected by Young Adults," *Journal of American Dietetic Association* 106, no. 9 (2006): 1412–1418.

3. Associated Press, "All-You-Can-Eat Seats Fill Fans Up—and Out," MSNBC.com, March 21, 2008, http://www.msnbc.msn.com/id/23746923/ (accessed September 17, 2009).

4. S. J. Nielsen et al., "Patterns of Food Portion Sizes, 1997-1998," *Journal of the American Medical Association* 289 (2003): 450–453.

5. Brian Wansick, "Can Package Size Accelerate Usage Volume?" *Journal of Marketing* 60 (1996): 1–14.

6. The National Alliance for Nutrition and Activity, "From Wallet to Waistline: The Hidden Costs of 'Super Sizing,'" PreventionInstitute.org, http://www.preventioninstitute.org/portionsizerept.html (accessed September 17, 2009).

7. American Institute for Cancer Research, "Drop Out of the Clean Plate Club," January 5, 2005, http://www.aicr.org/site/News2?page=NewsArticle&id=7718&news_iv_ctrl=0&abbr=pr_hf_ (accessed September 17, 2009).

8. HealthDay News, "Mom Was Right: Eating Soup Cuts Calorie Intake," May 1, 2007, WTHR.com, http://www.wthr.com/Global/story.asp?S=6454706 (accessed September 17, 2009).

9. Barbara Rolls, *The Volumetrics Eating Plan* (HarperCollins: New York, 2005), 93–94.

12—YOU HAVE A CHOICE

1. Lauren Muney, "Top 10 Excuses for Falling Off the Diet/Fitness Wagon—and Answers for Them," PhysicalMind.com, http://www.physicalmind.com/top_excuses.htm (accessed April 21, 2008).

13—ALL ABOUT COMMITMENT

1. Kansas Sports Hall of Fame, "Cunningham, Glenn V." http://www.kshof.org/siteresources/apps/records/halloffamer.asp?id=34 (accessed September 18, 2009).

2. Matthew Phillips, "Health Clubs Flatten Out Bulge in January Membership Sales," *The Business Review*, January 10, 2003, http://www.bizjournals.com/albany/stories/2003/01/13/story6.html (accessed September 18, 2009).

14—SETTING REACHABLE GOALS

1. Stephen B. Halls, "About Arithmetic Formulas for Calculating Ideal Body Weight," http://www.halls.md/ideal-weight/devine.htm (accessed September 17, 2009).

2. Roni Caryn Rabin, "Excess Pounds, but Not Too Many, May Lead to Longer Life," *New York Times*, June 26, 2009, http://www.nytimes. Com/2009/06/26/health/26weight.html (accessed September 18, 2009).

3. Amanda Spake, "The Belly Burden," *U.S. News & World Report*, November 20, 2005, http://health.usnews.com/usnews/health/articles/051128/28waist_print.htm (accessed September 18, 2009).

4. Krisha McCoy, "Your Body Fat Percentage: What Does It Mean?" Swedish.org. http://www.swedish.org/17390.cfm (accessed October 26, 2009).

5. Youfa Wang et al., "Comparison of Abdominal Adiposity and Overall Obesity in Predicting Risk of Type 2 Diabetes Among Men," *American Journal of Clinical Nutrition* 81, no. 3 (2005): 555–563.

15—The Eating Plan

1. Sharon Cohen, "Breakfast Out Adds Pounds—Eat Right," *Shape*, February 2004, http://findarticles.com/p/articles/mi_m0846/is_6_23/ai_112318550/ (accessed September 21, 2009).

2. University of Minnesota School of Public Health, "Teens Who Eat Breakfast Daily Are Healthier," March 3, 2008, http://www.sph.umn.edu/about/news/releases/breakfast 030308.html (accessed September 21, 2009).

3. Kellogg USA, "Study Shows Skipping Breakfast Is Not an Effective Way to Manage Weight Eating Cereal for Breakfast Leads to an Overall Healthier Diet And Lower Body Weight as Reported By Block Dietary Data Systems and Kellogg," April 2001, http://thyroid.about.com/library/news/blbreakfast.htm (accessed September 21, 2009).

4. Zinczenko, *Eat This, Not That!* 12.

16—Mix-a-Meal

1. MrBreakfast.com, "The Early Days of Breakfast Cereal."

2. UPI News Track, "Soup Cuts Calories," May 2, 2007, http://www.accessmylibrary.com/coms2/summary_0286-30667671_ITM (accessed September 21, 2009).

17—The Power of Snacking

1. Jennie Brand-Miller, Thomas M. S. Wolever, Kaye Foster-Powell, and Stephen Colagiuri, *The New Glucose Revolution*, 3rd ed., (New York: Marlow & Co., 2007), 86.

2. Charles Stuart Platkin, *The Automatic Diet* (New York: Hudson Street Press, 2005), 92.

3. Maria Conceição de Oliveira et al., "Weight Loss Association With a Daily Intake of Three Apples or Three Pears Among Overweight Women," *Nutrition* 19, no. 3 (2003): 253–256.

4. Judith J. Wurtman and Nina Frusztajer Marquis, *The Serotonin Power Diet* (New York: Rodale, 2006), 15.

5. Ibid., 66–68.

18—Gut Check: Keeping Tabs on What You're Really Eating

1. Laura Bruce, "John Harrison—The Face of Identity Theft," Bankrate.com, August 18, 2004, http://www.bankrate.com/brm/news/advice/IDTheft/ID-home.asp (accessed September 21, 2009).

2. Andrea A. Canning, "How to Keep a Successful Food Diary," ABCNews.com, July 22, 2008, http://abcnews.go.com/GMA/Diet/story?id=5421350 (accessed November 2, 2009).

3. National Heart, Lung and Blood Institute, "Portion Distortion: Spaghetti and Meatballs," http://hp2010.nhlbihin.net/portion/portion.cgi?action=question&number=3 (accessed September 21, 2009).

4. Zinczenko, *Eat This, Not That!* 35.

19—Mindful Eating

1. Zinczenko, *Eat This, Not That!* 47.

2. Elisabeth Rosenthal, "Even the French Are Fighting Obesity," *New York Times*, May 4, 2005, http://www.nytimes.com/2005/05/03/world/europe/03iht-obese.html?_r=1 (accessed September 21, 2009).

3. Tim Lobstein et al., *EU Platform on Diet, Physical Activity and Health,* International Obesity Task Force, Brussels, Germany, March 15, 2005, http://www.iotf.org/media/euobesity3.pdf (accessed September 21, 2009).

4. Shape Up America! "About Shape Up America!" http://www.shapeup.org/general/index.html (accessed September 29, 2009).

5. Victoria Lambert, "The French Children Learning to Fight Obesity," Telegraph
.co.uk, March 3, 2008, http://www.telegraph.co.uk/health/dietandfitness/3353715/The
-French-children-learning-to-fight-obesity.html (accessed September 21, 2009).

6. Rosenthal, "Even the French Are Fighting Obesity."

7. Ibid.

8. Hubert Vigilla, "A Short History of Diet Pills and Weight Loss Drugs," DocShop.com,
February 11, 2008, http://www.docshop.com/2008/02/11/a-short-history-of
-diet-pills-and-weight-loss-drugs-part-one/ (accessed September 21, 2009).

9. *Business Wire*, "Americans Need Help Managing 'Mealtime Multitasking';
American Dietetic Association/ConAgra Foods Share Pointers for September
National Food Safety Month," September 8, 2004, http://findarticles.com/p/articles/
mi_m0EIN/is_2004_Sept_8/ai_n6185136/ (accessed September 21, 2009).

10. Tesh, *Intelligence for Your Life*, 5.

11. Ibid., 103.

12. Benson-Henry Institute for Mind Body Medicine, "Mindfulness," Massachusetts
General Hospital, http://www.mbmi.org/basics/mstress_M.asp (accessed September 21, 2009).

20—ACTIVITY TIME

1. TMZ.com, "Janet In Shape and In 'Control'" July 17, 2006, http://www.tmz
.com/2006/07/17/janet-in-shape-and-in-control/ (accessed March 15, 2008).

2. Rob Carnevale, "Bruce Willis: Die Hard 4.0," BBC.com, July 2, 2007, http://www.bbc
.co.uk/films/2007/07/02/bruce_willis_die_hard_4_2007_interview.shtml (accessed September
21, 2009).

3. Mirelle Argaman, "Exclusive: Serena Williams Talks to *Star!*" *Star*, May 4,
2007, http://www.starmagazine.com/news/11945 (accessed March 15, 2008).

4. Sal Morgan, "Colin Farrell: The Bad Boy's a Gentleman," NineMSN, July 20, 2006,
http://news.ninemsn.com.au/article.aspx?id=121614 (accessed March 15, 2008).

5. Starpulse.com, "Memorable Celebrity Quotes," January 16, 2008, http://www.starpulse
.com/news/index.php/2008/01/16/memorable_celebrity_quotes_118 (accessed March 15, 2008).

6. Centers for Disease Control and Prevention, "U.S. Physical Activity Statistics,"
CDC.gov, http://apps.nccd.cdc.gov/PASurveillance/StateSumResultV.asp (accessed
September 21, 2009).

7. Jacqueline Stenson, "Excuses, Excuses," MSNBC.com, Dec. 16, 2004, http://www.msnbc
.msn.com/id/6391079/ (accessed September 21, 2009); Chad Clark, "Functional Exercises: Top
10 List of Reasons Why People Don't Exercise," http://pt-connections.com/topfit/publish
/printer_Functional_Exercise_Top_10_reasons.shtml (accessed September 21, 2009).

8. Zinczenko, *Eat This, Not That!* 113.

9. Lindsay Bergstrom, "70-Year-Old Swims English Channel to Promote Church's
Ministry in Haiti," *Associated Baptist Press*, September 2, 2004, http://www.abpnews
.com/index.php?option=com_content&task=view&id=1863&Itemid=117
(accessed September 21, 2009).

10. Levine, "Interindividual Variation in Posture Allocation: Possible Role in Human
Obesity."

11. Cris A. Slentz et al., "Effects of the Amount of Exercise on Body Weight, Body
Composition, and Measures of Central Obesity," *Archives of Internal Medicine* 164 (2004):
31–39.

12. Caroline J. Cedarquist, "Fitness With Fido: A Healthy Pastime for Dog Owners," NewsBlaze.com, http://newsblaze.com/story/20060110091932nnnn.nb/topstory.html (accessed September 21, 2009).

13. Berit L. Heitmann and Peder Fredericksen, "Thigh Circumference and Risk of Heart Disease and Premature Death: Prospective Cohort Study," *BMJ* 339 (September 3, 2009): abstract viewed at http://www.bmj.com/cgi/content/abstract/339/sep03_2/b3292 (accessed September 21, 2009).

14. Peter Jaret, "A Healthy Mix of Rest and Motion," *New York Times*, May 3, 2007, http://www.nytimes.com/2007/05/03/fashion/03Fitness.html?adxnnl=1&adxnnlx=1253561931-OZY42iiNSU3WgNPEf4OoxA (accessed September 21, 2009).

15. K. Boutelle and D. Kirschenbaum, "Further Support for Consistent Self-Monitoring as a Vital Component of Successful Weight Control," *Obesity Research* 6 (1998): 219–224.

16. Ibid.

17. NWCR.ws, "NWCR Facts."

21—Supplementing Your Weight Loss

1. National Toxicology Program, "CAS Registry Number: 299-42-3 Toxicity Effects," http://ntp.niehs.nih.gov/index.cfm?objectid=E87F352F-BDB5-82F8-F07D41E8B443A532 (accessed October 1, 2009).

2. Associated Press, "Drugmakers Vie for Magic Weight-Loss Pill," MSNBC.com, January 3, 2008, http://www.msnbc.msn.com/id/22490513/ (accessed September 22, 2009).

3. USAToday.com, "FDA Warns Consumers to Avoid Brazilian Diet Pills," January 14, 2006, http://www.usatoday.com/news/health/2006-01-13-brazilian-diet-pills_x.htm (accessed September 22, 2009).

4. Ano Lobb, "Hepatoxicity Associated With Weight-Loss Supplements: A Case for Better Post-Marketing Surveillance," *World Journal of Gastroenterology* 15, no. 14 (April 14, 2009): 1786–1787, http://www.pubmedcentral.nih.gov/articlerender.fcgi?artid=2668789 (accessed September 22, 2009).

5. Julius Goepp, "Critical Need for a Multi-Model Approach to Combat Obesity," *Life Extension Magazine*, June 2009, http://www.lef.org/magazine/mag2009/jun2009_Multi-Modal-Approach-To-Combat-Obesity_01.htm (accessed September 22, 2009).

6. P. Chantre and D. Lairon, "Recent Findings of Green Tea Extract AR25 (Exolise) and Its Activity for the Treatment of Obesity," *Phytomedicine* 9, no. 1 (2002): 3–8.

7. Goepp, "Critical Need for a Multi-Model Approach to Combat Obesity," citing *Integr Nutr.* 11, no. 2 (2008): 1–14.

8. Z. Ramazanov, "Effect of Fucoxanthin and Xanthigen, A Phytomedicine Containing Fucoxanthin and Pomegranate Seed Oil, on Energy Expenditure in Obese Non-Diabetic Female Volunteers: A Double-Blind, Randomized and Placebo-Controlled Trial." Submitted for publication 2008.

9. Ibid.

10. Judith A. Marlett et al., "Position of the American Dietetic Association: Health Implications of Dietary Fiber," *Journal of the American Dietetic Association* 102, no. 7 (2002): 993–1000.

11. Lisa Bolton et al., "How Does Drug and Supplement Marketing Affect a Healthy Lifestyle?" *Journal of Consumer Research* 34 (2008).

12. N. C. Howarth et al., "Dietary Fiber and Weight Regulation," *Nutrition Review* 59, no. 5 (2001): 129–139.

13. LifeSpanMD.com, "The Magic of Soluble Fiber," http://www.lifespanmd.com /articles-weight-solublefiber.html (accessed September 22, 2009).

14. Judith L. Ngondi at al., "IGOB131, a Novel Seed Extract of the West African Plant *Irvingia Gabonensis*, Significantly Reduces Body Weight and Improves Metabolic Parameters in Overweight Humans in a Randomized Double-blind Placebo Controlled Investigation," *Lipids in Health and Disease* 8, no. 7 (March 2009): http://www.lipidworld.com/content/8/1/7 (accessed September 22, 2009).

15. Hoodia Advice, "The Science of Hoodia," http://www.hoodia-advice.org/hoodia-plant .html (accessed September 22, 2009).

16. Tom Mangold, "Sampling the Kalahari Hoodia Diet," BBC News, May 30, 2003, http:// news.bbc.co.uk/2/hi/programmes/correspondent/2947810.stm (accessed September 22, 2009).

23—When Weight Loss Stalls or Stops

1. Tanya E. Froehlich et al., "Prevalence, Recognition, and Treatment of Attention-Deficit/ Hyperactivity Disorder in a National Sample of U.S. Children," *Archives of Pediatrics and Adolescent Medicine* 161, no. 9 (2007): 857–864.

2. L. B. Silver, "Attention-Deficit Hyperactivity Disorder in Adult Life," *Child and Adolescent Psychiatric Clinics of North America* 9, no. 3 (2000): 411–523.

3. L. Breum et al., "Twenty-Four-Hour Plasma Tryptophan Concentrations and Ratios Are Below Normal in Obese Subjects and Are Not Normalized by Substantial Weight Reduction," *American Journal of Clinical Nutrition* 77, no. 5 (2003): 1112–1118.

4. Ibid.

5. J. G. Hollowell et al., "Serum Thyrotropin, Thyroxine, and Thyroid Antibodies in the United States Population (1988 to 1994): National Health and Nutrition Examination Survey (NHANES III)," *Journal of Clinical Endocrinology & Metabolism* 87, no. 2 (2002): 489–99.

6. M. P. Vanderpump and W.M. Turnbridge, "Epidemiology and Prevention of Clinical and Subclinical Hypothyroidism," *Thyroid* 12, no. 10 (2002): 839–47.

7. U.S. Department of Health and Human Services and National Institutes of Health, *Food Allergy: An Overview* (Washington DC: 2007).

8. Deborah P. Whitman, "Genetically Modified Foods: Harmful or Helpful?" April 2000, htto://www.csa.com/discoveryguide/gmfood/overview.php (accessed October 13, 2009).

9. Phul Froom et al., "Smoking Cessation and Weight Gain," *Journal of Family Practice* 46, no. 6 (1998): 460–464.

Appendix G—Body Mass Index Chart

1. Adapted from the National Heart, Lung, and Blood Institute's body mass index table in the *Clinical Guidelines on the Identification, Evaluation, and Treatment of Overweight and Obesity in Adults*. Used by permission.

INDEX

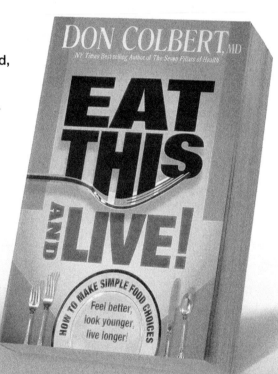